D1325629

Type 1 Diabetes

Clinical Management of the Athlete

Ian Gallen

Editor

Type 1 Diabetes

Clinical Management of the Athlete

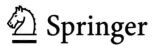 Springer

Editor
Ian Gallen
Diabetes Centre
Wycombe Hospital
High Wycombe
UK

ISBN 978-0-85729-753-2   e-ISBN 978-0-85729-754-9
DOI 10.1007/978-0-85729-754-9
Springer London Dordrecht Heidelberg New York

British Library Cataloguing in Publication Data
A catalogue record for this book is available from the British Library

Library of Congress Control Number: 2012934821

Printed on acid-free paper

Springer is part of Springer Science+Business Media (www.springer.com)

This book is dedicated to my parents Louis and Barbara for their lifelong love, encouragement and support, to my wife Susan for our happy life together and to our children Robert and Hannah who make my life meaningful. I thank all my outstanding and inspirational medical teachers, the many colleagues with whom I have been privileged to work and the people with diabetes who have trusted me to help them.

Foreword

I was diagnosed with diabetes at the start of training for the 2000 Sydney Olympic Games, having won gold medals in rowing events at the previous four Olympic Games. The diagnosis was a shock, and I felt my sporting world was over. I had a grandfather who had the condition in his late 60s, and even though I was very young at the time and didn't know very much about diabetes, I felt I knew enough to know that I wouldn't be able to carry on my sporting path. I was sent up to my local diabetic center where my diabetes was confirmed, and I was taught to inject insulin and all the life-changing routines and dietary adjustments that needed to be implemented immediately. At the end of the consultation when I was expecting to be told that this was it, my sporting career was over, my consultant said to me, "I can't see any reason why you can't still achieve your dreams in 3 years time by competing at the Sydney Olympics in 2000." This was a bigger shock to me than being told I wouldn't be able to compete. All my instincts and limited knowledge as a newly diagnosed diabetic told me otherwise. He did say it would be a tough path, but immediately I thought if he thinks I can do it, I will give it my best shot.

The path over the next few months was very traumatic. Firstly, of coming to terms with the condition and, secondly, as an athlete with a certain pride in your performance at the highest level is about consistency within training and racing. In the early days of my diabetes, it was the consistency that had gone. The main issue was not actually the controlling of the diabetes; it had more to do with the refueling of my body. To compete in rowing at Olympic level, you have to train somewhere in the region of 18–24 sessions a week, averaging about 1½h a session of intensive endurance work, splitting these sessions between three and four a day. There is very little time to regain the energy when you are limited to the insulin you can take because of the fear of hypoglycemia. I was put onto the normal diabetic diet, and session after session I was not gaining the energy to perform. The way I felt after each session was convincing me I was never going to be the athlete that I was.

Over time, my consultant changed the patterns of refueling. In fact, this meant going back to my old diet. He knew that I had been successful on this before, but he had to come up with a regime that allowed me to eat 6–7,000 cal a day and still control my diabetes. When you are first diagnosed, you are given so much information, and this is so difficult to take on board – even as an athlete when you need to have the freshness of mind to adapt to your needs. I feel that if you could be drip-fed information over time, this would be a better process. There wasn't any information for athletes to achieve at the highest level, and books like this really do help the athlete and give the consultants a good foresight. Since I was diagnosed in 1997, the world looks at diabetes and elite sport in a very different way, and there are so many more diabetic athletes achieving their dreams now. With all the help I was given, I decided very early on that diabetes was going to live with me, not me live with diabetes.

I very much welcome this book, in which leading experts highlight the many advances in the understanding of the effects of diabetes and insulin treatment during and following exercise, and on how diabetes management can be optimized. This will help clinicians in turn help those people with diabetes who want to play sport, and even for some like me achieve the highest level of sporting success.

Sir Steve Redgrave

Preface

In this year of the London Olympic Games, our attention is drawn to sport and physical performance. Type 1 diabetes is initially a disorder of the young, and in this age group and for many older people physical activity is a very important component of lifestyle. Whilst it is of undoubted importance for physicians to optimize insulin therapy programs and other treatments to avoid or treat the chronic complications of type 1 diabetes, people with diabetes also seek to normalize their lifestyle. Some will want to advance their sporting ambitions, and the examples of outstanding sportsmen with diabetes, such the rower Sir Stephen Redgrave, or the Rugby Union player Chris Pennell, show us that type 1 diabetes per se is not a barrier to maximum physical performance in sport. These examples encourage people with type 1 diabetes to engage in all types of physical activity, and they will seek best advice on how to manage their diabetes with exercise.

There are some significant barriers for people with type 1 diabetes performing sports and exercise. They are likely to experience marked fluctuations in blood glucose control and frequent hypoglycaemia with exercise. The occurrence of hypoglycaemia may seem both unpredictable and inexplicable to the person with diabetes, which may force the response of excess replacement of carbohydrate before and following exercise, with resultant hyperglycaemia, adding to the burden of dysglycaemia. Perhaps of more concern to people with diabetes is the risk of hypoglycaemia during and nocturnal hypoglycaemia following exercise. When hypoglycaemia is severe, requiring assistance from another person, it may cause embarrassment to people with diabetes, and is likely to cause concern to parents, teachers and coaching staff as to the safety of physical activity. Excessive fatigue and weakness during prolonged exercise compared with peers without diabetes may be experienced, and this may reduce the wish to continue in sport. For the outstanding athlete with diabetes, there is potential that diabetes and insulin treatment may cause loss of maximum physical performance, which also may discourage progression in sport. We now know many of the causes of impaired physical performance and how these may be rectified through augmented diabetes management strategies.

Evidence from people with type 1 diabetes suggests that advice from healthcare professionals to people with type 1 diabetes on the management of physical exercise may be simplistic. Over the last decade, we have established a specialist clinic to help sportspeople and athletes manage their diabetes and physical activity success-fully to reduce dysglycaemia with and following exercise, and to normalize physical performance. Athletes and sports people explained in our clinic what problems they had found during exercise, and how they had tried to overcome those difficulties. This experiential evidence has produced many effective clinical strategies. These are now strongly supported by the growth in the clinical research knowledge base of the effects of diabetes on the physiological response to exercise, on the effect of exercise on the response to hypoglycaemia and on effective dietetic and insulin management of diabetes during and following exercise. There have also been sig-nificant technological improvements in the support of the management of type 1 diabetes with continuously infused insulin infusion pump therapy and continuous sub-cutaneous glucose monitoring equipment.

People with type 1 diabetes will seek to be effectively supported in any sporting ambition, presenting an interesting challenge to healthcare professionals. This book aims to provide the evidence on the management of type 1 diabetes and exercise, bringing together outstanding clinical science, clinical practice from experts in the field and the evidence of the real experts, the athletes themselves. The book outlines potential dietetic and therapeutic strategies which may be employed to promote these aims. Our aim is that if applied, the evidence will equip the healthcare profes-sional with the knowledge base to support the development of clinical skills to sup-port any person with type 1 diabetes perform physical activity safely and for some talented individuals to pursue their sporting ambitions to the highest level.

Contents

1 Endocrine and Metabolic Responses to Exercise 1
   Kostas Tsintzas and Ian A. MacDonald

2 The Impact of Type 1 Diabetes on the Physiological
   Responses to Exercise 29
   Michael C. Riddell

3 Pre-exercise Insulin and Carbohydrate Strategies
   in the Exercising T1DM Individual 47
   Richard M. Bracken, Daniel J. West, and Stephen C. Bain

4 Physical Activity in Childhood Diabetes 73
   Krystyna A. Matyka and S. Francesca Annan

5 The Role of Newer Technologies (CSII and CGM)
   and Novel Strategies in the Management of Type 1
   Diabetes for Sport and Exercise 101
   Alistair N. Lumb

6 Hypoglycemia and Hypoglycemia Unawareness
   During and Following Exercise 115
   Lisa M. Younk and Stephen N. Davis

7 Fueling the Athlete with Type 1 Diabetes 151
   Carin Hume

8 Diabetes and Doping 167
   Richard I.G. Holt

9 Synthesis of Best Practice 193
   Ian Gallen

10 The Athlete's Perspective 203

Index 219

Contributors

Jen Alexander, B.Math., Bed Halifax, NS, Canada

S. Francesca Annan, B.Sc. (Hons), PGCert Department of Nutrition and Dietetics, Alder Hey Children's NHS Foundation Trust, West Derby, Liverpool, Merseyside, UK

Stephen C. Bain, M.A., M.D., FRCP Institute of Life Sciences, College of Medicine, Swansea University, Swansea, Wales, UK

Mark S. Blewitt, M.A. Forton, Lancashire, UK

Richard M. Bracken, B.Sc., M.Sc., PGCert, Ph.D. Health and Sport Science, College of Engineering, Swansea University, Swansea, UK

Russell D. Cobb, B.Sc. (Hons), DMS Department of Supply Chain, Coco-Cola Enterprises, Uxbridge, Middlesex, UK

Stephen N. Davis, M.B.B.S., FRCP, FACP Department of Medicine, University of Maryland School of Medicine, Baltimore, MD, USA

Ian Gallen, B.Sc., M.D., FRCP Diabetes Centre, Wycombe Hospital, High Wycombe, UK

Fred H.R. Gill, B.A. (Cantab) Deloitte, Reading, Buckinghamshire, UK

Monique S. Hanley HypoActive, North Fitzroy, VIC, Australia

Richard I.G. Holt, M.A., M.B., B.Chir., Ph.D., FRCP, FHEA Human Development and Health Academic Unit, University of Southampton, Faculty of Medicine, Southampton General Hospital, Southampton, Hampshire, UK

Carin Hume, B.Sc., M.Sc. Department of Nutrition and Dietetics, Buckinghamshire Hospitals NHS Trust, High Wycombe, Buckinghamshire, UK

Alistair N. Lumb, B.A., Ph.D., M.B.B.S., MRCP Diabetes Centre, Wycombe Hospital, Buckinghamshire Healthcare NHS Trust, High Wycombe, Buckinghamshire, UK

Ian A. MacDonald, Ph.D. School of Biomedical Sciences, Queen's Medical Centre, University of Nottingham Medical School, Nottingham, Nottinghamshire, UK

Krystyna A. Matyka, M.B.B.S., M.D., M.R.C.P.C.H. Division of Metabolic and Vascular Health, Warwick Medical School, Clinical Sciences Research Laboratories, University Hospital, Coventry, UK

Christopher J. Pennell Sixways Stadium, Worcester, Worcestershire, UK

Michael C. Riddell, Ph.D. Physical Activity and Diabetes Unit, School of Kinesiology and Health Science, Muscle Health Research Centre, York University, Toronto, ON, Canada

Sébastien Sasseville Quebec City, QC, Canada

Kostas Tsintzas, B.Sc., M.Sc., Ph.D. School of Biomedical Sciences, Queen's Medical Centre, University of Nottingham Medical School, Nottingham, Nottinghamshire, UK

Daniel J. West, B.Sc., Ph.D. Department of Sport and Exercise, Northumbria University, Newcastle upon Tyne, Tyne and Wear, UK

Lisa M. Younk, B.S. Department of Medicine, University of Maryland School of Medicine, Baltimore, MD, USA

Chapter 1
Endocrine and Metabolic Responses to Exercise

Kostas Tsintzas and Ian A. MacDonald

1.1 Introduction

The successful completion of any human physical movement requires the transformation of chemical energy into mechanical energy in skeletal muscles at rates appropriate to their needs. The source of this chemical energy is the hydrolysis of adenosine triphosphate (ATP). However, the amount of ATP stored in skeletal muscle is limited and would only last for a few seconds of contraction. Therefore, the ATP must be regenerated continuously at the same rate as it is broken down if the work rate is to be maintained for a prolonged period of time. Generating this continuous supply of energy places a great demand on the capacity of the human body to mobilize and utilize the energy substrates required for muscle contraction and to maintain blood glucose homeostasis in the face of substantial increases in both muscle glucose utilization and hepatic glucose production during exercise. In fact, blood glucose concentrations are normally maintained within a narrow physiological range during exercise as the central nervous system (CNS) relies heavily upon continuous blood glucose supply to meet its energy requirements. In order to achieve this, a decrement in blood glucose concentration during exercise is counteracted by a complex and well-coordinated neuroendocrine and autonomic nervous system response. This counterregulatory response aims to prevent and, when necessary, correct any substantial decreases in blood glucose concentration and thus the development of hypoglycemia. This chapter will describe the main metabolic and neuroendocrine responses to exercise of varying intensity and focus on factors affecting blood glucose utilization in humans. It will also examine gender differences in the

K. Tsintzas, B.Sc., M.Sc., Ph.D. (✉) • I.A. MacDonald, Ph.D.
School of Biomedical Sciences,
Queen's Medical Centre, University of Nottingham Medical School,
Nottingham, Nottinghamshire NG7 2UH, UK
e-mail: kostas.tsintzas@nottingham.ac.uk; ian.macdonald@nottingham.ac.uk

I. Gallen (ed.), *Type 1 Diabetes*,
DOI 10.1007/978-0-85729-754-9_1, © Springer-Verlag London Limited 2012

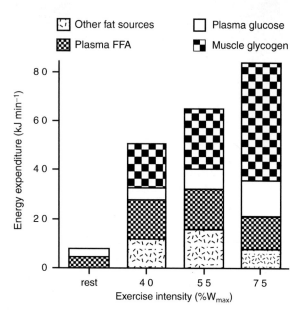

Fig. 1.1 Energy expenditure and the contribution of different metabolic fuels during exercise of varying intensity in humans (Reprinted by permission of the publisher from van Loon et al. [2], John Wiley & Sons)

endocrine response and substrate utilization during exercise and examine how these responses might be altered in exercising children and adolescents. Finally, this chapter will describe the effects of glucose ingestion before and during exercise on counterregulatory responses, substrate utilization, and exercise performance.

1.2 Energy Metabolism and Fuel Utilization During Exercise

Carbohydrate (blood glucose and muscle glycogen) and fat [plasma free fatty acids (FFA) and intramuscular triglycerides (TGs)] are the main energy substrates for aerobic synthesis of ATP during exercise. Both muscle glycogen and blood glucose oxidation rates are markedly increased with increasing exercise intensity (Fig. 1.1). The rate of fat oxidation also increases up to about 60% of maximal oxygen consumption ($\dot{V}O_{2\,max}$) [1, 2]. However, a reduction in the rate of fat oxidation is observed at higher exercise intensities. This decrease in fat contribution to energy metabolism is a result of a significant decline in the oxidation rate of both plasma FFAs and intramuscular TGs and is not entirely related to a decline in plasma FFA availability that normally occurs at high exercise intensities [2].

Pioneering studies in the 1960s and 1970s showed that fatigue during prolonged exercise at intensities between 65% and 85% $\dot{V}O_{2\,max}$ is associated with depletion of glycogen in active skeletal muscle [3, 4]. Although the precise mechanism by which glycogen depletion causes fatigue is still unclear, it appears to be related to a decrease in the rate of oxidative ATP production [5, 6]. The ATP concentrations in skeletal muscle at the point of fatigue are usually maintained at their preexercise levels

[6–9], but a decline in phosphocreatine (PCr) concentration is normally observed. The extent of PCr decline during prolonged, constant intensity exercise, which leads to muscle glycogen depletion, reflects the extent of the inability of the working muscles to maintain oxidative ATP production [10, 11]. Indeed, a strong positive correlation is observed between changes in PCr and glycogen concentrations in skeletal muscle, which supports the presence of a close functional link between oxidative ATP production and glycogen depletion during prolonged exercise [6].

Human skeletal muscles are composed of at least two major fiber types, which differ in their physiological, metabolic, and contractile characteristics [12, 13]. Using a quantitative biochemical method to examine the glycogen changes in pools of muscle fibers of different types, Tsintzas et al. [9] showed that glycogen depletion occurs exclusively in type I (slow-twitch) fibers during running exercise at ~70% $\dot{V}O_{2\,max}$ performed in the fasted (postabsorptive) state. It appears that relatively little glycogen is utilized in type II (fast-twitch) fibers during the first hour of submaximal exercise [7, 9, 14–16]. In contrast, a substantial breakdown of glycogen occurs in type II fibers toward the end of exercise, at a time when an increase in the recruitment of type II fibers occurs to compensate for loss of recruitment of type I fibers as a result of glycogen depletion in the latter fiber type.

Apart from muscle glycogen, blood glucose is also an important energy substrate during exercise. The liver is the only significant source of blood glucose both at rest and during exercise performed in the fasted (postabsorptive) state. Indeed, the contribution of kidney to glucose production during exercise is minimal [17]. Blood glucose utilization in the fasted (postabsorptive) state is mainly a function of the intensity and duration of exercise [17–19] and, in particular, shows a positive curvilinear relationship with exercise intensity [20]. Hence, the liver plays a key role in the maintenance of blood glucose homeostasis during exercise in humans by increasing its glucose production by two- to threefold (when compared to rest) to match the increase in glucose utilization during low- and moderate-intensity exercise (up to 70% $\dot{V}O_{2\,max}$) (Fig. 1.2) [17, 21]. During intense exercise (>80% $\dot{V}O_{2\,max}$), hepatic glucose production may increase up to eightfold [22]. A mismatch between hepatic glucose production and utilization may occur during intense exercise (>80% $\dot{V}O_{2\,max}$), in which the increase in hepatic glucose output exceeds the increase in glucose utilization by skeletal muscle (Fig. 1.2), leading to transient hyperglycemia [22].

Blood glucose utilization also increases with the duration of exercise [18]. Therefore, toward the latter stages of prolonged exercise [23, 24], at a time when muscle glycogen levels are very low, the contribution from blood glucose could account for the majority of total CHO oxidation rate. Furthermore, when endogenous liver glycogen stores are becoming depleted during prolonged exercise continued to the point of fatigue, a mismatch between the glucose production and glucose utilization may occur (Fig. 1.3), resulting in a decrease in blood glucose concentration [25].

Both hepatic glycogenolysis and gluconeogenesis (glucose formed from noncarbohydrate sources such as glycerol, lactate, and amino acids) contribute to the body's ability to maintain blood glucose homeostasis during exercise [26]. During

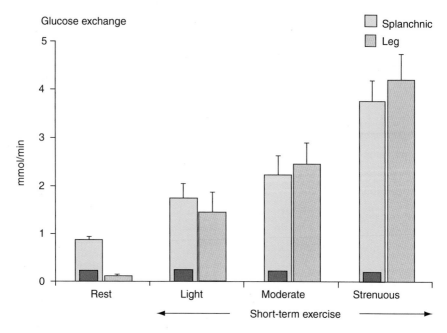

Fig. 1.2 Splanchnic (*yellow*) and leg (*gray*) glucose exchange during exercise of varying intensity in healthy subjects. Gluconeogenesis is indicated in *green* (Reprinted by permission of the publisher from Wahren and Ekberg [182], *Annual Reviews*)

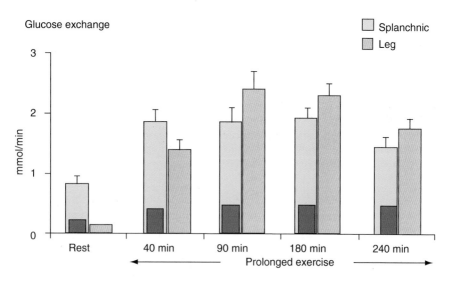

Fig. 1.3 Splanchnic (*yellow*) and leg (*gray*) glucose exchange during prolonged exercise. Gluconeogenesis is indicated in *green* (Reprinted by permission of the publisher from Wahren and Ekberg [182], *Annual Reviews*)

acute exercise of varying intensity, hepatic glycogenolysis is the main source of endogenous glucose production (Fig. 1.2). As liver glycogen stores are becoming depleted during prolonged submaximal exercise, the contribution of hepatic gluconeogenesis increases and may account for up to 50% of total hepatic glucose output after 4 h of low intensity exercise (Fig. 1.3). Furthermore, during prolonged exercise under fasting conditions, a much greater contribution of hepatic glucose output is derived from gluconeogenesis [27, 28]. These findings further emphasize the importance of blood glucose as an energy substrate during exercise. Apart from the intensity and duration of exercise, other factors that can affect the rate of blood glucose utilization during exercise include antecedent nutritional status (see also last section in this chapter), endurance training, and muscle mass involved in exercise. In particular, glucose uptake is inversely related to muscle mass involved [29], which may explain the higher occurrence of hypoglycemic episodes during cycling when compared with running. Conversely, a diet rich in CHO may increase blood glucose utilization, whereas a low CHO diet would lower it [30]. Endurance training decreases blood glucose utilization [31] but has no effect on exogenous glucose utilization [32].

1.3 Exercise and Hyperinsulinemia Stimulate Glucose Uptake in Skeletal Muscle

Both muscle contraction and insulin stimulate muscle glucose uptake through a rapid increase in the translocation of the glucose transporter protein GLUT4 from intracellular vesicle compartments to both the sarcolemma and transverse tubules at the plasma membrane using distinct, at least proximally, signaling pathways [33–35]. Interestingly, in response to insulin, there is a delay in GLUT4 translocation and its reinternalization from the transverse tubules when compared with the sarcolemma [34, 36], whereas the kinetics of contraction-stimulated GLUT4 translocation and reinternalization are similar for the two compartments [35].

The effect of insulin on GLUT4 translocation is mediated through a well-described intracellular signaling pathway that involves tyrosine phosphorylation of insulin receptor substrate-1 (IRS-1), activation of IRS-1-associated phosphatidylinositol 3-kinase (PI3K), and phosphorylation of Akt/PKB and TBC14D/AS160 (a downstream target of Akt in the distal insulin signaling pathway) [37–42]. The signaling pathway underlying the exercise-induced translocation of GLUT4 is less defined, and it appears to include factors such as LKB1, Ca^{2+}/calmodulin-dependent protein kinase II (CaMKII), and their downstream target AMP-activated protein kinase (AMPK) [33, 43, 44]. The TBC14D/AS160 protein may also play a role in exercise-induced GLUT4 translocation and appears to be the point of convergence for the two signaling pathways [45]. More recently, Myo1c, an actin-associated motor protein that is part of the GLUT4 vesicle carrier complex that mediates GLUT4 translocation to the plasma membrane, was shown to mediate both insulin and exercise-induced glucose uptake in skeletal muscle [46].

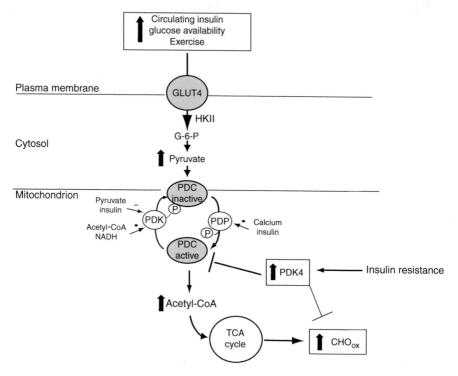

Fig. 1.4 Schematic diagram of hyperinsulinemia, hyperglycemia, and exercise-induced increase in pyruvate flux, stimulation of PDC, the formation of acetyl-CoA, and a concomitant increase in CHO oxidation. In insulin-resistant states, skeletal muscle PDC activation, which controls the rate-limiting step in CHO oxidation, is impaired through a selective upregulation of PDK4 [55, 56, 183]

Superimposing hyperinsulinemia on muscle contraction exerts a synergistic stimulatory effect on glucose uptake and oxidation [47, 48]. Skeletal muscle is the primary tissue responsible for this synergism, which might be explained, at least in part, by an increase in blood flow and hence glucose delivery to the tissue [47, 49]. Indeed, both insulin and muscle contraction can increase blood flow to skeletal muscle [50], although a debate exists whether this is mediated by increasing the number of perfused capillaries (capillary recruitment) [50] or simply an increase in capillary blood flow [51]. Regardless of the mechanism involved, an augmented increase in tissue perfusion will further increase insulin and glucose delivery and/ or fractional glucose extraction by the exercising muscle. Unlike resting conditions, the primary route of insulin-stimulated glucose metabolism during exercise is oxidative metabolism [48]. The pyruvate dehydrogenase complex (PDC) controls the rate-limiting step in CHO oxidation, the oxidative decarboxylation of pyruvate to acetyl-CoA (Fig. 1.4). The activity of PDC increases during exercise in a calcium-dependent manner resulting in an increase in pyruvate flux, the formation of acetyl-CoA, and a concomitant increase in CHO oxidation [52]. Both hyperglycemia and hyperinsulinemia increase the activity of PDC in resting human skeletal muscle [53–56]. Hyperglycemia is thought to stimulate PDC through an increase in pyruvate availability as a result of increases in glucose uptake and glycolysis [53]. On the other hand, an increase in circulating insulin concentration has been shown to activate the PDC phosphatase (PDP), the regulatory enzyme responsible for the dephosphorylation and hence activation of PDC [54, 57]. Interestingly, the stimulatory effect of insulin on skeletal muscle PDC activation is impaired in insulin-resistant states through a selective upregulation of pyruvate dehydrogenase kinase 4 (PDK4), one of the four isoforms of the kinase responsible for the phosphorylation and hence inactivation of PDC [55, 56]. Carbohydrate ingestion immediately before exercise (resulting in increased blood glucose and insulin concentrations) augments the exercise-induced activation of PDC in human skeletal muscle [58], which facilitates the increase in insulin-stimulated glucose oxidation under those conditions.

1.4 Effect of Acute Exercise on Insulin Action in Human Skeletal Muscle

Exercise is beneficial in the treatment of diabetes, and a single bout of exercise was shown to increase insulin sensitivity in insulin-resistant individuals by reversing a defect in insulin-stimulated glucose transport and phosphorylation [59]. However, despite a plethora of studies in this area, the exact cellular mechanisms underlying the well-documented increase in insulin-stimulated skeletal muscle glucose uptake and glycogen synthesis observed up to 2 days following a single bout of exercise [60, 61] remain unresolved.

It is well established that a single bout of exercise increases the transcription [62] and protein content of both whole muscle [63, 64] and plasma membrane [62, 65, 66] fractions of glucose transporter GLUT4. A single bout of exercise also increases skeletal muscle hexokinase II (HKII) activity, transcription, and protein content for a number of hours after the end of exercise [67–70]. HKII is the predominant hexokinase isoform in skeletal muscle, where it phosphorylates internalized glucose, thus ensuring a concentration gradient across the plasma membrane and sustained glucose transport into muscle. Exercise also increases glycogen synthase (GS) activity [40], and it appears that exercise-induced depletion of muscle glycogen content plays a role in enhancing postexercise insulin sensitivity as it is tightly coupled with GS activity [71].

Postexercise augmentation of the classical insulin signaling cascade may not be involved in this positive effect of exercise on insulin action, as many studies have demonstrated that a single bout of exercise does not increase IRS-1 tyrosine phosphorylation, IRS-1-associated PI3K activity, serine phosphorylation of Akt, and glycogen synthase kinase 3 (GSK3) in response to insulin for up to 1 day after exercise [37–41, 70]. Therefore, the enhanced insulin action observed after exercise may involve signaling proteins downstream of Akt, enhanced activation of GS, and/or increased glucose transport and phosphorylation capacity. Indeed, Treebak et al. [72] demonstrated increased phosphorylation of TBC14D/AS160 (a downstream target of Akt) in response to insulin 4 h following a single bout of one-legged exercise compared to the nonexercised leg, suggesting it may play a role in increased postexercise insulin sensitivity. Recently, it was also shown that acute exercise enhances insulin action in skeletal muscle by increasing its capacity to phosphorylate glucose (via upregulation of HKII) and divert it toward glycogen synthesis rather than oxidize it [70]. Although the molecular mechanisms responsible for the upregulation of HK and GLUT4 content following an acute bout of exercise are unclear, possible candidates include the activation of transcription factors such as the peroxisome proliferator-activated receptor-γ (PPARγ) coactivator 1α (PGC1α) [73], sterol regulatory binding protein 1c (SREBP1c) [74, 75], and peroxisome proliferator-activated receptor-δ (PPARδ) [76].

1.5 Hormonal Regulation of Glucose Metabolism

As discussed previously, the liver plays a key role in the maintenance of blood glucose homeostasis during exercise by increasing its glucose production (through increased glycogenolysis and gluconeogenesis) in response to the increase in glucose utilization by the contracting skeletal muscles. Hepatic glycogenolysis is regulated by allosteric factors acting upon the hepatic phosphorylase and glycogen synthase enzymes, whereas hepatic gluconeogenesis is controlled by factors that affect the delivery of gluconeogenic precursors to the liver, their extraction by the tissue, and the activation of key intracellular gluconeogenic enzymes (such as the phosphoenolpyruvate carboxykinase; PEPCK). In general, a number of circulating hormones (insulin, glucagon, catecholamines, cortisol, and growth hormone) and autonomic nerve impulses to the liver are implicated in the regulation of hepatic glucose production during exercise.

The typical hormonal response to exercise is characterized by a reduction in plasma insulin concentration [17, 77] and an increase in the levels of glucagon, catecholamines (both adrenaline and noradrenaline), cortisol, and growth hormone [78]. These hormonal effects are more pronounced during prolonged or high-intensity exercise [79, 80] and collectively facilitate the increase in hepatic glucose production required to counteract the stimulation of muscle glucose uptake that occurs during exercise. The decrease in insulin levels during exercise appears to be due to inhibition in its secretion by the pancreas, which is mediated by activation of the sympathetic nervous system and, in particular, increased α-adrenergic stimulation of the pancreatic β cells [17, 81]. The greater catecholamine stimulation at higher exercise intensities results in greater suppression of insulin secretion compared with low exercise intensities. A decrease in insulin secretion augments the liver's sensitivity to the actions of glucagon, and even a small increase in plasma glucagon is sufficient to increase hepatic glucose output under those conditions [82]. Plasma glucagon levels increase with the duration and intensity of exercise, and this response is augmented in the presence of hypoglycemia [79].

Insulin suppresses both net hepatic glycogenolysis (through an increase in GSK3-mediated activation of glycogen synthase activity) and gluconeogenesis, although the former effect is more potent [83, 84]. Insulin can suppress hepatic gluconeogenesis directly by decreasing the delivery and extraction of gluconeogenic precursors (such as amino acids, lactate, and glycerol) and indirectly by suppressing lipolysis in adipose tissue and thus circulating FFAs, which provide the energy source required to support gluconeogenesis [85].

Glucagon exerts a rapid and potent increase in hepatic glucose production possibly through an AMPK-mediated increase in the hepatic glycogen phosphorylase to glycogen synthase activity ratio, which favors an increase in net hepatic glycogenolysis [86]. Glucagon can also increase hepatic gluconeogenesis through an increase in gluconeogenic precursor (such as lactate) extraction by the liver and their conversion to glucose [87], although this process is modest and slower when compared with the effect of glucagon on hepatic glycogenolysis [88]. Given the antagonistic effects of insulin and glucagon on hepatic glycogenolysis and gluconeogenesis, it is not surprising that glucagon and insulin concentrations in the portal vein [87] and, in particular, the glucagon-to-insulin ratio are important regulators of hepatic glucose production during low and moderate intensity exercise [89, 90]. Indeed, an increase in glucagon is required for the maximum stimulation of hepatic glycogenolysis and gluconeogenesis [87], whereas a reduction in circulating insulin is necessary for the full increase in hepatic glycogenolysis [91]. Prevention of this physiological response of the islet hormones with somatostatin infusion attenuates the normal exercise-induced increase in hepatic glucose output [92, 93].

In addition to glucagon and insulin, small changes in arterial blood glucose concentration and in particular portal vein glucose concentration can also alter hepatic glucose output. Indeed, during prolonged exercise, the decline in both circulating glucose and insulin appears to play a major role in preserving glucose homeostasis by facilitating an increase in hepatic glucose output [94]. Conversely, hyperglycemia and hyperinsulinemia inhibit hepatic glucose output [84, 95]. Indeed, carbohydrate ingestion during exercise and the associated increases in blood glucose and insulin concentrations can completely suppress hepatic glucose production [96].

It must be pointed out however that under normal physiological conditions, the liver extracts a great proportion (up to 50–60%) of insulin secreted in the portal vein, and therefore, the insulin concentration in the latter can be two- to threefold higher than peripheral arterial insulin concentration [97]. However, only about a fifth of secreted glucagon is extracted by the liver [97]. Therefore, arterial insulin concentrations underestimate those in the portal vein to a greater extent than the corresponding glucagon concentrations. Furthermore, the gradient of portal to arterial concentrations for both hormones is widened during exercise because of a reduction in hepatic blood flow and, in the case of glucagon, increased secretion [98]. This is important not only because the glucagon-to-insulin ratio is an important regulator of hepatic glucose production during exercise, but also because portal venous hyperinsulinemia appears to be more potent than peripheral hyperinsulinemia in suppressing hepatic glucose production during the early stages of exercise. In contrast, peripheral arterial hyperinsulinemia becomes more important as the duration of exercise increases through suppression of lipolysis in adipose tissue and hence reduction in circulating glycerol and FFAs, which will further suppress hepatic glucose output [99].

Studies in humans [92, 93] and dogs [87] have clearly demonstrated the importance of increased circulating glucagon levels in the stimulation of hepatic glucose production during exercise. Although the rise in glucagon can account for ~60% of total splanchnic glucose output during exercise [100], other factors also seem to play important roles [101]. Catecholamine (adrenaline and noradrenaline) plasma concentrations increase with exercise intensity and duration, and these changes coincide with increased hepatic glucose output, although a causal relationship between these parameters has not been established. It should be noted that a large proportion of circulating catecholamines are extracted by the gut [102], which suggest that the liver is exposed to portal vein concentrations that are considerably lower than the corresponding levels in peripheral circulation. Catecholamines can enhance both hepatic glycogenolysis by stimulating glycogen phosphorylase and adipose tissue lipolysis by activating hormone-sensitive lipase, resulting in increased levels of circulating glycerol and FFAs [103–105]. However, it appears that adrenaline is significantly more potent than noradrenaline in stimulating hepatic glucose output [106]. At rest under conditions of basal circulating insulin and glucagon concentrations, a 20-fold increase in plasma adrenaline concentration in humans (through infusion of adrenaline for 90 min) resulted in a biphasic increase in hepatic glucose production; during the first hour of infusion, an increase in hepatic glycogenolysis was responsible for the majority (~60%) of the increase in glucose production, whereas during the last 30 min of infusion, the rate of hepatic glucose production declined and the contribution of hepatic gluconeogenesis increased 2.5-fold accounting for 80% of glucose production [107]. It is also well established that adrenaline inhibits insulin-stimulated glucose uptake and that skeletal muscle appears to be the major site of this temporary insulin-resistant state [108].

The role of the neural input to the liver and catecholamine stimulation in the regulation of hepatic glucose production during exercise has been questioned [109]. Indeed, combined α-and β-adrenergic blockade in healthy humans, in contrast to type I diabetics, failed to demonstrate an important role for adrenergic nervous system in controlling exercise-induced hepatic glucose output [110]. Further evidence that catecholamines may not be important in stimulating the exercise-induced increase in hepatic glucose output (at least during low and moderate intensity exercise) comes from animal studies that used pharmacological blockade of the sympathetic nervous system [102] and studies on adrenalectomized humans [111], in which a normal increase in hepatic glucose output was observed during moderate exercise.

In contrast, during high-intensity exercise, there is rapid and marked elevation in circulating catecholamine levels [112–115]. Interestingly, infusion of both adrenaline and noradrenaline during moderate intensity exercise (designed to reproduce the pattern of catecholamine release during intense exercise) resulted in an augmented hepatic glucose output of the same magnitude as during intense exercise [116].

This suggests that, unlike light and moderate exercise, catecholamines may play an important role in the regulation of glucose homeostasis during high-intensity exercise.

However, it should be noted that in humans, there appears to be some redundancy in the hormonal regulation of hepatic glucose production. For example, when both the fall in insulin and rise in glucagon concentrations were prevented during 60 min of moderate exercise by infusion of somatostatin along with insulin and glucagon replacement at fixed rates (islet clamp technique), hepatic glucose production did not increase, and plasma glucose initially decreased from 5.5 to 3.4 mmol/l (from 100 to ~62 mg/dl) and then leveled off and was 3.3 mmol/l (~60 mg/dl) at the end of exercise [93]. In contrast, when insulin was allowed to decrease and glucagon to increase simultaneously (which represents the normal response to exercise), there was an increase in hepatic glucose production and the plasma glucose level was 4.5 mmol/l (~80 mg/ml) at the end of exercise [93]. Since hypoglycemia did not occur when the normal insulin and glucagon response was prevented, it is likely that other counterregulatory hormones (such as adrenaline) play a more important role in the regulation of hepatic glucose production during exercise when the islet hormone responses are disturbed. Indeed, if changes in circulating glucagon and insulin levels are prevented in the presence of adrenergic blockade during exercise, progressive hypoglycemia (2.6 mmol/l or < 50 mg/dl) will ensue [117].

Growth hormone (GH), secreted from the anterior pituitary gland, and cortisol, secreted from the adrenal cortex, appear to play a minor role in the regulation of glucose homeostasis during short-term exercise, but as the duration of exercise increases, they contribute to the stimulation of whole body lipolysis (and therefore release of FFAs and glycerol into the circulation) and the increase in hepatic gluconeogenesis [118, 119]. During moderate-intensity running exercise to exhaustion in humans, plasma GH concentrations may increase by up to tenfold above postabsorptive levels, whereas cortisol concentrations may double [120, 121]. This increase occurs in the absence of a decrease in blood glucose concentration, which suggests that blood glucose concentration is not the sole determinant of hormonal response to prolonged exercise [122]. Carbohydrate ingestion or infusion during prolonged exercise suppresses the increase in cortisol secretion usually observed during exercise without exogenous carbohydrate supply [123]. Interestingly, carbohydrate ingestion immediately before and during the first hour of prolonged running exercise also attenuated the normal increase in GH concentration (along with suppression of lipolysis and attenuation of plasma glycerol and FFA levels) [121]. However, when carbohydrate ingestion was discontinued after the first hour of exercise, plasma GH and FFA levels were quickly increased and at exhaustion reached levels comparable with those observed in the control (nonsupplemented) trial [121]. Since the changes in GH paralleled those in FFA and glycerol, it appears that during prolonged exercise continued to the point of exhaustion, secretion of GH is important for fat mobilization from adipose tissue and therefore, indirectly, for glucose metabolism by enhancing liver glucose output during exercise performed in the postabsorptive state.

1.6 Counterregulatory Responses to Hypoglycemia During Exercise

Blood glucose concentration is normally maintained within a narrow physiological range during exercise. It may fall however during prolonged exercise performed in the fasted state and continued to the point of fatigue when endogenous muscle and liver glycogen stores are becoming depleted, resulting in a mismatch between hepatic glucose production and working muscle glucose utilization.

In resting healthy humans, even a small decrement in blood glucose concentration to ~80 mg/dl (~4.4 mmol/l) would provoke a reduction in insulin secretion in an initial effort to counteract the fall in blood glucose [124]. There is a hierarchy of glycemic thresholds for activation of counterregulatory hormone secretion, autonomic symptoms, and cerebral dysfunction, which allows for a more effective and redundant response to hypoglycemia [125]. Increased secretion of glucagon and adrenaline occurs at blood glucose concentration of ~68–70 mg/dl (3.8–3.9 mmol/l), secretion of noradrenaline and growth hormone at ~65–67 mg/dl (3.6–3.7 mmol/l), and secretion of cortisol at ~ 55 mg/dl (3.0 mmol/l). Autonomic symptoms begin to develop at ~58 mg/dl (3.2 mmol/l), whereas deterioration in cognitive function is observed at glucose concentrations of around 50–55 mg/dl (2.8–3.0 mmol/l) [125, 126].

As discussed in the previous section, insulin, glucagon, and catecholamines also respond in a hierarchical fashion to regulate hepatic glucose production and prevent exercise-induced hypoglycemia. However, the normal counterregulatory hormone (catecholamines, glucagon, cortisol, and GH) response to exercise is amplified by simultaneous hypoglycemia in nondiabetic individuals [127]. In fact, the counterregulatory hormone response to exercise and insulin-induced hypoglycemia is synergistic when the two stimuli are combined [128]. Furthermore, it appears that the catecholamine (and in particular adrenaline) response to hypoglycemia can be dissociated from the corresponding response to exercise [127]. It appears that exercise augments the adrenaline response to hypoglycemia in an effort to reduce glucose utilization by peripheral tissues [89]. Therefore, the potent effect of exercise on the counterregulatory hormone response to hypoglycemia is important in both increasing hepatic glucose output and limiting peripheral glucose utilization in a coordinated effort to minimize the magnitude of hypoglycemia during exercise.

During exercise, hepatic glucose output is very sensitive to small changes in plasma glucose concentration resulting from changes in the balance between glucose supply and utilization [95]. Indeed, in both humans and dogs, the normal exercise-induced increase in hepatic glucose output can be completely prevented when glucose is infused in an attempt to match systemic glucose supply with the increase in glucose utilization by skeletal muscle [95, 129]. Interestingly, although this suppression of hepatic glucose output occurred in the presence of elevated portal vein insulin levels when compared with those seen in the control trial, the response of glucagon, catecholamines, and cortisol was not altered, indicating that the counterregulatory hormone response to exercise is less sensitive than hepatic glucose output to changes in glucose supply [129]. Based on human and animal studies that observed reduced counterregulatory response to induced systemic hypoglycemia

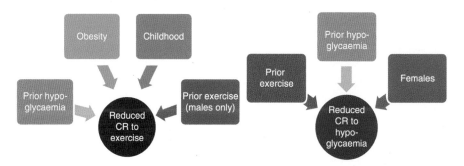

Fig. 1.5 Factors blunting the normal counterregulatory hormone response (CR) to subsequent exercise (*left*) and hypoglycemia (*right*) (Data taken from [2, 134, 135, 137, 138, 153–155, 184])

when portal vein glucose concentrations were elevated (through local infusion or oral ingestion of glucose), it appears that, in addition to glucose-responsive neurons in the brain, glucose-sensitive neurons in the portal vein or the liver itself may also play an important role in mediating glucose-induced changes in hepatic glucose output [130–132]. However, the extent to which this feedback mechanism operates in humans during exercise requires further investigation.

Interestingly, the occurrence of preexercise hypoglycemia is associated with blunted counterregulation and impaired hepatic glycogenolysis during subsequent exercise [133]. Conversely, prior exercise also blunts the counterregulatory hormone response to subsequent hypoglycemia [134]. In healthy humans, two prior episodes of moderate hypoglycemia (~2.9 mmol/l or ~50 mg/dl) for 120 min result in considerable attenuation (~50%) of the neuroendocrine (glucagon, insulin, and catecholamines) and metabolic (hepatic glucose production, lipolysis, and ketogenesis) responses to moderate exercise (~50% $\dot{V}O_{2\,max}$) performed the next day [133]. This blunted response became more apparent after the first 30 min of exercise and hepatic glucose production, despite an initial increase, declined to basal levels by the end of exercise (90 min). However, the opposite is also true, as two 90-min bouts of exercise at 50% $\dot{V}O_{2\,max}$, separated by 3 h, were shown to markedly blunt (by ~30–60%) the counterregulatory hormone response (adrenaline, noradrenaline, glucagon, pancreatic polypeptide, ACTH, and GH but surprisingly not cortisol), hepatic glucose production (by ~60%), and muscle sympathetic nerve activity (by ~90%) response to a 2-h bout of moderate hypoglycemia (~3.0 mmol/l or ~54 mg/dl) the day after [134].

The similarity between the latter responses and those reported after antecedent hypoglycemia led to the hypothesis that a common mechanism underlies both set of responses. A number of factors including elevations in circulating cortisol, ketone bodies, and lactate levels have been proposed as mediators of the hypoglycemia-induced blunting effect on glucose counterregulation during a subsequent episode of hypoglycemia [134–136]. Whether this is the case in exercise-induced responses requires further investigation.

In addition to antecedent exercise and hypoglycemia, other factors that can also modulate the normal counterregulatory response to exercise are obesity and maturation (Fig. 1.5). Obesity blunts catecholamine and growth hormone responses to acute intense and submaximal exercise in both adults [137, 138] and children [139].

Despite this blunting effect on counterregulatory response to exercise and higher circulating insulin levels during exercise, none of the studies reported any incidents of hypoglycemia, possibly because of a concurrent decrease in peripheral glucose utilization during exercise in the obese population as a result of insulin resistance.

In general, when compared with adults, children (both boys and girls) rely more on fat and less on carbohydrate as a metabolic fuel during exercise of similar relative intensity performed both in the fasting state and with carbohydrate feeding [140, 141]. Although the typically observed decrease in circulating insulin and increase in glucagon during exercise in adults occurs in children too, other responses (such as catecholamine and cortisol secretion) appear to be blunted in children; however, this is a not a uniform finding in the literature (for extensive review on this topic see Riddell [140]). Despite potential differences in the hormonal response to exercise between children and adults, there is no evidence that children are at greater risk for developing hypoglycemia during prolonged exercise, perhaps because they rely less on carbohydrate as a metabolic fuel at a given exercise intensity, which compensates for any deficiency in glucose counterregulation.

1.7   Gender Differences in the Endocrine and Metabolic Responses to Exercise

During moderate- and high-intensity exercise (60–85% $\dot{V}O_{2\,max}$) performed in the postabsorptive (fasting) state, women oxidize more lipid and less CHO than men [142–144]. This may explain the greater plasma glucose clearance rate and tendency for a decline in plasma glucose concentration during exercise in the fasting state in men compared with women [144]. However, this gender difference is relatively small during low intensity (~40% $\dot{V}O_{2\,max}$) exercise [145], and therefore, exercising at moderate to high intensity, which is known to increase muscle glucose uptake and oxidation [1, 2, 19], may present a greater challenge for glucose counterregulation in men than women.

Interestingly, studies that compared the metabolic responses to exercise performed with CHO ingestion in men and women reported that the contribution of exogenous CHO to energy production was either similar [146] or slightly higher in women than men [147]. In support of this, moderate exercise performed in the postprandial state resulted in similar glycemic response and substrate oxidation rates during exercise after either oral (high glycemic index meal) or intravenous CHO (glucose) loads in men and women [148]. This may, at least in part, have been due to the similar pancreatic insulin secretory response and whole body insulin sensitivity observed in the men and women studied. However, it should be noted that there is no consensus in the literature with regard to insulin sensitivity differences in men and women. Indeed, although some studies demonstrated greater whole body insulin sensitivity in women than in men [149, 150], others did not observe a gender difference in this parameter [151]. Regardless of the mechanism involved, it appears that moderate exercise performed in the postprandial state abolishes the gender difference in substrate utilization normally observed during exercise in the fasting state and appears to present a similar challenge to the ability of healthy men and women to perform exercise without a substantial decline in plasma glucose concentration.

Higher adrenaline, noradrenaline, and pancreatic polypeptide responses have been reported in men than women during 90 min of cycling exercise at approximately 50% $\dot{V}O_{2\,max}$ (with euglycemia maintained through an exogenous glucose infusion). However, insulin, glucagon, cortisol, and GH levels responded similarly in both genders, which may have accounted for the absence of a gender difference in hepatic glucose production [152].

Interestingly, in healthy humans, exercise performed in the morning can suppress the counterregulatory response to exercise performed in the afternoon, and this effect appears to be gender specific [153]. Indeed, 90 min of cycling at 50% $\dot{V}O_{2\,max}$ blunts the adrenaline, noradrenaline, cortisol, and GH responses to subsequent exercise of similar duration and intensity performed 3 h later in men but not women. Despite this differential neuroendocrine response between the two genders, the exogenous glucose infusion rate required to maintain euglycemia was fivefold higher during the second bout of exercise (most likely as a result of decreased hepatic glucose production) and no gender difference was observed [153]. The gender difference in the counterregulatory responses to exercise is also present after two episodes of antecedent hypoglycemia in individuals with type I diabetes [154]. Furthermore, there is also a gender difference in the counterregulatory responses to moderately controlled hypoglycemia at rest, with women showing lower catecholamine responses when compared with men [155].

The functional significance and origin of this gender difference in the neuroendocrine response to exercise after either antecedent exercise or hypoglycemia is not clear (Fig. 1.5), but it is possible that antecedent exercise may present a greater risk for developing hypoglycemia during subsequent exercise in men than women by shifting the glycemic threshold for the initiation of counterregulatory responses to lower plasma glucose concentrations.

1.8 Glucose Ingestion During Exercise and Effects on Counterregulatory Responses, Substrate Utilization, and Exercise Performance

Fatigue during prolonged intense exercise in a thermoneutral environment appears to be associated with either glycogen depletion in working muscles [3, 4, 25] or hypoglycemia [156]. However, it is possible that during exhaustive intense exercise, volitional fatigue is a multifactorial process that involves both peripheral and central mechanisms. When the endogenous carbohydrate stores are severely reduced during the latter stages of prolonged exercise, a reduction in plasma glucose concentration may pose a threat to cerebral metabolism (which depends on constant glucose supply). This threat to normal cerebral function may be prevented by discontinuing exercise as a result of impaired mental drive for motor performance [157, 158]. However, the extent to which a central mechanism operates during exercise in humans remains to be elucidated.

It should be noted that moderate exercise to exhaustion can be continued in the presence of hypoglycemia [25]. Furthermore, plasma glucose concentrations do not consistently fall during prolonged exhaustive exercise in the absence of CHO supplementation. Indeed, a 30-km running race, and even marathon running, performed after an overnight fast and without CHO supplementation may not always challenge euglycemia [120, 159]. This may not be surprising given that glucose uptake is inversely related to the amount of muscle mass involved during exercise [29]. A greater active muscle mass is involved during running when compared with cycling, and this may explain the higher occurrence of hypoglycemic episodes during the latter when compared with the former mode of exercise. It is well established that oral CHO ingestion during prolonged glycogen-depleting exercise can delay the onset of fatigue and thus substantially increase endurance performance in humans [160]. The typical metabolic response to exercise with oral CHO ingestion is characterized by elevated plasma glucose and insulin concentrations, an increase in exogenous glucose uptake and utilization, suppression in hepatic glucose output, and a reduction in plasma FFA and glycerol concentrations [96, 120, 121, 161].

In healthy subjects, carbohydrate ingestion or glucose infusion before or during exercise suppresses the increase in cortisol [123, 162], adrenaline [25], glucagon [30, 163], and growth hormone [121] secretion usually observed during prolonged exercise without exogenous CHO supply. These reciprocal changes in insulin on one hand and glucagon, cortisol, adrenaline, and growth hormone on the other hand during exercise with CHO ingestion are important in facilitating suppression in both hepatic glucose output and adipose tissue lipolysis under conditions of increased exogenous glucose supply and utilization.

Exogenous CHO administration may either spare endogenous muscle glycogen utilization during prolonged continuous or intermittent exercise [6, 9, 164, 165] or better maintain blood glucose concentration and whole body CHO oxidation rate late in exercise at a time when a significant reduction in muscle glycogen stores occurs [166]. The sparing of muscle glycogen occurs in type I slow-twitch fibers during continuous exercise [6, 9] and mainly in type II fast-twitch muscle fibers during high-intensity intermittent exercise [164]. During exhaustive continuous exercise, this ergogenic effect of CHO ingestion is associated with attenuated decline in oxidative ATP resynthesis in type I fibers [6].

It is important however that CHO ingestion starts immediately before or as early as possible during exercise. Once muscle glycogen concentrations are depleted and fatigue is imminent, the provision of exogenous CHO cannot sustain exercise at high intensity ($>70\%$ $\dot{V}O_{2\,max}$) [30], possibly as a result of a mismatch between the rate of blood glucose uptake by the working muscles and the rate of CHO utilization required to meet the metabolic demand of exercise.

The metabolic effects of CHO ingestion during exercise depend on factors such as the type and intensity of exercise, type and timing of CHO ingestion, preexercise nutritional and training status of the subjects, and the magnitude of the associated perturbation in insulin secretion. Although endurance training reduces the contribution of endogenous CHO utilization to energy expenditure, it does not diminish the exogenous glucose utilization during submaximal exercise [32], possibly because the sensitivity and responsiveness of insulin-stimulated glucose uptake is increased in the trained compared with the untrained human muscle [167]. An antecedent CHO-rich diet that elevates resting muscle glycogen concentrations preserves the ergogenic effect of CHO solutions ingested during high-intensity intermittent running by better maintaining plasma glucose concentrations toward the end of exercise but without affecting muscle glycogen utilization [168].

The intensity and/or type of exercise and their effect on blood glucose, plasma insulin, and catecholamine responses may play a major role in determining the contribution of blood glucose and muscle glycogen utilization to energy metabolism when CHO is ingested during exercise. Indeed, CHO ingestion during high-intensity cycling ($>70\%$ $\dot{V}O_{2\,max}$) results in modest increases in circulating glucose and insulin levels [169, 170], whereas during low intensity cycling (30–50% $\dot{V}O_{2\,max}$), it amplifies the glycemic and insulinemic responses [171, 172]. Therefore, changes in exercise intensity and the associated catecholamine responses may have a profound impact on glycemic responses to exercise, which in turn may have important implications for choice of metabolic fuel (i.e., endogenous and exogenous CHO) during exercise.

There are a number of differences in the responses of blood glucose and insulin to oral CHO ingestion between cycling and running, the most frequently used exercise modes in the study of energy metabolism in humans [160]. These apparent differences between cycling and running are likely to result from differences in glucose uptake into active muscle tissue. Although exogenous CHO oxidation rates were reported to be similar between prolonged running and cycling at the same relative exercise intensity [173], in healthy individuals, the rate of whole body glucose uptake during physiological hyperinsulinemia (maintained by constant infusion of insulin at a fixed rate) is greater during running than cycling performed at the same relative intensity [174]. In humans, skeletal muscle accounts for almost all the glucose uptake during exercise performed under euglycemic-hyperinsulinemic conditions. Under those conditions, the increase in muscle glucose uptake when compared with hyperinsulinemia alone appears to be due to a stimulatory effect of contractile activity and an increase in muscle blood flow and, hence, glucose delivery [49]. Therefore, the greater insulin-stimulated glucose disposal during running than cycling might be explained by a higher contractile activity as a result of a greater active muscle mass in the former compared with the latter exercise mode. Alternatively, a difference in the pattern of muscle fiber type recruitment and/or glycogen utilization between running and cycling might also explain the difference in glucose disposal between the two exercise modes. Regardless of the mechanism involved, exercise mode differences in glucose uptake may have important implications for control of blood glucose concentration and choice of metabolic fuel during exercise performed under hyperinsulinemic conditions (i.e., postprandial state) in both healthy and diabetic individuals.

Carbohydrate ingestion during the hour before the onset of exercise may result in transient hypoglycemia during subsequent exercise. Contrary to popular belief, this transient hypoglycemia (which may or may not be accompanied by relevant symptoms) does not appear to adversely affect subsequent exercise performance, which may actually improve when compared with exercise in the fasting state [175]. It should be noted that hypoglycemia is not always observed following CHO ingestion during the hour before the onset of exercise and some individuals appear to be more prone than others, although the factors that determine this susceptibility are not clear [175].

Ingestion of CHO-rich meals 3–4 h before exercise also improves endurance performance when compared to exercise after an overnight fast [176–178]. However, large glycemic and insulinemic perturbations are normally associated with such practice, which may result in a sharp decline in blood glucose concentration during the early stages of subsequent exercise, increased muscle glycogenolysis, and reduced plasma FFA availability and oxidation [179, 180]. The low glucagon-to-insulin ratio during exercise under those conditions is expected to suppress hepatic glucose output. As the effect of insulin and contraction on muscle glucose uptake is synergistic, the sharp decline in plasma glucose concentration under those conditions may be a reflection of insufficient blood glucose supply in the face of increased muscle glucose uptake.

One way to ameliorate such large glycemic and insulinemic perturbations is to consume a meal that consists of low glycemic index (GI) foods, which would provoke smaller metabolic disturbances during both the postprandial period and subsequent exercise, as well as result in lower CHO oxidation rates during exercise when compared with a meal consisting of high GI foods [163, 181]. The lower glycemic and insulinemic responses to low GI meals (secondary to slow digestion and absorption of the ingested foods) prevent a sharp decline in blood glucose concentration during the early stages of exercise and maintain higher glucagon-to-insulin ratio and plasma FFA availability and fat oxidation rates, together with a sparing of muscle glycogen utilization and lower muscle lactate accumulation [163].

Despite the profound glycemic and insulinemic perturbations associated with ingestion of high glycemic index (GI) foods or meals, there is no consensus in the literature on whether they adversely affect subsequent exercise performance when compared with low GI meals [175]. It is likely that any profound glycemic effects of high GI meals observed early in exercise might be offset by the fact that high GI foods (if consumed sufficiently in advance to the start of exercise, i.e., 3–4 h) confer an advantage in terms of muscle and liver glycogen storage compared to low GI foods [163].

1.9 Summary

Exercise exerts a great demand on the capacity of the human body to maintain blood glucose homeostasis. Blood glucose utilization by skeletal muscle increases with increasing intensity and duration of exercise, and a decrement in blood glucose concentration is counteracted by a complex and well-coordinated neuroendocrine response. The liver plays a key role in the maintenance of blood glucose homeostasis during exercise by increasing its glucose production (through increased glycogenolysis and gluconeogenesis). An increase in glucagon and a fall in insulin concentrations in the portal vein are important stimulators of hepatic glucose production during low and moderate intensity exercise, whereas catecholamines may play an important role during high-intensity exercise or when the islet hormone responses are disturbed. The normal counterregulatory hormone response to exercise is amplified by simultaneous hypoglycemia in nondiabetic individuals. However, occurrence of preexercise hypoglycemia is associated with blunted counterregulation during subsequent exercise. Conversely, prior exercise blunts the counterregulatory response to a subsequent episode of hypoglycemia. The normal counterregulatory response to exercise is also blunted in obese individuals, and there is evidence that at least part of the response might be impaired in children, although their risk for developing hypoglycemia during prolonged exercise is similar to that of adults. Moderate exercise performed in the postprandial state abolishes the gender difference in substrate utilization normally observed during exercise in the fasting state. However, prior exercise performed in the morning can suppress the counterregulatory response to exercise performed in the afternoon in men but not women. Therefore, it is possible that antecedent exercise may present a greater risk for developing hypoglycemia during subsequent exercise in men than women. Oral CHO ingestion during prolonged exercise can delay the onset of fatigue in humans by either sparing muscle glycogen utilization or better maintaining blood glucose concentration and CHO oxidation late in exercise. The metabolic effects of CHO ingestion during exercise depend on factors such as the type and intensity of exercise, type and timing of CHO ingestion, preexercise nutritional status, and the magnitude of the associated perturbation in insulin secretion. Carbohydrate ingestion in the minutes and hours before the onset of exercise is associated with profound glycemic and insulinemic perturbations which may result in transient hypoglycemia and increased reliance on muscle glycogen during subsequent exercise. Consumption of low glycemic index foods or meals ameliorates these metabolic perturbations, but there is inconclusive evidence on whether they confer an advantage in terms of exercise performance.

References

1. Romijn JA, Coyle EF, Sidossis LS, et al. Regulation of endogenous fat and carbohydrate metabolism in relation to exercise intensity and duration. Am J Physiol. 1993;265:E380–91.
2. van Loon LJ, Greenhaff PL, Constantin-Teodosiu D, Saris WH, Wagenmakers AJ. The effects of increasing exercise intensity on muscle fuel utilisation in humans. J Physiol. 2001;536: 295–304.
3. Hermansen L, Hultman E, Saltin B. Muscle glycogen during prolonged severe exercise. Acta Physiol Scand. 1967;71:129–39.
4. Karlsson J, Saltin B. Diet, muscle glycogen, and endurance performance. J Appl Physiol. 1971;31:203–6.

5. Broberg S, Sahlin K. Adenine nucleotide degradation in human skeletal muscle during prolonged exercise. J Appl Physiol. 1989;67:116–22.
6. Tsintzas K, Williams C, Constantin-Teodosiu D, et al. Phosphocreatine degradation in type I and type II muscle fibres during submaximal exercise in man: effect of carbohydrate ingestion. J Physiol. 2001;537:305–11.
7. Ball-Burnett M, Green HJ, Houston ME. Energy metabolism in human slow and fast twitch fibres during prolonged cycle exercise. J Physiol. 1991;437:257–67.
8. Norman B, Sollevi A, Kaijser L, Jansson E. ATP breakdown products in human skeletal muscle during prolonged exercise to exhaustion. Clin Physiol. 1987;7:503–10.
9. Tsintzas OK, Williams C, Boobis L, Greenhaff P. Carbohydrate ingestion and single muscle fiber glycogen metabolism during prolonged running in men. J Appl Physiol. 1996;81:801–9.
10. Hultman E, Bergstrom J, Anderson NM. Breakdown and resynthesis of phosphorylcreatine and adenosine triphosphate in connection with muscular work in man. Scand J Clin Lab Invest. 1967;19:56–66.
11. Sahlin K, Soderlund K, Tonkonogi M, Hirakoba K. Phosphocreatine content in single fibers of human muscle after sustained submaximal exercise. Am J Physiol. 1997;273:C172–8.
12. Essen B, Jansson E, Henriksson J, Taylor AW, Saltin B. Metabolic characteristics of fibre types in human skeletal muscle. Acta Physiol Scand. 1975;95:153–65.
13. Schiaffino S, Reggiani C. Molecular diversity of myofibrillar proteins: gene regulation and functional significance. Physiol Rev. 1996;76:371–423.
14. Gollnick PD, Piehl K, Saltin B. Selective glycogen depletion pattern in human muscle fibres after exercise of varying intensity and at varying pedalling rates. J Physiol. 1974;241:45–57.
15. Tsintzas OK, Williams C, Boobis L, Greenhaff P. Carbohydrate ingestion and glycogen utilization in different muscle fibre types in man. J Physiol. 1995;489(Pt 1):243–50.
16. Vollestad NK, Blom PC. Effect of varying exercise intensity on glycogen depletion in human muscle fibres. Acta Physiol Scand. 1985;125:395–405.
17. Wahren J, Felig P, Ahlborg G, Jorfeldt L. Glucose metabolism during leg exercise in man. J Clin Invest. 1971;50:2715–25.
18. Ahlborg G, Felig P. Lactate and glucose exchange across the forearm, legs, and splanchnic bed during and after prolonged leg exercise. J Clin Invest. 1982;69:45–54.
19. Katz A, Broberg S, Sahlin K, Wahren J. Leg glucose uptake during maximal dynamic exercise in humans. Am J Physiol. 1986;251:E65–70.
20. Coggan AR. Plasma glucose metabolism during exercise in humans. Sports Med. 1991;11: 102–24.
21. Bergeron R, Kjaer M, Simonsen L, Bulow J, Galbo H. Glucose production during exercise in humans: a-hv balance and isotopic-tracer measurements compared. J Appl Physiol. 1999;87: 111–5.
22. Marliss EB, Vranic M. Intense exercise has unique effects on both insulin release and its roles in glucoregulation: implications for diabetes. Diabetes. 2002;51 Suppl 1:S271–83.
23. Coggan AR, Coyle EF. Reversal of fatigue during prolonged exercise by carbohydrate infusion or ingestion. J Appl Physiol. 1987;63:2388–95.
24. Coggan AR, Spina RJ, Kohrt WM, Bier DM, Holloszy JO. Plasma glucose kinetics in a well-trained cyclist fed glucose throughout exercise. Int J Sport Nutr. 1991;1:279–88.
25. Felig P, Cherif A, Minagawa A, Wahren J. Hypoglycemia during prolonged exercise in normal men. N Engl J Med. 1982;306:895–900.
26. Petersen KF, Price TB, Bergeron R. Regulation of net hepatic glycogenolysis and gluconeogenesis during exercise: impact of type 1 diabetes. J Clin Endocrinol Metab. 2004;89: 4656–64.
27. Bjorkman O, Eriksson LS. Splanchnic glucose metabolism during leg exercise in 60-hour-fasted human subjects. Am J Physiol. 1983;245:E443–8.
28. Lavoie C, Ducros F, Bourque J, Langelier H, Chiasson JL. Glucose metabolism during exercise in man: the role of insulin and glucagon in the regulation of hepatic glucose production and gluconeogenesis. Can J Physiol Pharmacol. 1997;75:26–35.

29. Richter EA, Kiens B, Saltin B, Christensen NJ, Savard G. Skeletal muscle glucose uptake during dynamic exercise in humans: role of muscle mass. Am J Physiol. 1988;254:E555–61.

30. Galbo H, Holst JJ, Christensen NJ. The effect of different diets and of insulin on the hormonal response to prolonged exercise. Acta Physiol Scand. 1979;107:19–32.

31. Coggan AR, Kohrt WM, Spina RJ, Bier DM, Holloszy JO. Endurance training decreases plasma glucose turnover and oxidation during moderate-intensity exercise in men. J Appl Physiol. 1990;68:990–6.

32. Jeukendrup AE, Mensink M, Saris WH, Wagenmakers AJ. Exogenous glucose oxidation during exercise in endurance-trained and untrained subjects. J Appl Physiol. 1997;82: 835–40.

33. Jessen N, Goodyear LJ. Contraction signaling to glucose transport in skeletal muscle. J Appl Physiol. 2005;99:330–7.

34. Lauritzen HP, Galbo H, Brandauer J, Goodyear LJ, Ploug T. Large GLUT4 vesicles are stationary while locally and reversibly depleted during transient insulin stimulation of skeletal muscle of living mice: imaging analysis of GLUT4-enhanced green fluorescent protein vesicle dynamics. Diabetes. 2008;57:315–24.

35. Lauritzen HP, Galbo H, Toyoda T, Goodyear LJ. Kinetics of contraction-induced GLUT4 translocation in skeletal muscle fibers from living mice. Diabetes. 2010;59:2134–44.

36. Lauritzen HP, Ploug T, Prats C, Tavare JM, Galbo H. Imaging of insulin signaling in skeletal muscle of living mice shows major role of T-tubules. Diabetes. 2006;55:1300–6.

37. Frosig C, Roepstorff C, Brandt N, et al. Reduced malonyl-CoA content in recovery from exercise correlates with improved insulin-stimulated glucose uptake in human skeletal muscle. Am J Physiol Endocrinol Metab. 2009;296:E787–95.

38. Goodyear LJ, Giorgino F, Balon TW, Condorelli G, Smith RJ. Effects of contractile activity on tyrosine phosphoproteins and PI 3-kinase activity in rat skeletal muscle. Am J Physiol. 1995; 268:E987–95.

39. Hansen PA, Nolte LA, Chen MM, Holloszy JO. Increased GLUT-4 translocation mediates enhanced insulin sensitivity of muscle glucose transport after exercise. J Appl Physiol. 1998; 85:1218–22.

40. Wojtaszewski JF, Hansen BF, Gade J, et al. (2000) Insulin signaling and insulin sensitivity after exercise in human skeletal muscle. Diabetes 49:325–331

41. Wojtaszewski JF, Hansen BF, Kiens B, Richter EA. Insulin signaling in human skeletal muscle: time course and effect of exercise. Diabetes. 1997;46:1775–81.

42. Treebak JT, Taylor EB, Witczak CA, et al. Identification of a novel phosphorylation site on TBC1D4 regulated by AMP-activated protein kinase in skeletal muscle. Am J Physiol Cell Physiol. 2010;298:C377–85.

43. Koh HJ, Toyoda T, Fujii N, et al. Sucrose nonfermenting AMPK-related kinase (SNARK) mediates contraction-stimulated glucose transport in mouse skeletal muscle. Proc Natl Acad Sci USA. 2010;107:15541–6.

44. Witczak CA, Jessen N, Warro DM, et al. CaMKII regulates contraction- but not insulin-induced glucose uptake in mouse skeletal muscle. Am J Physiol Endocrinol Metab. 2010;298: E1150–60.

45. Taylor EB, An D, Kramer HF, et al. Discovery of TBC1D1 as an insulin-, AICAR-, and contraction-stimulated signaling nexus in mouse skeletal muscle. J Biol Chem. 2008;283: 9787–96.

46. Toyoda T, An D, Witczak CA, et al. Myo1c regulates glucose uptake in mouse skeletal muscle. J Biol Chem. 2011;286:4133–40.

47. DeFronzo RA, Ferrannini E, Sato Y, Felig P, Wahren J. Synergistic interaction between exercise and insulin on peripheral glucose uptake. J Clin Invest. 1981;68:1468–74.

48. Wasserman DH, Geer RJ, Rice DE, et al. Interaction of exercise and insulin action in humans. Am J Physiol. 1991;260:E37–45.

49. Hespel P, Vergauwen L, Vandenberghe K, Richter EA. Important role of insulin and flow in stimulating glucose uptake in contracting skeletal muscle. Diabetes. 1995;44:210–5.

50. Newman JM, Ross RM, Richards SM, Clark MG, Rattigan S. Insulin and contraction increase nutritive blood flow in rat muscle in vivo determined by microdialysis of L-[14C]glucose. J Physiol. 2007;585:217–29.
51. Poole DC, Copp SW, Hirai DM, Musch TI. Dynamics of muscle microcirculatory and blood-myocyte O(2) flux during contractions. Acta Physiol (Oxf). 2011;202:293–310.
52. Constantin-Teodosiu D, Cederblad G, Hultman E. PDC activity and acetyl group accumulation in skeletal muscle during prolonged exercise. J Appl Physiol. 1992;73:2403–7.
53. Mandarino LJ, Consoli A, Jain A, Kelley DE. Differential regulation of intracellular glucose metabolism by glucose and insulin in human muscle. Am J Physiol. 1993;265:E898–905.
54. Mandarino LJ, Wright KS, Verity LS, et al. Effects of insulin infusion on human skeletal muscle pyruvate dehydrogenase, phosphofructokinase, and glycogen synthase. Evidence for their role in oxidative and nonoxidative glucose metabolism. J Clin Invest. 1987;80: 655–63.
55. Tsintzas K, Chokkalingam K, Jewell K, Norton L, Macdonald IA, Constantin-Teodosiu D. Elevated free fatty acids attenuate the insulin-induced suppression of PDK4 gene expression in human skeletal muscle: potential role of intramuscular long-chain acyl-coenzyme A. J Clin Endocrinol Metab. 2007;92:3967–72.
56. Chokkalingam K, Jewell K, Norton L, et al. High-fat/low-carbohydrate diet reduces insulin-stimulated carbohydrate oxidation but stimulates nonoxidative glucose disposal in humans: an important role for skeletal muscle pyruvate dehydrogenase kinase 4. J Clin Endocrinol Metab. 2007;92:284–92.
57. Patel MS, Roche TE. Molecular biology and biochemistry of pyruvate dehydrogenase complexes. FASEB J. 1990;4:3224–33.
58. Tsintzas K, Williams C, Constantin-Teodosiu D, Hultman E, Boobis L, Greenhaff P. Carbohydrate ingestion prior to exercise augments the exercise-induced activation of the pyruvate dehydrogenase complex in human skeletal muscle. Exp Physiol. 2000;85:581–6.
59. Perseghin G, Price TB, Petersen KF, et al. Increased glucose transport-phosphorylation and muscle glycogen synthesis after exercise training in insulin-resistant subjects. N Engl J Med. 1996;335:1357–62.
60. Mikines KJ, Sonne B, Farrell PA, Tronier B, Galbo H. Effect of physical exercise on sensitivity and responsiveness to insulin in humans. Am J Physiol. 1988;254:E248–59.
61. Dela F, Mikines KJ, Sonne B, Galbo H. Effect of training on interaction between insulin and exercise in human muscle. J Appl Physiol. 1994;76:2386–93.
62. Kraniou GN, Cameron-Smith D, Hargreaves M. Acute exercise and GLUT4 expression in human skeletal muscle: influence of exercise intensity. J Appl Physiol. 2006;101:934–7.
63. Kuo CH, Browning KS, Ivy JL. Regulation of GLUT4 protein expression and glycogen storage after prolonged exercise. Acta Physiol Scand. 1999;165:193–201.
64. Greiwe JS, Holloszy JO, Semenkovich CF. Exercise induces lipoprotein lipase and GLUT-4 protein in muscle independent of adrenergic-receptor signaling. J Appl Physiol. 2000;89:176–81.
65. Ren JM, Semenkovich CF, Gulve EA, Gao J, Holloszy JO. Exercise induces rapid increases in GLUT4 expression, glucose transport capacity, and insulin-stimulated glycogen storage in muscle. J Biol Chem. 1994;269:14396–401.
66. Hansen PA, Wang W, Marshall BA, Holloszy JO, Mueckler M. Dissociation of GLUT4 translocation and insulin-stimulated glucose transport in transgenic mice overexpressing GLUT1 in skeletal muscle. J Biol Chem. 1998;273:18173–9.
67. O'Doherty RM, Bracy DP, Osawa H, Wasserman DH, Granner DK. Rat skeletal muscle hexokinase II mRNA and activity are increased by a single bout of acute exercise. Am J Physiol. 1994;266:E171–8.
68. Koval JA, DeFronzo RA, O'Doherty RM, et al. Regulation of hexokinase II activity and expression in human muscle by moderate exercise. Am J Physiol. 1998;274:E304–8.
69. Pilegaard H, Osada T, Andersen LT, Helge JW, Saltin B, Neufer PD. Substrate availability and transcriptional regulation of metabolic genes in human skeletal muscle during recovery from exercise. Metabolism. 2005;54:1048–55.

70. Stephens FB, Norton L, Jewell K, Chokkalingam K, Parr T, Tsintzas K. Basal and insulin-stimulated pyruvate dehydrogenase complex activation, glycogen synthesis and metabolic gene expression in human skeletal muscle the day after a single bout of exercise. Exp Physiol. 2010;95:808–18.
71. Nielsen JN, Derave W, Kristiansen S, Ralston E, Ploug T, Richter EA. Glycogen synthase localization and activity in rat skeletal muscle is strongly dependent on glycogen content. J Physiol. 2001;531:757–69.
72. Treebak JT, Frosig C, Pehmoller C, et al. Potential role of TBC1D4 in enhanced post-exercise insulin action in human skeletal muscle. Diabetologia. 2009;52:891–900.
73. Wende AR, Schaeffer PJ, Parker GJ, et al. A role for the transcriptional coactivator PGC-1alpha in muscle refueling. J Biol Chem. 2007;282:36642–51.
74. Ikeda S, Miyazaki H, Nakatani T, et al. Up-regulation of SREBP-1c and lipogenic genes in skeletal muscles after exercise training. Biochem Biophys Res Commun. 2002;296:395–400.
75. Boonsong T, Norton L, Chokkalingam K, et al. Effect of exercise and insulin on SREBP-1c expression in human skeletal muscle: potential roles for the ERK1/2 and Akt signalling pathways. Biochem Soc Trans. 2007;35:1310–1.
76. Burkart EM, Sambandam N, Han X, et al. Nuclear receptors PPARbeta/delta and PPARalpha direct distinct metabolic regulatory programs in the mouse heart. J Clin Invest. 2007; 117:3930–9.
77. Hunter WM, Sukkar MY. Changes in plasma insulin levels during muscular exercise. J Physiol. 1968;196:110P–2.
78. Hartley LH, Mason JW, Hogan RP, et al. Multiple hormonal responses to prolonged exercise in relation to physical training. J Appl Physiol. 1972;33:607–10.
79. Felig P, Wahren J, Hendler R, Ahlborg G. Plasma glucagon levels in exercising man. N Engl J Med. 1972;287:184–5.
80. Ahlborg G, Felig P, Hagenfeldt L, Hendler R, Wahren J. Substrate turnover during prolonged exercise in man. Splanchnic and leg metabolism of glucose, free fatty acids, and amino acids. J Clin Invest. 1974;53:1080–90.
81. Hermansen L, Pruett ED, Osnes JB, Giere FA. Blood glucose and plasma insulin in response to maximal exercise and glucose infusion. J Appl Physiol. 1970;29:13–6.
82. Lins PE, Wajngot A, Adamson U, Vranic M, Efendic S. Minimal increases in glucagon levels enhance glucose production in man with partial hypoinsulinemia. Diabetes. 1983;32:633–6.
83. Edgerton DS, Cardin S, Emshwiller M, et al. Small increases in insulin inhibit hepatic glucose production solely caused by an effect on glycogen metabolism. Diabetes. 2001;50:1872–82.
84. Petersen KF, Laurent D, Rothman DL, Cline GW, Shulman GI. Mechanism by which glucose and insulin inhibit net hepatic glycogenolysis in humans. J Clin Invest. 1998;101:1203–9.
85. Edgerton DS, Ramnanan CJ, Grueter CA, et al. Effects of insulin on the metabolic control of hepatic gluconeogenesis in vivo. Diabetes. 2009;58:2766–75.
86. Rivera N, Ramnanan CJ, An Z, et al. Insulin-induced hypoglycemia increases hepatic sensitivity to glucagon in dogs. J Clin Invest. 2010;120:4425–35.
87. Wasserman DH, Spalding JA, Lacy DB, Colburn CA, Goldstein RE, Cherrington AD. Glucagon is a primary controller of hepatic glycogenolysis and gluconeogenesis during muscular work. Am J Physiol. 1989;257:E108–17.
88. Cherrington AD, Williams PE, Shulman GI, Lacy WW. Differential time course of glucagon's effect on glycogenolysis and gluconeogenesis in the conscious dog. Diabetes. 1981;30:180–7.
89. Wasserman DH, Lickley HL, Vranic M. Interactions between glucagon and other counterregulatory hormones during normoglycemic and hypoglycemic exercise in dogs. J Clin Invest. 1984;74:1404–13.
90. Miles PD, Finegood DT, Lickley HL, Vranic M. Regulation of glucose turnover at the onset of exercise in the dog. J Appl Physiol. 1992;72:2487–94.
91. Wasserman DH, Williams PE, Lacy DB, Goldstein RE, Cherrington AD. Exercise-induced fall in insulin and hepatic carbohydrate metabolism during muscular work. Am J Physiol. 1989;256:E500–9.

92. Wolfe RR, Nadel ER, Shaw JH, Stephenson LA, Wolfe MH. Role of changes in insulin and glucagon in glucose homeostasis in exercise. J Clin Invest. 1986;77:900–7.
93. Hirsch IB, Marker JC, Smith LJ, et al. Insulin and glucagon in prevention of hypoglycemia during exercise in humans. Am J Physiol. 1991;260:E695–704.
94. Issekutz Jr B. Effects of glucose infusion on hepatic and muscle glycogenolysis in exercising dogs. Am J Physiol. 1981;240:E451–7.
95. Jenkins AB, Chisholm DJ, James DE, Ho KY, Kraegen EW. Exercise-induced hepatic glucose output is precisely sensitive to the rate of systemic glucose supply. Metabolism. 1985;34:431–6.
96. Jeukendrup AE, Wagenmakers AJ, Stegen JH, Gijsen AP, Brouns F, Saris WH. Carbohydrate ingestion can completely suppress endogenous glucose production during exercise. Am J Physiol. 1999;276:E672–83.
97. Rojdmark S, Bloom G, Chou MC, Jaspan JB, Field JB. Hepatic insulin and glucagon extraction after their augmented secretion in dogs. Am J Physiol. 1978;235:E88–96.
98. Wasserman DH, Lacy DB, Bracy DP. Relationship between arterial and portal vein immunoreactive glucagon during exercise. J Appl Physiol. 1993;75:724–9.
99. Camacho RC, Pencek RR, Lacy DB, James FD, Wasserman DH. Suppression of endogenous glucose production by mild hyperinsulinemia during exercise is determined predominantly by portal venous insulin. Diabetes. 2004;53:285–93.
100. Wasserman DH. Regulation of glucose fluxes during exercise in the postabsorptive state. Annu Rev Physiol. 1995;57:191–218.
101. Coker RH, Simonsen L, Bulow J, Wasserman DH, Kjaer M. Stimulation of splanchnic glucose production during exercise in humans contains a glucagon-independent component. Am J Physiol Endocrinol Metab. 2001;280:E918–27.
102. Coker RH, Krishna MG, Lacy DB, Allen EJ, Wasserman DH. Sympathetic drive to liver and nonhepatic splanchnic tissue during heavy exercise. J Appl Physiol. 1997;82:1244–9.
103. Issekutz Jr B. Role of beta-adrenergic receptors in mobilization of energy sources in exercising dogs. J Appl Physiol. 1978;44:869–76.
104. Wahrenberg H, Engfeldt P, Bolinder J, Arner P. Acute adaptation in adrenergic control of lipolysis during physical exercise in humans. Am J Physiol. 1987;253:E383–90.
105. Wasserman DH, Lacy DB, Goldstein RE, Williams PE, Cherrington AD. Exercise-induced fall in insulin and increase in fat metabolism during prolonged muscular work. Diabetes. 1989;38:484–90.
106. Connolly CC, Steiner KE, Stevenson RW, et al. Regulation of glucose metabolism by norepinephrine in conscious dogs. Am J Physiol. 1991;261:E764–72.
107. Dufour S, Lebon V, Shulman GI, Petersen KF. Regulation of net hepatic glycogenolysis and gluconeogenesis by epinephrine in humans. Am J Physiol Endocrinol Metab. 2009;297:E231–5.
108. Han XX, Bonen A. Epinephrine translocates GLUT-4 but inhibits insulin-stimulated glucose transport in rat muscle. Am J Physiol. 1998;274:E700–7.
109. Wasserman DH, Williams PE, Lacy DB, Bracy D, Cherrington AD. Hepatic nerves are not essential to the increase in hepatic glucose production during muscular work. Am J Physiol. 1990;259:E195–203.
110. Simonson DC, Koivisto V, Sherwin RS, et al. Adrenergic blockade alters glucose kinetics during exercise in insulin-dependent diabetics. J Clin Invest. 1984;73:1648–58.
111. Howlett K, Galbo H, Lorentsen J, et al. Effect of adrenaline on glucose kinetics during exercise in adrenalectomised humans. J Physiol. 1999;519(Pt 3):911–21.
112. Calles J, Cunningham JJ, Nelson L, et al. Glucose turnover during recovery from intensive exercise. Diabetes. 1983;32:734–8.
113. Marliss EB, Simantirakis E, Miles PD, et al. Glucose turnover and its regulation during intense exercise and recovery in normal male subjects. Clin Invest Med. 1992;15:406–19.
114. Marliss EB, Simantirakis E, Miles PD, et al. Glucoregulatory and hormonal responses to repeated bouts of intense exercise in normal male subjects. J Appl Physiol. 1991;71:924–33.

115. Purdon C, Brousson M, Nyveen SL, et al. The roles of insulin and catecholamines in the glucoregulatory response during intense exercise and early recovery in insulin-dependent diabetic and control subjects. J Clin Endocrinol Metab. 1993;76:566–73.

116. Kreisman SH, Halter JB, Vranic M, Marliss EB. Combined infusion of epinephrine and norepinephrine during moderate exercise reproduces the glucoregulatory response of intense exercise. Diabetes. 2003;52:1347–54.

117. Marker JC, Hirsch IB, Smith LJ, Parvin CA, Holloszy JO, Cryer PE. Catecholamines in prevention of hypoglycemia during exercise in humans. Am J Physiol. 1991;260:E705–12.

118. Hartley LH. Growth hormone and catecholamine response to exercise in relation to physical training. Med Sci Sports. 1975;7:34–6.

119. Bak JF, Moller N, Schmitz O. Effects of growth hormone on fuel utilization and muscle glycogen synthase activity in normal humans. Am J Physiol. 1991;260:E736–42.

120. Tsintzas OK, Williams C, Singh R, Wilson W, Burrin J. Influence of carbohydrate-electrolyte drinks on marathon running performance. Eur J Appl Physiol Occup Physiol. 1995;70:154–60.

121. Tsintzas OK, Williams C, Wilson W, Burrin J. Influence of carbohydrate supplementation early in exercise on endurance running capacity. Med Sci Sports Exerc. 1996;28:1373–9.

122. Galbo H, Holst JJ, Christensen NJ. Glucagon and plasma catecholamine responses to graded and prolonged exercise in man. J Appl Physiol. 1975;38:70–6.

123. Deuster PA, Singh A, Hofmann A, Moses FM, Chrousos GC. Hormonal responses to ingesting water or a carbohydrate beverage during a 2 h run. Med Sci Sports Exerc. 1992;24:72–9.

124. Fanelli C, Pampanelli S, Epifano L, et al. Relative roles of insulin and hypoglycaemia on induction of neuroendocrine responses to, symptoms of, and deterioration of cognitive function in hypoglycaemia in male and female humans. Diabetologia. 1994;37:797–807.

125. Mitrakou A, Ryan C, Veneman T, et al. Hierarchy of glycemic thresholds for counterregulatory hormone secretion, symptoms, and cerebral dysfunction. Am J Physiol. 1991;260:E67–74.

126. Heller SR, Macdonald IA. The measurement of cognitive function during acute hypoglycaemia: experimental limitations and their effect on the study of hypoglycaemia unawareness. Diabet Med. 1996;13:607–15.

127. Sotsky MJ, Shilo S, Shamoon H. Regulation of counterregulatory hormone secretion in man during exercise and hypoglycemia. J Clin Endocrinol Metab. 1989;68:9–16.

128. Zinker BA, Allison RG, Lacy DB, Wasserman DH. Interaction of exercise, insulin, and hypoglycemia studied using euglycemic and hypoglycemic insulin clamps. Am J Physiol. 1997;272:E530–42.

129. Berger CM, Sharis PJ, Bracy DP, Lacy DB, Wasserman DH. Sensitivity of exercise-induced increase in hepatic glucose production to glucose supply and demand. Am J Physiol. 1994;267:E411–21.

130. Niijima A. Glucose-sensitive afferent nerve fibres in the hepatic branch of the vagus nerve in the guinea-pig. J Physiol. 1982;332:315–23.

131. Smith D, Pernet A, Reid H, et al. The role of hepatic portal glucose sensing in modulating responses to hypoglycaemia in man. Diabetologia. 2002;45:1416–24.

132. Donovan CM, Halter JB, Bergman RN. Importance of hepatic glucoreceptors in sympathoadrenal response to hypoglycemia. Diabetes. 1991;40:155–8.

133. Davis SN, Galassetti P, Wasserman DH, Tate D. Effects of antecedent hypoglycemia on subsequent counterregulatory responses to exercise. Diabetes. 2000;49:73–81.

134. Galassetti P, Mann S, Tate D, et al. Effects of antecedent prolonged exercise on subsequent counterregulatory responses to hypoglycemia. Am J Physiol Endocrinol Metab. 2001;280:E908–17.

135. Davis SN, Shavers C, Mosqueda-Garcia R, Costa F. Effects of differing antecedent hypoglycemia on subsequent counterregulation in normal humans. Diabetes. 1997;46:1328–35.

136. Veneman T, Mitrakou A, Mokan M, Cryer P, Gerich J. Effect of hyperketonemia and hyperlacticacidemia on symptoms, cognitive dysfunction, and counterregulatory hormone responses during hypoglycemia in normal humans. Diabetes. 1994;43:1311–7.

137. Vettor R, Macor C, Rossi E, Piemonte G, Federspil G. Impaired counterregulatory hormonal and metabolic response to exhaustive exercise in obese subjects. Acta Diabetol. 1997;34:61–6.
138. Gustafson AB, Farrell PA, Kalkhoff RK. Impaired plasma catecholamine response to submaximal treadmill exercise in obese women. Metabolism. 1990;39:410–7.
139. Eliakim A, Nemet D, Zaldivar F, et al. Reduced exercise-associated response of the GH-IGF-I axis and catecholamines in obese children and adolescents. J Appl Physiol. 2006;100: 1630–7.
140. Riddell MC. The endocrine response and substrate utilization during exercise in children and adolescents. J Appl Physiol. 2008;105:725–33.
141. Martinez LR, Haymes EM. Substrate utilization during treadmill running in prepubertal girls and women. Med Sci Sports Exerc. 1992;24:975–83.
142. Steffensen CH, Roepstorff C, Madsen M, Kiens B. Myocellular triacylglycerol breakdown in females but not in males during exercise. Am J Physiol Endocrinol Metab. 2002;282: E634–42.
143. Tarnopolsky LJ, MacDougall JD, Atkinson SA, Tarnopolsky MA, Sutton JR. Gender differences in substrate for endurance exercise. J Appl Physiol. 1990;68:302–8.
144. Carter SL, Rennie C, Tarnopolsky MA. Substrate utilization during endurance exercise in men and women after endurance training. Am J Physiol Endocrinol Metab. 2001;280:E898–907.
145. Horton TJ, Pagliassotti MJ, Hobbs K, Hill JO. Fuel metabolism in men and women during and after long-duration exercise. J Appl Physiol. 1998;85:1823–32.
146. M'Kaouar H, Peronnet F, Massicotte D, Lavoie C. Gender difference in the metabolic response to prolonged exercise with [13C]glucose ingestion. Eur J Appl Physiol. 2004; 92:462–9.
147. Riddell MC, Partington SL, Stupka N, Armstrong D, Rennie C, Tarnopolsky MA. Substrate utilization during exercise performed with and without glucose ingestion in female and male endurance trained athletes. Int J Sport Nutr Exerc Metab. 2003;13:407–21.
148. Leelayuwat N, Tsintzas K, Patel K, Macdonald IA. Metabolic responses to exercise after carbohydrate loads in healthy men and women. Med Sci Sports Exerc. 2005;37:1721–7.
149. Nuutila P, Knuuti MJ, Maki M, et al. Gender and insulin sensitivity in the heart and in skeletal muscles. Studies using positron emission tomography. Diabetes. 1995;44:31–6.
150. Robertson MD, Livesey G, Mathers JC. Quantitative kinetics of glucose appearance and disposal following a 13C-labelled starch-rich meal: comparison of male and female subjects. Br J Nutr. 2002;87:569–77.
151. Perseghin G, Scifo P, Pagliato E, et al. Gender factors affect fatty acids-induced insulin resistance in nonobese humans: effects of oral steroidal contraception. J Clin Endocrinol Metab. 2001;86:3188–96.
152. Davis SN, Galassetti P, Wasserman DH, Tate D. Effects of gender on neuroendocrine and metabolic counterregulatory responses to exercise in normal man. J Clin Endocrinol Metab. 2000;85:224–30.
153. Galassetti P, Mann S, Tate D, Neill RA, Wasserman DH, Davis SN. Effect of morning exercise on counterregulatory responses to subsequent, afternoon exercise. J Appl Physiol. 2001;91:91–9.
154. Galassetti P, Tate D, Neill RA, Morrey S, Wasserman DH, Davis SN. Effect of sex on counterregulatory responses to exercise after antecedent hypoglycemia in type 1 diabetes. Am J Physiol Endocrinol Metab. 2004;287:E16–24.
155. Amiel SA, Maran A, Powrie JK, Umpleby AM, Macdonald IA. Gender differences in counterregulation to hypoglycaemia. Diabetologia. 1993;36:460–4.
156. Pruett ED. Glucose and insulin during prolonged work stress in men living on different diets. J Appl Physiol. 1970;28:199–208.
157. Lambert EV, St Clair Gibson A, Noakes TD. Complex systems model of fatigue: integrative homoeostatic control of peripheral physiological systems during exercise in humans. Br J Sports Med. 2005;39:52–62.

158. Nybo L, Secher NH. Cerebral perturbations provoked by prolonged exercise. Prog Neurobiol. 2004;72:223–61.
159. Tsintzas K, Liu R, Williams C, Campbell I, Gaitanos G. The effect of carbohydrate ingestion on performance during a 30-km race. Int J Sport Nutr. 1993;3:127–39.
160. Tsintzas K, Williams C. Human muscle glycogen metabolism during exercise. Effect of carbohydrate supplementation. Sports Med. 1998;25:7–23.
161. McConell G, Fabris S, Proietto J, Hargreaves M. Effect of carbohydrate ingestion on glucose kinetics during exercise. J Appl Physiol. 1994;77:1537–41.
162. Tabata I, Ogita F, Miyachi M, Shibayama H. Effect of low blood glucose on plasma CRF, ACTH, and cortisol during prolonged physical exercise. J Appl Physiol. 1991;71: 1807–12.
163. Wee SL, Williams C, Tsintzas K, Boobis L. Ingestion of a high-glycemic index meal increases muscle glycogen storage at rest but augments its utilization during subsequent exercise. J Appl Physiol. 2005;99:707–14.
164. Nicholas CW, Tsintzas K, Boobis L, Williams C. Carbohydrate-electrolyte ingestion during intermittent high-intensity running. Med Sci Sports Exerc. 1999;31:1280–6.
165. Yaspelkis 3rd BB, Patterson JG, Anderla PA, Ding Z, Ivy JL. Carbohydrate supplementation spares muscle glycogen during variable-intensity exercise. J Appl Physiol. 1993;75: 1477–85.
166. Coyle EF, Hagberg JM, Hurley BF, Martin WH, Ehsani AA, Holloszy JO. Carbohydrate feeding during prolonged strenuous exercise can delay fatigue. J Appl Physiol. 1983;55: 230–5.
167. Dela F, Mikines KJ, von Linstow M, Secher NH, Galbo H. Effect of training on insulin-mediated glucose uptake in human muscle. Am J Physiol. 1992;263:E1134–43.
168. Foskett A, Williams C, Boobis L, Tsintzas K. Carbohydrate availability and muscle energy metabolism during intermittent running. Med Sci Sports Exerc. 2008;40:96–103.
169. Mitchell JB, Costill DL, Houmard JA, Fink WJ, Pascoe DD, Pearson DR. Influence of carbohydrate dosage on exercise performance and glycogen metabolism. J Appl Physiol. 1989;67:1843–9.
170. Hargreaves M, Briggs CA. Effect of carbohydrate ingestion on exercise metabolism. J Appl Physiol. 1988;65:1553–5.
171. Yaspelkis 3rd BB, Ivy JL. Effect of carbohydrate supplements and water on exercise metabolism in the heat. J Appl Physiol. 1991;71:680–7.
172. Ahlborg G, Felig P. Influence of glucose ingestion on fuel-hormone response during prolonged exercise. J Appl Physiol. 1976;41:683–8.
173. Pfeiffer B, Stellingwerff T, Zaltas E, Hodgson AB, Jeukendrup AE. Carbohydrate oxidation from a drink during running compared with cycling exercise. Med Sci Sports Exerc. 2011;43:327–34.
174. Tsintzas K, Simpson EJ, Seevaratnam N, Jones S. Effect of exercise mode on blood glucose disposal during physiological hyperinsulinaemia in humans. Eur J Appl Physiol. 2003;89: 217–20.
175. Jeukendrup AE, Killer SC. The myths surrounding pre-exercise carbohydrate feeding. Ann Nutr Metab. 2010;57 Suppl 2:18–25.
176. Neufer PD, Costill DL, Flynn MG, Kirwan JP, Mitchell JB, Houmard J. Improvements in exercise performance: effects of carbohydrate feedings and diet. J Appl Physiol. 1987;62:983–8.
177. Schabort EJ, Bosch AN, Weltan SM, Noakes TD. The effect of a preexercise meal on time to fatigue during prolonged cycling exercise. Med Sci Sports Exerc. 1999;31:464–71.
178. Sherman WM, Brodowicz G, Wright DA, Allen WK, Simonsen J, Dernbach A. Effects of 4 h preexercise carbohydrate feedings on cycling performance. Med Sci Sports Exerc. 1989; 21:598–604.
179. Coyle EF, Jeukendrup AE, Wagenmakers AJ, Saris WH. Fatty acid oxidation is directly regulated by carbohydrate metabolism during exercise. Am J Physiol. 1997;273:E268–75.

180. Coyle EF, Coggan AR, Hemmert MK, Lowe RC, Walters TJ. Substrate usage during prolonged exercise following a preexercise meal. J Appl Physiol. 1985;59:429–33.
181. Wee SL, Williams C, Gray S, Horabin J. Influence of high and low glycemic index meals on endurance running capacity. Med Sci Sports Exerc. 1999;31:393–9.
182. Wahren J, Ekberg K. Splanchnic regulation of glucose production. Annu Rev Nutr. 2007;27:329–45.
183. Tsintzas K, Jewell K, Kamran M, et al. Differential regulation of metabolic genes in skeletal muscle during starvation and refeeding in humans. J Physiol. 2006;575:291–303.
184. Davis SN, Fowler S, Costa F. Hypoglycemic counterregulatory responses differ between men and women with type 1 diabetes. Diabetes. 2000;49:65–72.

Chapter 2
The Impact of Type 1 Diabetes on the Physiological Responses to Exercise

Michael C. Riddell

2.1 Brief Overview of the Normal Endocrine Response to Exercise

To provide energy in the form of carbohydrates, lipids, and protein in the face of increased energy demands during exercise, the healthy body must orchestrate a complex neuroendocrine response that starts at the onset of the activity. This response is continuously modulated as the duration of the exercise increases and as the intensity of the activity changes. Since one of the main fuels for exercise is carbohydrate, glucose utilization by the working muscle must be matched equally by glucose provision, predominantly by the liver, or hypoglycemia will ensue. If the liver cannot keep up with glucose utilization, then carbohydrate intake is critical to maintain performance. Glucose homeostasis during prolonged moderate-intensity exercise (~40–60% maximal oxygen uptake [VO_2max]) is primarily regulated by a reduction in insulin secretion and an increase in glucagon release from the pancreatic islets, which together helps to increase liver glucose production [1]. The increase in the glucagon-to-insulin ratio raises the rate of glucose appearance (Ra) to match almost perfectly the increased rate of peripheral glucose disposal (Rd) into working muscle (Fig. 2.1).

Increased hepatic glucose production during exercise occurs primarily through enhanced glycogenolysis and gluconeogenesis, with a greater reliance on the latter pathway as the duration of exercise increases [2]. Hypoglycemia can occur, even in nondiabetic individuals, when hepatic glucose production fails to match the elevated glucose uptake by working muscle, which is particularly pronounced during prolonged exercise (usually >3 h of activity), if not enough carbohydrate is consumed [3]. If hepatic glycogen stores are depleted during prolonged exercise,

M.C. Riddell, Ph.D.
Physical Activity and Diabetes Unit, School of Kinesiology and Health Science,
Muscle Health Research Centre, York University,
4700 Keele Street, M3J1P3 Toronto, ON, Canada
e-mail: mriddell@yorku.ca

I. Gallen (ed.), *Type 1 Diabetes*,
DOI 10.1007/978-0-85729-754-9_2, © Springer-Verlag London Limited 2012

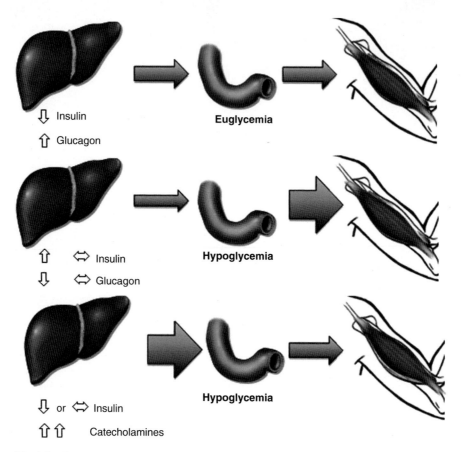

Fig. 2.1 Blood glucose responses to exercise in nondiabetic or ideally controlled patient with type 1 diabetes (*upper panel*), overinsulinized patient (*middle panel*), and underinsulinized patient or patient performing high-intensity exercise under competition stress (*lower panel*). The thicknesses of the *arrows* represent glucose flux. In the *upper panel*, hepatic glucose production is balanced with muscle glucose uptake and normal blood glucose levels are maintained. In the middle panel, high circulating insulin levels reduce hepatic glucose production and increase muscle glucose uptake, thereby resulting in hypoglycemia. In the *lower panel*, low circulating insulin levels and/ or elevated counterregulatory hormones increase hepatic glucose production and decrease muscle glucose uptake, resulting in hyperglycemia (Reprinted by permission of the publisher from Chu et al. [94], JTE Multimedia)

gluconeogenesis alone is unable to provide adequate glucose to supply the working muscles. To help reduce the reliance on endogenous carbohydrate as a fuel source, reductions in insulin levels and increases in growth hormone along with increases in sympathoadrenal activity and other factors help promote increased lipid provision for oxidation by muscle [4]. Even with very prolonged exercise, when reliance on lipid as a primary fuel source is maximal, carbohydrate provision, either by the liver through gluconeogenesis or by oral ingestion, is essential to prevent hypoglycemia even in nondiabetics [5].

In healthy individuals, several glucose counterregulatory mechanisms (i.e., anti-hypoglycemic actions) exist to help limit hypoglycemia, both when fasting occurs at rest and when prolonged exercise is performed. For example, [6] a slight decrease in glycemia from normal (normal being ~90 mg/dL or 5 mmol/L) lowers insulin secretion and activates the release of various counterregulatory hormones including glucagon, catecholamines, growth hormone, and cortisol in a stepwise and hierarchical fashion [7]. During exercise, other humoral and muscle factors also likely help augment glucose production [100]. All of these hormones act to increase hepatic glucose production and lower peripheral glucose disposal, thereby defending against ensuing hypoglycemia. As such, several safeguards need to be breached before hypoglycemia occurs in nondiabetic individuals.

Interestingly, heavy aerobic exercise (>80% $VO_{2\,max}$) also generates a complex neuroendocrine response, similar to that of acute stress, perhaps as a means of elevating glucose provision for "fight or flight". In intense exercise, glucose is the exclusive muscle fuel, and it must be mobilized from muscle and liver glycogen in the fed and fasted state. This process is largely governed by increases in catecholamines, which facilitate glucose production but limit glucose uptake. As such, in healthy individuals, insulin secretion actually increases post-exercise to help normalize this transient hyperglycemia caused by intense exercise [8]. This complex neurohormonal regulation during exercise, performed at a wide range of differing intensities and durations and at different environmental conditions, makes it nearly impossible to mimic in the patient with type 1 diabetes.

2.2 Abnormalities in the Endocrine Responses to Acute Exercise in Type 1 Diabetes

The blood glucose response to exercise in patients with type 1 diabetes varies considerably both between and within individuals, likely depending on several factors including the type and intensity of exercise performed, the duration of the activity, and the level of circulating "on board" insulin during and after the exercise. Even if all of these variables are taken into consideration, the blood glucose response differs markedly between individuals but has some reproducibility within an individual [9]. One of the key determinates of the glycemic response to exercise is the general classification of the exercise (i.e., aerobic vs. anaerobic).

2.2.1 Aerobic Exercise

Aerobic exercise may be defined as any activity that uses large muscle groups at relatively low rates of muscular contraction. This type of activity can be maintained continuously (or rhythmically) for prolonged periods (minutes to hours) through oxidative metabolism of various fuel sources including carbohydrates, fats, and some protein. Moderate-intensity aerobic exercise generally involves continuous, aerobic activity between 40% and 59% of VO$_2$max or 55–69% of maximal heart rate (HRmax) [10]. Examples of moderate-intensity exercise include continuous aerobic activities such as jogging, cycling, and swimming. Typically, this type of exercise promotes a lowering of blood glucose concentration, both during and after the end of the activity, and thus requires nutritional intervention and/or adjustments in insulin dosages to limit hypoglycemia. The physiological mechanisms by which aerobic exercise causes undesirable alterations in glycemia in individuals with type 1 diabetes are detailed below and highlighted in Fig. 2.1.

2.2.1.1 Hypoglycemia

For individuals with type 1 diabetes, the inability to reduce exogenous insulin levels during aerobic exercise is a key factor that contributes to an increased risk of exercise-induced hypoglycemia [11]. As discussed above, insulin levels in the portal circulation normally drop after the onset of aerobic exercise, and this drop helps to sensitize the liver to increasing glucagon concentrations [2, 12]. Since, in the insulin-dependent type 1 patient, exercise is often performed in a 0–4-h time frame post-insulin injection, concentrations of insulin typically do not decrease during exercise and may actually increase just because of the kinetics of peak insulin action [13, 14]. A second related factor that increases the risk of hyperinsulinemia and hypoglycemia is the accelerated absorption of insulin from subcutaneous tissues, once it has been injected or infused [15]. Even if no bolus insulin has been injected or infused in the hours preceding exercise, it is still possible, but less likely to have hypoglycemia because of elevated basal insulin concentrations, compared to nondiabetics who are exercising [13]. Relative hyperinsulinemia during exercise in the patient with type 1 diabetes limits the effect of glucagon on hepatic glucose production and promotes insulin-induced peripheral glucose uptake, further decreasing blood glucose levels. A third factor that may contribute to an increased risk for exercise-associated hypoglycemia in patients with type 1 diabetes may be the loss in glucagon response to developing hypoglycemia [16] or an impaired stimulation of hepatic glucose output in response to glucagon secretion [17]. Although it has been established that the glucagon response to exercise may be intact in people with type 1 diabetes, if they are not hypoglycemic [18], there may be deficiencies in the glucagon response during exercise if the patients were previously exposed to hypoglycemia [19] or perhaps if they are, in fact, exercising while hypoglycemic. Moreover, there may also be impaired adrenergic responses to exercise in patients with type 1 diabetes under hypoglycemic conditions [18]. Finally, other factors such as a low level of hepatic glycogen content in poorly controlled diabetes [20] and/or reduced gluconeogenesis and/or increased peripheral glucose disposal in the face of hyperinsulinemia [21] may contribute to exercise-induced hypoglycemia in patients with type 1 diabetes. A summary of the factors that may predispose the patient to hypoglycemia during aerobic exercise is shown in Table 2.1.

Table 2.1 Factors that can affect changes in blood glucose levels during exercise

Drop in blood glucose	Blood glucose unchanged	Increase in blood glucose
Hyperinsulinemia due to usual insulin injection (or infusion) prior to exercise and increased insulin absorption kinetics and action	Pre-exercise insulin adjusted appropriately	Hypoinsulinemia and ketoacidosis prior to exercise
Prolonged aerobic type activity with no carbohydrate intake or without a reduction in insulin administration	Appropriate consumption of carbohydrate before and during exercise	Prolonged pump disconnect
Unfamiliarity with the activity		Very vigorous aerobic exercise (>80% of maximal oxygen consumption)
Defective glucose counterregulation to hypoglycemia and/or exercise		Repeated or intermittent anaerobic exercise
		Excessive carbohydrate consumption
		Post-exercise when glucose production or carbohydrate feeding exceeds disposal

2.2.1.2 Hyperglycemia

Although aerobic exercise is typically associated with an increased risk for hypoglycemia, certain types of activity may promote hyperglycemia. Specifically, high-intensity aerobic exercise (i.e., above the lactate threshold) tends to increase blood glucose levels because insulin levels do not rise in the portal circulation of the patient with diabetes to compensate for the normal increase in circulating catecholamine levels. It is well established that heavy aerobic exercise (short- and middle-distance running, short track cycling, some other individual and team sports, etc.) induce increases in catecholamines that increase hepatic glucose production and limit peripheral disposal (Fig. 2.1). In individuals who do not have diabetes, the increase in catecholamines and hyperglycemia is compensated for by increases in insulin secretion, usually at the end of the activity. If hyperglycemia occurs post-exercise, this phenomenon is usually transient in the individual with diabetes, lasting for 1–2 h in recovery. No current guidelines are available on the amount of insulin to administer in the presence of hyperglycemia after high-intensity exercise for patients with type 1 diabetes. Although some limited experimental data suggests that a doubling in insulin levels relative to when the vigorous exercise was performed may be needed to counter this transient hyperglycemia [22].

Patients and caregivers should be aware of the potential for a rise in blood glucose before "stressful" competition. Even if blood glucose levels are normal in the hours before exercise, anticipatory stress increases counterregulatory hormones and hyperglycemia can occur. Typically, this "stress-related" increase in glycemia at the onset of exercise does not need to be corrected for since the increased glucose utilization rate during the activity, as long as it is aerobic in nature, will often lower blood glucose levels. However, frequent self-monitoring of blood glucose is needed to make sure that any pre-exercise hyperglycemia is not worsened during the exercise, to which continuous glucose monitoring (CGM) may be an asset.

In situations of prolonged and severe hypoinsulinemia (missed insulin injections, blocked insulin pump, illness, etc.), patients may have elevations in circulating and urinary ketone bodies. In these situations, vigorous exercise may cause further increases in hyperglycemia and ketoacidosis, particularly if elevated blood ketones are present at the time of exercise. In these situations, hepatic glucose production continues to rise, while glucose utilization remains impaired and glycemic control deteriorates even further. For these reasons, it is recommended to delay exercise if blood glucose is higher than 14 mmol/L and if blood or urinary ketones are also elevated [23, 24]. A summary of the possible reasons for exercise-associated hyperglycemia during sport is shown in Table 2.1.

For patients on insulin pump devices with hyperglycemia and elevated ketone levels, infusion sets should be changed, and individuals may need to temporarily change to needles, with rapid-acting insulin injected until glucose is restored. Hyperglycemia and ketoacidosis may cause dehydration and decrease blood pH, resulting in impaired performance and severe illness. Rapid ketone production can precipitate ketoacidotic abdominal pain and vomiting. In these situations, patients are advised to seek emergency care for intravenous insulin and rehydration protocols.

2.2.2 Anaerobic Exercise

Anaerobic activities are characterized by high rates of intense muscular contraction. With purely anaerobic exercise, muscle contractions are sustained by the phosphagen and anaerobic glycolytic systems to produce lactic acid and energy in the form of adenosine triphosphate (ATP). Anaerobic activities include sprinting, power lifting, hockey, and some motions during basketball and racquet sports. In reality, however, most of the sports and physical activities that athletes perform are a mix of both anaerobic and aerobic actions (soccer, basketball, mountain biking, squash, football, etc.). Anaerobic fitness refers to the ability to work at a very high level during these activities for relatively short periods (5–30 s).

With anaerobic exercise, lactate production within the muscle rises dramatically. This lactate, which is a glycolytic end product, can either be used within the cells of formation or transported through the interstitium and vasculature to adjacent and anatomically distributed cells for utilization by other tissues [25]. Elevations in lactate and catecholamines during anaerobic exercise are known to lower the uptake of plasma glucose and free fatty acids into skeletal muscle [26] and increase hepatic glucose production [27], thereby increasing the likelihood of hyperglycemia in patients with type 1 diabetes. Moreover, anaerobic flux of muscle glycogen also lowers skeletal muscle glucose uptake [26], which could contribute to hyperglycemia in persons with diabetes if hepatic glucose production is elevated.

Interestingly, just a 10-s high-intensity anaerobic sprint has been shown to help prevent early post-exercise hypoglycemia in persons with type 1 diabetes [28, 29]. In addition, performing weight training before the onset of aerobic exercise may also attenuate the drop in blood glucose levels in patients with type 1 diabetes [30]. Similarly, performing intermittent high-intensity exercise (with repeated anaerobic work) may be superior over continuous moderate-intensity aerobic exercise for glycemic stability, particularly in early and late recovery [31, 32].

2.2.3 Early Post-exercise Hyperglycemia

Just after the end of either vigorous aerobic or anaerobic work, individuals with type 1 diabetes may experience increases in blood glucose levels through a number of mechanisms. First, any reduction in insulin dosage prior to exercise might promote hyperglycemia once the activity is finished, since glucose disposal will eventually return toward pre-exercise levels but glucose production will remain elevated because of the reduction in circulating insulin concentration. If the individual wears an insulin infusion device (insulin pump) and has removed the pump altogether, then circulating insulin levels may be very low by the end of prolonged exercise and hyperglycemia is likely [33]. In addition, some individuals may be motivated to consume carbohydrates early in recovery, which may drive up blood glucose levels. In addition, as mentioned above, very vigorous aerobic exercise with a heavy anaerobic (producing catecholamines and lactate) component will increase glycemia for 1–2 h in recovery [8]. In these situations, it may be necessary (or desirable) to lower glycemia by injecting rapid-acting insulin analogs or by increasing the basal infusion rates to normal (or slightly above normal) early in recovery.

2.2.4 Late Post-exercise Hypoglycemia

Post-exercise late-onset hypoglycemia has long been a complaint of patients with type 1 diabetes [34]. If patients develop hypoglycemia during sleep, it may go unnoticed. If patients perform just 45 min of moderate-intensity exercise during the day, then the risk of nocturnal hypoglycemia may be as high as 30–40% in the evening following exercise [35–39]. An investigation in children with type 1 diabetes indicates that increased insulin sensitivity occurs immediately after exercise and again 7–11 h later [40], which may further elevate their risk for late-onset post-exercise (nocturnal) hypoglycemia.

This is particularly problematic as patients may not perceive hypoglycemia during sleep, and the hypoglycemic duration may last for just a few minutes or for several hours. In these situations, a reduction in bedtime basal insulin by ~20% is recommended, with a reduction in basal infusion rate from bedtime to ~4 AM if on a pump [35]. Otherwise, a complex carbohydrate snack with some protein is advised, either without an insulin bolus at all or with a drastically reduced bolus dose.

2.3   Abnormalities in Fuel Utilization During Exercise in Type 1 Diabetes

A number of subtle alterations in fuel metabolism during exercise have been noted in persons with type 1 diabetes [41–45]. In patients deprived of insulin for 12–24 h, prolonged moderate-intensity exercise is associated with a lower respiratory exchange ratio, and thus a reduced rate of carbohydrate oxidation, than that shown in control subjects at the same exercise intensity [42, 46]. As such, it would appear that a patient with type 1 diabetes who is underinsulinized would have a greater reliance on lipid oxidation during exercise compared to when they have elevated insulin levels. When insulin is administered to the patient, to levels somewhat representative of nondiabetics, the overall ratio of carbohydrate to lipid utilization during exercise performed in the postprandial state looks remarkably normal [43, 44, 47, 48]. Indeed, in a study conducted by Francescato et al. [44], which was conducted at various time intervals after insulin injection and with different amounts of glucose ingested, fat oxidation and CHO oxidation were not significantly different from those observed in control subjects.

The ingestion of fast-acting carbohydrate during exercise clearly helps to limit the hypoglycemic effect of endurance type exercise in individuals with type 1 diabetes [49, 50]. Largely, the oxidation of orally ingested carbohydrate is normal in those with diabetes, if the circulating insulin levels are elevated, although the rate of oxidation may be initially slightly impaired [41, 43, 45]. Moreover, rates of plasma glucose disappearance during exercise in patients with diabetes are comparable to control subjects [11, 51–53] or just slightly impaired [48].

Although total fat and carbohydrate oxidation rates may be normal during exercise in persons with type 1 diabetes who are well insulinized, some evidence does exist to suggest that muscle glycogen utilization rates may be higher and plasma glucose oxidation rates lower during prolonged exercise than in nondiabetic individuals [21]. Unfortunately, a greater reliance on limited endogenous muscle fuels (i.e., muscle glycogen) may put the individual at risk of early fatigue.

A recent study has shown that a low-glycemic-index carbohydrate and reduced insulin dose administered 30 min before running maintains control of both pre- and post-exercise blood glucose responses in type 1 diabetes [54]. The amount of carbohydrate needed to limit hypoglycemia is at least partly related to the proximity of the last insulin injection [44]. As such, anywhere from 1.0 to 1.5 g of carbohydrate per kilogram body mass per hour of exercise is required when the exercise is within 1–2 h of insulin administration [24], but this amount drops to about 0.2 g/kg by about 5.5 h postinjection [44]. Estimating glucose utilization rates during exercise, either via respiratory exchange ratio or via heart rate, appears to be an effective means for determining the appropriate carbohydrate feeding regimen to help prevent hypoglycemia [50, 55].

2.4 Effects of Type 1 Diabetes on Performance

Normally, insulin therapy is rapidly initiated at the time of diagnosis in patients with type 1 diabetes, and dramatic metabolic improvements are achievable within a fairly short time frame (days to weeks after the initiation of treatment) [56]. However, clinical diagnosis may be delayed and the overall management in youth with the disease is usually suboptimal for a variety of physiological and psychosocial reasons [57]. It should also be noted that normal restoration in glucose homeostasis is nearly impossible in type 1 diabetes since the sophisticated control system is no longer in place that maintains a small, but critical, amount of blood glucose constant [2]. As such, a number of physiological challenges in substrate metabolism exist that places the individual with type 1 diabetes at risk for suboptimal exercise performance.

Overall, aerobic capacity can be impaired significantly in young patients with type 1, particularly if they are in suboptimal glycemic control. For example, in one large study of healthy and diabetic adolescents/young adults, matched similarly in age, weight, height, and body composition, aerobic capacity was shown to be about 20% lower in those with type 1 diabetes [58]. Several cardiovascular, muscular, and metabolic impairments in type 1 diabetes might help to explain their potential decrement in aerobic and anaerobic performance. A number of studies report reduced physical work capacity or maximal aerobic capacity (VO_2max) in young patients with type 1 diabetes, despite insulin therapy, when compared to their nondiabetic peers [58–64]. Both end diastolic volume and left ventricular ejection fraction fail to increase normally during exercise in young adults with type 1 diabetes compared with controls [65]. In contrast, Nugent and colleagues [66] report no difference in VO_2 peak during a progressive incremental exercise test in adults with long-standing diabetes, while Veves et al. [67] found that only inactive adults with demonstrated neuropathic complications had reduced VO_2max. Taken together, these studies suggest that if one is physically active with type 1 diabetes, then aerobic capacity can be normal, at least if neuropathy has not yet developed.

Impairments in physical work capacity in those with type 1 diabetes, if observed, appear to be related to the level of glycemic control in the patient. For example, Poortmans et al. [64] and Huttunen et al. [61] both reported that physical capacities were inversely related to the level of metabolic control, as measured by HbA1c. It is unclear, however, if a reduced work capacity in youth with type 1 diabetes is a result of poorer oxygenation of muscle [68], a lower amount of muscle capillarization [69], or if poorer metabolic control is a function of lower amounts of habitual physical activity [70]. In an experimentally induced murine model of diabetes, there is altered expression of several genes involved in angiogenesis and reduced muscle capillarization which could not be normalized even by high-volume endurance exercise training [69].

Studies investigating muscular strength and endurance in individuals with type 1 diabetes have shown mixed results, although a recent review by Krause and colleagues has indicated that a myopathy may exist in type 1 diabetes [71]. A number of investigators report decrements in strength [72–77], while others have shown no strength deficit, but slower rates of muscular recruitment during isometric contraction [78]. Although fatigue is a common complaint of patients with diabetes [79, 80], the effect of type 1 diabetes on endurance capacity during exercise is not well documented. Compared to controls, patients with type 1 diabetes have been reported to have both impaired [78] and enhanced [74] capacity during relatively brief bouts of intense exercise. Ratings of perceived exertion during prolonged exercise have been reported to be higher in boys with type 1 diabetes compared to age, weight, and aerobic fitness matched controls [81]. Also during prolonged exercise, those with type 1 diabetes who are under good glycemic control have a higher glycolytic flux [82] and tend to rely considerably more on muscle glycogen utilization as an energy source [45], which might reduce endurance capacity, although this hypothesis has yet to be tested. Moreover, exercising while hyperglycemic has been shown to increase reliance on muscle glycogen compared to exercising while euglycemic [83], and the individual who is exercising while hypoinsulinemic/hyperglycemic would be expected to be prone to early dehydration and acidosis [84], all factors that might promote early fatigue. Moreover, increasing blood glucose levels to 16 mmol/L has been shown to reduce isometric muscle strength, but not maximal isokinetic muscle strength, compared with strength measured at glycemia clamped at 5 mmol/L in patients with type 1 diabetes [85]. This reduction in isometric strength might play a role in the development of early fatigue during certain types of resistance exercise.

If individuals with type 1 diabetes are actively engaged in regular exercise, they can clearly achieve a normal, or even an elite, level of sport performance. In one German study of ten middle-aged long-distance triathletes with type 1 diabetes studied over 3 years, overall endurance performance was said to be "normal" despite documented hyperglycemia during the early part of a race, then hypoglycemia during the marathon leg [86]. The degree to which acute changes in blood glucose levels influence sports performance remains somewhat unclear, however. Unfortunately, very few studies have been conducted in which exercise performance is examined during differing levels of blood glucose concentrations in those with type 1 diabetes. Circumstantial evidence suggests that an increase in plasma glucose availability might improve the exercise capacity perhaps because more fuel is readily available for muscle contraction. However, this hypothesis has not been supported by one study that "clamped" nondiabetic cyclists at hyperglycemia and euglycemia and found no difference in endurance performance [87]. Similarly, in one study of prepubertal boys with type 1 diabetes ($n = 16$), lowering the insulin dose prior to exercise to reduce the likelihood of hypoglycemia did not influence aerobic capacity during cycling compared to the usual insulin dose [88]. In eight endurance-trained adults with type 1 diabetes, elevating blood glucose levels from 5.3 ± 0.6 mmol/L to 12.4 ± 2.1 mmol/L, via hyperinsulinemic glucose clamp technique, also failed to change peak power output or other physiological endpoints such as lactate, heart rate, or respiratory exchange ratio [89].

In contrast to mild hyperglycemia, mild hypoglycemia probably lowers exercise capacity and sport performance in individuals with type 1 diabetes. For example, capacity was reduced and ratings of perceived exertion increased with hypoglycemia in a group of youth with type 1 diabetes [50, 81], although the exercise was always stopped by the research investigators rather than the subjects for safety reasons. In a recent sports camp field study of 28 youth with type 1 diabetes, Kelly et al. [90] found that the ability to carry out fundamental sports skills was markedly reduced by mild hypoglycemia compared with either euglycemia or hyperglycemia. Importantly, this finding of significantly impaired sports performance with hypoglycemia appeared universally across nearly all subjects and is similar to the well-documented detrimental effects of hypoglycemia on cognitive processing [91].

Profound or sustained hyperglycemia also likely impairs endurance performance in those with type 1 diabetes, although the evidence for this statement is somewhat limited. Prolonged hypoinsulinemia/hyperglycemia would be expected to lower muscle glycogen levels, reduce muscle strength, and predispose the individual to dehydration and electrolyte imbalance [92]. As mentioned above, exercising while hyperglycemic has been shown to increase the reliance on muscle glycogen as a fuel source and limit the capacity to switch from carbohydrate to lipid energy sources [83]. Importantly, substrate oxidation during prolonged endurance exercise can be similar to what is observed in nondiabetics if diabetic subjects are clamped euglycemic [83]. Taken together, it is likely that there is an inverted-U shape relationship between glycemia and exercise/sport performance, with the best performance in the euglycemic range.

2.5   Adaptations to Exercise Training in Type 1 Diabetes

Individuals with type 1 diabetes appear to respond normally to both endurance- and resistance type training, from an adaptive point of view, particularly if they are in good glycemic control.

Endurance training in humans normally results in numerous beneficial adaptations in skeletal muscles, including an increase in GLUT4 expression and glucose transport capacity, resulting in increased insulin sensitivity [93]. Paradoxically; however, despite these adaptations, improvements in glycemic control are not always observed with regular exercise in this patient population [94]. The physiological adaptations to regular exercise are clearly beneficial for patients, even if glycemic control is not improved. For example, in response to endurance training, children with type 1 diabetes have improved vascular function [95] and an improved cardiovascular risk profile [96], which will likely enhance long-term health. Interval sprint training has been shown to reduce metabolic acidosis and enhance oxidative capacity and fitness [97]. Some have even speculated that regular exercise may attenuate the autoimmune event that causes beta cell death [98]. Overall, life expectancy appears to increase with regular activity in this patient population [99].

2.6 Summary

In summary, a number of neuroendocrine disturbances can influence glucose regulation during exercise, making the management of glycemia challenging for the patient and caregiver. In general, aerobic exercise promotes a reduction in blood glucose concentration, while anaerobic exercise can promote transient hyperglycemia. Although individuals with type 1 diabetes can achieve excellence in sport, rigorous glycemic control and the appropriate insulin modifications on exercise days and appropriate nutritional intake is likely critical for maximizing individual performance. Overall, improvements in various health metrics clearly indicate that regular exercise should remain at the cornerstone of clinical care for patients with type 1 diabetes.

References

1. Wasserman DH. Regulation of glucose fluxes during exercise in the postabsorptive state. Annu Rev Physiol. 1995;57:191–218.
2. Wasserman DH. Berson award lecture 2008 four grams of glucose. Am J Physiol Endocrinol Metab. 2009;296(1):E11–21.
3. Levine SA, Gordon B, Derick CL. Some changes in the chemical constituents of the blood following a marathon race: with special reference to the development of hypoglycemia. J Am Med Assoc. 1924;82(22):1778–9.
4. Frayn KN. Fat as a fuel: emerging understanding of the adipose tissue-skeletal muscle axis. Acta Physiol (Oxf). 2010;199(4):509–18.
5. Dennis SC, Noakes TD, Hawley JA. Nutritional strategies to minimize fatigue during prolonged exercise: fluid, electrolyte and energy replacement. J Sports Sci. 1997;15(3):305–13.
6. Cryer PE. Hypoglycemia: still the limiting factor in the glycemic management of diabetes. Endocr Pract. 2008;14(6):750–6.
7. Cryer PE. Hierarchy of physiological responses to hypoglycemia: relevance to clinical hypoglycemia in type I (insulin dependent) diabetes mellitus. Horm Metab Res. 1997;29(3):92–6.
8. Marliss EB, Vranic M. Intense exercise has unique effects on both insulin release and its roles in glucoregulation: implications for diabetes. Diabetes. 2002;51 Suppl 1:S271–83.
9. Temple MY, Bar-Or O, Riddell MC. The reliability and repeatability of the blood glucose response to prolonged exercise in adolescent boys with IDDM. Diabetes Care. 1995;18(3):326–32.
10. Warburton DE, Nicol CW, Bredin SS. Prescribing exercise as preventive therapy. CMAJ. 2006;174(7):961–74.
11. Zinman B, Murray FT, Vranic M, Albisser AM, Leibel BS, Mc Clean PA, et al. Glucoregulation during moderate exercise in insulin treated diabetics. J Clin Endocrinol Metab. 1977;45(4):641–52.
12. Camacho RC, Galassetti P, Davis SN, Wasserman DH. Glucoregulation during and after exercise in health and insulin-dependent diabetes. Exerc Sport Sci Rev. 2005;33(1):17–23.
13. Tuominen JA, Karonen SL, Melamies L, Bolli G, Koivisto VA. Exercise-induced hypoglycaemia in IDDM patients treated with a short-acting insulin analogue. Diabetologia. 1995;38(1):106–11.
14. Rabasa-Lhoret R, Bourque J, Ducros F, Chiasson JL. Guidelines for premeal insulin dose reduction for postprandial exercise of different intensities and durations in type 1 diabetic subjects treated intensively with a basal-bolus insulin regimen (ultralente-lispro). Diabetes Care. 2001;24(4):625–30.

15. Berger M, Halban PA, Assal JP, Offord RE, Vranic M, Renold AE. Pharmacokinetics of sub-cutaneously injected tritiated insulin: effects of exercise. Diabetes. 1979;28 Suppl 1:53–7.
16. Gerich JE, Langlois M, Noacco C, Karam JH, Forsham PH. Lack of glucagon response to hypoglycemia in diabetes: evidence for an intrinsic pancreatic alpha cell defect. Science. 1973;182(108):171–3.
17. Orskov L, Alberti KG, Mengel A, Moller N, Pedersen O, Rasmussen O, et al. Decreased hepatic glucagon responses in type 1 (insulin-dependent) diabetes mellitus. Diabetologia. 1991;34(7):521–6.
18. Schneider SH, Vitug A, Ananthakrishnan R, Khachadurian AK. Impaired adrenergic response to prolonged exercise in type I diabetes. Metabolism. 1991;40(11):1219–25.
19. Galassetti P, Tate D, Neill RA, Morrey S, Wasserman DH, Davis SN. Effect of antecedent hypoglycemia on counterregulatory responses to subsequent euglycemic exercise in type 1 diabetes. Diabetes. 2003;52(7):1761–9.
20. Cline GW, Rothman DL, Magnusson I, Katz LD, Shulman GI. 13C-nuclear magnetic reso-nance spectroscopy studies of hepatic glucose metabolism in normal subjects and subjects with insulin-dependent diabetes mellitus. J Clin Invest. 1994;94(6):2369–76.
21. Chokkalingam K, Tsintzas K, Snaar JE, Norton L, Solanky B, Leverton E, et al. Hyperinsulinaemia during exercise does not suppress hepatic glycogen concentrations in patients with type 1 dia-betes: a magnetic resonance spectroscopy study. Diabetologia. 2007;50(9):1921–9.
22. Sigal RJ, Purdon C, Fisher SJ, Halter JB, Vranic M, Marliss EB. Hyperinsulinemia prevents prolonged hyperglycemia after intense exercise in insulin-dependent diabetic subjects. J Clin Endocrinol Metab. 1994;79(4):1049–57.
23. Sigal R, Kenny G, Oh P, Perkins BA, Plotnikoff RC, Prud'homme D, et al. Physical activity and diabetes. Canadian diabetes association clinical practice guidelines expert committee. Canadian diabetes association 2008 clinical practice guidelines for the prevention and man-agement of diabetes in Canada. Can J Diabetes. 2008;32(1):S37–9.
24. Robertson K, Adolfsson P, Scheiner G, Hanas R, Riddell MC. Exercise in children and adoles-cents with diabetes. Pediatr Diabetes. 2009;10 Suppl 12:154–68.
25. Brooks GA. Cell-cell and intracellular lactate shuttles. J Physiol. 2009;587(Pt 23):5591–600.
26. Lee AD, Hansen PA, Schluter J, Gulve EA, Gao J, Holloszy JO. Effects of epinephrine on insulin-stimulated glucose uptake and GLUT-4 phosphorylation in muscle. Am J Physiol. 1997;273(3 Pt 1):C1082–7.
27. Purdon C, Brousson M, Nyveen SL, Miles PD, Halter JB, Vranic M, et al. The roles of insulin and catecholamines in the glucoregulatory response during intense exercise and early recovery in insulin-dependent diabetic and control subjects. J Clin Endocrinol Metab. 1993;76(3):566–73.
28. Bussau VA, Ferreira LD, Jones TW, Fournier PA. A 10-s sprint performed prior to moderate-intensity exercise prevents early post-exercise fall in glycaemia in individuals with type 1 diabetes. Diabetologia. 2007;50(9):1815–8.
29. Bussau VA, Ferreira LD, Jones TW, Fournier PA. The 10-s maximal sprint: a novel approach to counter an exercise-mediated fall in glycemia in individuals with type 1 diabetes. Diabetes Care. 2006;29(3):601–6.
30. Yardley JE, Sigal RJ, Perkins BA, Riddell M. Performing resistance exercise before aerobic exercise reduces the risk of hypoglycemia in type 1 diabetes: a study using continuous glucose monitoring. Can J Diabetes. 2010;34(3):247.
31. Guelfi KJ, Ratnam N, Smythe GA, Jones TW, Fournier PA. Effect of intermittent high-inten-sity compared with continuous moderate exercise on glucose production and utilization in individuals with type 1 diabetes. Am J Physiol Endocrinol Metab. 2007;292(3):E865–70.
32. Iscoe KE, Riddell MC. Continuous moderate-intensity exercise with or without intermittent high-intensity work: effects on acute and late glycaemia in athletes with type 1 diabetes mel-litus. Diabet Med. 2011;28(7):824–32.
33. Delvecchio M, Zecchino C, Salzano G, Faienza MF, Cavallo L, De Luca F, et al. Effects of moderate-severe exercise on blood glucose in type 1 diabetic adolescents treated with insulin pump or glargine insulin. J Endocrinol Invest. 2009;32(6):519–24.

34. MacDonald MJ. Post-exercise late-onset hypoglycemia in insulin-dependent diabetic patients. Diabetes Care. 1987;10(5):584–8.
35. Taplin CE, Cobry E, Messer L, McFann K, Chase HP, Fiallo-Scharer R. Preventing post-exercise nocturnal hypoglycemia in children with type 1 diabetes. J Pediatr. 2010;157(5):784–8.e1.
36. Iscoe KE, Campbell JE, Jamnik V, Perkins BA, Riddell MC. Efficacy of continuous real-time blood glucose monitoring during and after prolonged high-intensity cycling exercise: spinning with a continuous glucose monitoring system. Diabetes Technol Ther. 2006;8(6):627–35.
37. Iscoe KE, Corcoran M, Riddell MC. High rates of nocturnal hypoglycemia in a unique sports camp for athletes with type 1 diabetes: lessons learned from continuous glucose monitoring. Can J Diabetes. 2008;32(3):182–9.
38. Tsalikian E, Mauras N, Beck RW, Tamborlane WV, Janz KF, Chase HP, et al. Impact of exercise on overnight glycemic control in children with type 1 diabetes mellitus. J Pediatr. 2005;147(4):528–34.
39. Maran A, Pavan P, Bonsembiante B, Brugin E, Ermolao A, Avogaro A, et al. Continuous glucose monitoring reveals delayed nocturnal hypoglycemia after intermittent high-intensity exercise in nontrained patients with type 1 diabetes. Diabetes Technol Ther. 2010;12(10):763–8.
40. McMahon SK, Ferreira LD, Ratnam N, Davey RJ, Youngs LM, Davis EA, et al. Glucose requirements to maintain euglycemia after moderate-intensity afternoon exercise in adolescents with type 1 diabetes are increased in a biphasic manner. J Clin Endocrinol Metab. 2007;92(3):963–8.
41. Krzentowski G, Pirnay F, Pallikarakis N, Luyckx AS, Lacroix M, Mosora F, et al. Glucose utilization during exercise in normal and diabetic subjects. The role of insulin. Diabetes. 1981;30(12):983–9.
42. Ramires PR, Forjaz CL, Strunz CM, Silva ME, Diament J, Nicolau W, et al. Oral glucose ingestion increases endurance capacity in normal and diabetic (type I) humans. J Appl Physiol. 1997;83(2):608–14.
43. Riddell MC, Bar-Or O, Hollidge-Horvat M, Schwarcz HP, Heigenhauser GJ. Glucose ingestion and substrate utilization during exercise in boys with IDDM. J Appl Physiol. 2000;88(4):1239–46.
44. Francescato MP, Geat M, Fusi S, Stupar G, Noacco C, Cattin L. Carbohydrate requirement and insulin concentration during moderate exercise in type 1 diabetic patients. Metabolism. 2004;53(9):1126–30.
45. Robitaille M, Dube MC, Weisnagel SJ, Prud'homme D, Massicotte D, Peronnet F, et al. Substrate source utilization during moderate intensity exercise with glucose ingestion in type 1 diabetic patients. J Appl Physiol. 2007;103(1):119–24.
46. Wahren J, Hagenfeldt L, Felig P. Splanchnic and leg exchange of glucose, amino acids, and free fatty acids during exercise in diabetes mellitus. J Clin Invest. 1975;55(6):1303–14.
47. Murray FT, Zinman B, McClean PA, Denoga A, Albisser AM, Leibel BS, et al. The metabolic response to moderate exercise in diabetic man receiving intravenous and subcutaneous insulin. J Clin Endocrinol Metab. 1977;44(4):708–20.
48. Raguso CA, Coggan AR, Gastaldelli A, Sidossis LS, Bastyr 3rd EJ, Wolfe RR. Lipid and carbohydrate metabolism in IDDM during moderate and intense exercise. Diabetes. 1995;44(9):1066–74.
49. Nathan DM, Madnek SF, Delahanty L. Programming pre-exercise snacks to prevent post-exercise hypoglycemia in intensively treated insulin-dependent diabetics. Ann Intern Med. 1985;102(4):483–6.
50. Riddell MC, Bar-Or O, Ayub BV, Calvert RE, Heigenhauser GJ. Glucose ingestion matched with total carbohydrate utilization attenuates hypoglycemia during exercise in adolescents with IDDM. Int J Sport Nutr. 1999;9(1):24–34.
51. Shilo S, Shamoon H. Abnormal growth hormone responses to hypoglycemia and exercise in adults with type I diabetes. Isr J Med Sci. 1990;26(3):136–41.
52. Shilo S, Sotsky M, Shamoon H. Islet hormonal regulation of glucose turnover during exercise in type 1 diabetes. J Clin Endocrinol Metab. 1990;70(1):162–72.

53. Simonson DC, Koivisto V, Sherwin RS, Ferrannini E, Hendler R, Juhlin-Dannfelt A, et al. Adrenergic blockade alters glucose kinetics during exercise in insulin-dependent diabetics. J Clin Invest. 1984;73(6):1648–58.
54. West DJ, Stephens JW, Bain SC, Kilduff LP, Luzio S, Still R, et al. A combined insulin reduction and carbohydrate feeding strategy 30 min before running best preserves blood glucose concentration after exercise through improved fuel oxidation in type 1 diabetes mellitus. J Sports Sci. 2011;29(3):279–89.
55. Francescato MP, Carrato S. Management of exercise-induced glycemic imbalances in type 1 diabetes. Curr Diabetes Rev. 2011;7(4):253–63.
56. Chase HP, Lockspeiser T, Peery B, Shepherd M, MacKenzie T, Anderson J, et al. The impact of the diabetes control and complications trial and humalog insulin on glycohemoglobin levels and severe hypoglycemia in type 1 diabetes. Diabetes Care. 2001;24(3):430–4.
57. Hamilton J, Daneman D. Deteriorating diabetes control during adolescence: physiological or psychosocial? J Pediatr Endocrinol Metab. 2002;15(2):115–26.
58. Komatsu WR, Gabbay MA, Castro ML, Saraiva GL, Chacra AR, de Barros Neto TL, et al. Aerobic exercise capacity in normal adolescents and those with type 1 diabetes mellitus. Pediatr Diabetes. 2005;6(3):145–9.
59. Baraldi E, Monciotti C, Filippone M, Santuz P, Magagnin G, Zanconato S, et al. Gas exchange during exercise in diabetic children. Pediatr Pulmonol. 1992;13(3):155–60.
60. Gusso S, Hofman P, Lalande S, Cutfield W, Robinson E, Baldi JC. Impaired stroke volume and aerobic capacity in female adolescents with type 1 and type 2 diabetes mellitus. Diabetologia. 2008;51(7):1317–20.
61. Huttunen NP, Kaar ML, Knip M, Mustonen A, Puukka R, Akerblom HK. Physical fitness of children and adolescents with insulin-dependent diabetes mellitus. Ann Clin Res. 1984;16(1):1–5.
62. Larsson Y, Persson B, Sterky G, Thoren C. Functional adaptation to rigorous training and exercise in diabetic and nondiabetic adolescents. J Appl Physiol. 1964;19:629–35.
63. Larsson YA, Sterky GC, Ekengren KE, Moller TG. Physical fitness and the influence of training in diabetic adolescent girls. Diabetes. 1962;11:109–17.
64. Poortmans JR, Saerens P, Edelman R, Vertongen F, Dorchy H. Influence of the degree of metabolic control on physical fitness in type I diabetic adolescents. Int J Sports Med. 1986;7(4):232–5.
65. Larsen S, Brynjolf I, Birch K, Munck O, Sestoft L. The effect of continuous subcutaneous insulin infusion on cardiac performance during exercise in insulin-dependent diabetics. Scand J Clin Lab Invest. 1984;44(8):683–91.
66. Nugent AM, Steele IC, al-Modaris F, Vallely S, Moore A, Campbell NP, et al. Exercise responses in patients with IDDM. Diabetes Care. 1997;20(12):1814–21.
67. Veves A, Saouaf R, Donaghue VM, Mullooly CA, Kistler JA, Giurini JM, et al. Aerobic exercise capacity remains normal despite impaired endothelial function in the micro- and macro-circulation of physically active IDDM patients. Diabetes. 1997;46(11):1846–52.
68. Ditzel J, Standl E. The problem of tissue oxygenation in diabetes mellitus. Acta Med Scand Suppl. 1975;578:59–68.
69. Kivela R, Silvennoinen M, Touvra AM, Lehti TM, Kainulainen H, Vihko V. Effects of experimental type 1 diabetes and exercise training on angiogenic gene expression and capillarization in skeletal muscle. FASEB J. 2006;20(9):1570–2.
70. Valerio G, Spagnuolo MI, Lombardi F, Spadaro R, Siano M, Franzese A. Physical activity and sports participation in children and adolescents with type 1 diabetes mellitus. Nutr Metab Cardiovasc Dis. 2007;17(5):376–82.
71. Krause MP, Riddell MC, Hawke TJ. Effects of type 1 diabetes mellitus on skeletal muscle: clinical observations and physiological mechanisms. Pediatr Diabetes. 2011;12(4 Pt 1):345–64.
72. Andersen H, Gadeberg PC, Brock B, Jakobsen J. Muscular atrophy in diabetic neuropathy: a stereological magnetic resonance imaging study. Diabetologia. 1997;40(9):1062–9.
73. Andersen H, Stalberg E, Gjerstad MD, Jakobsen J. Association of muscle strength and electrophysiological measures of reinnervation in diabetic neuropathy. Muscle Nerve. 1998;21(12):1647–54.

74. Andersen H. Muscular endurance in long-term IDDM patients. Diabetes Care. 1998;21(4):604–9.
75. Andersen H, Gjerstad MD, Jakobsen J. Atrophy of foot muscles: a measure of diabetic neuropathy. Diabetes Care. 2004;27(10):2382–5.
76. Andreassen CS, Jakobsen J, Ringgaard S, Ejskjaer N, Andersen H. Accelerated atrophy of lower leg and foot muscles–a follow-up study of long-term diabetic polyneuropathy using magnetic resonance imaging (MRI). Diabetologia. 2009;52(6):1182–91.
77. Andreassen CS, Jakobsen J, Flyvbjerg A, Andersen H. Expression of neurotrophic factors in diabetic muscle–relation to neuropathy and muscle strength. Brain. 2009;132(Pt 10):2724–33.
78. Almeida S, Riddell MC, Cafarelli E. Slower conduction velocity and motor unit discharge frequency are associated with muscle fatigue during isometric exercise in type 1 diabetes mellitus. Muscle Nerve. 2008;37(2):231–40.
79. Surridge DH, Erdahl DL, Lawson JS, Donald MW, Monga TN, Bird CE, et al. Psychiatric aspects of diabetes mellitus. Br J Psychiatry. 1984;145:269–76.
80. Van der Does FE, De Neeling JN, Snoek FJ, Kostense PJ, Grootenhuis PA, Bouter LM, et al. Symptoms and well-being in relation to glycemic control in type II diabetes. Diabetes Care. 1996;19(3):204–10.
81. Riddell MC, Bar-Or O, Gerstein HC, Heigenhauser GJ. Perceived exertion with glucose ingestion in adolescent males with IDDM. Med Sci Sports Exerc. 2000;32(1):167–73.
82. Crowther GJ, Milstein JM, Jubrias SA, Kushmerick MJ, Gronka RK, Conley KE. Altered energetic properties in skeletal muscle of men with well-controlled insulin-dependent (type 1) diabetes. Am J Physiol Endocrinol Metab. 2003;284(4):E655–62.
83. Jenni S, Oetliker C, Allemann S, Ith M, Tappy L, Wuerth S, et al. Fuel metabolism during exercise in euglycaemia and hyperglycaemia in patients with type 1 diabetes mellitus–a prospective single-blinded randomised crossover trial. Diabetologia. 2008;51(8):1457–65.
84. Magee MF, Bhatt BA. Management of decompensated diabetes. Diabetic ketoacidosis and hyperglycemic hyperosmolar syndrome. Crit Care Clin. 2001;17(1):75–106.
85. Andersen H, Schmitz O, Nielsen S. Decreased isometric muscle strength after acute hyperglycaemia in type 1 diabetic patients. Diabet Med. 2005;22(10):1401–7.
86. Boehncke S, Poettgen K, Maser-Gluth C, Reusch J, Boehncke WH, Badenhoop K. Endurance capabilities of triathlon competitors with type 1 diabetes mellitus. Dtsch Med Wochenschr. 2009;134(14):677–82.
87. Bosch AN, Kirkman MC. Maintenance of hyperglycaemia does not improve performance in a 100 km cycling time trial. S Afr J Sports Med. 2007;19(3):94–8.
88. Heyman E, Briard D, Dekerdanet M, Gratas-Delamarche A, Delamarche P. Accuracy of physical working capacity 170 to estimate aerobic fitness in prepubertal diabetic boys and in 2 insulin dose conditions. J Sports Med Phys Fitness. 2006;46(2):315–21.
89. Stettler C, Jenni S, Allemann S, Steiner R, Hoppeler H, Trepp R, et al. Exercise capacity in subjects with type 1 diabetes mellitus in eu- and hyperglycaemia. Diabetes Metab Res Rev. 2006;22(4):300–6.
90. Kelly D, Hamilton JK, Riddell MC. Blood glucose levels and performance in a sports camp for adolescents with type 1 diabetes mellitus: a field study. Int J Pediatr. 2010;2010. doi:10.1155/2010/216167. 216167. Epub 2010 Aug 2.
91. Gonder-Frederick LA, Zrebiec JF, Bauchowitz AU, Ritterband LM, Magee JC, Cox DJ, et al. Cognitive function is disrupted by both hypo- and hyperglycemia in school-aged children with type 1 diabetes: a field study. Diabetes Care. 2009;32(6):1001–6.
92. Jimenez CC, Corcoran MH, Crawley JT, Guyton Hornsby W, Peer KS, Philbin RD, et al. National athletic trainers' association position statement: management of the athlete with type 1 diabetes mellitus. J Athl Train. 2007;42(4):536–45.
93. Goodyear LJ, Kahn BB. Exercise, glucose transport, and insulin sensitivity. Annu Rev Med. 1998;49:235–61.
94. Chu L, Hamilton J, Riddell MC. Clinical management of the physically active patient with type 1 diabetes. Phys Sportsmed. 2011;39(2):64–77.

95. Seeger JP, Thijssen DH, Noordam K, Cranen ME, Hopman MT, Nijhuis-van der Sanden MW. Exercise training improves physical fitness and vascular function in children with type 1 diabetes. Diabetes Obes Metab. 2011;13(4):382–4.

96. Heyman E, Toutain C, Delamarche P, Berthon P, Briard D, Youssef H, et al. Exercise training and cardiovascular risk factors in type 1 diabetic adolescent girls. Pediatr Exerc Sci. 2007;19(4):408–19.

97. Harmer AR, Chisholm DJ, McKenna MJ, Hunter SK, Ruell PA, Naylor JM, et al. Sprint training increases muscle oxidative metabolism during high-intensity exercise in patients with type 1 diabetes. Diabetes Care. 2008;31(11):2097–102.

98. Krause Mda S, de Bittencourt Jr PI. Type 1 diabetes: can exercise impair the autoimmune event? The L-arginine/glutamine coupling hypothesis. Cell Biochem Funct. 2008;26(4):406–33.

99. Moy CS, Songer TJ, LaPorte RE, Dorman JS, Kriska AM, Orchard TJ, et al. Insulin-dependent diabetes mellitus, physical activity, and death. Am J Epidemiol. 1993;137(1):74–81.

100. Coker RH, Kjaer M. Glucoregulation during exercise: the role of the neuroendocrine system. Sports Med. 2005;35(7):575–83.

Chapter 3
Pre-exercise Insulin and Carbohydrate Strategies in the Exercising T1DM Individual

Richard M. Bracken, Daniel J. West, and Stephen C. Bain

3.1 Characteristics of Physical Exercise

Physical exercise is a potent stressor that causes large increases in the metabolic rate of the type 1 diabetes (T1DM) individual. The magnitude of the increase in fuel use above resting values is dependent on factors such as the duration, intensity, and type of exercise. Somewhat simplistically, an ability to perform exercise is dependent on the amount and rate of supply of carbohydrate and lipid fuel to facilitate completion of exercise. Deficiencies in carbohydrate availability will cause fatigue but from the viewpoint of the person with T1DM, aid the development of hypoglycemia.

Carbohydrate and fat represent the most abundant and available stores for the exercising type 1 athlete. Liver (80–110 g for a 70-kg male) and skeletal muscle (300–350 g) stores represent the main sites of endogenous carbohydrate. The meager amount of circulating glucose of 10–15 g represents the balance between glucose appearance into the circulation, released from the liver, and uptake by bodily tissues. With resting rates of whole-body carbohydrate use of ~0.25 g·min^{-1}, 1 day of starvation can significantly reduce carbohydrate stores, excepting for the body's ability to

R.M. Bracken, B.Sc., M.Sc., PGCert, Ph.D. (✉)
Health and Sport Science, College of Engineering, Swansea University,
Singleton Park, Swansea, SA2 8PP, UK
e-mail: r.m.bracken@swansea.ac.uk

D.J. West, B.Sc., Ph.D.
Department of Sport and Exercise, Northumbria University,
Northumberland Street, Newcastle upon Tyne, Tyne and Wear NE1 8ST, UK
e-mail: d.j.west@northumbria.ac.uk

S.C. Bain, M.A., M.D., FRCP
Institute of Life Sciences, College of Medicine, Swansea University,
Singleton Park, Swansea, Wales SA2 8PP, UK
e-mail: s.c.bain@swansea.ac.uk

I. Gallen (ed.), *Type 1 Diabetes*,
DOI 10.1007/978-0-85729-754-9_3, © Springer-Verlag London Limited 2012

minimize this loss through the manufacture of new glucose from, e.g., amino acids, keto acids, or lactate. Adipose tissue and skeletal muscle fat stores are more plentiful; so for a 70-kg male with an estimated 10% body fat, i.e., 7 kg, an energy density of 37.7 kJ per gram of fat provides an estimated potential energy store of 264 MJ – enough to run more than 20 marathons! Fats are used heavily in low-intensity exercise, but are rate limited to ~60–65% VO_2 peak. An ability to increase exercise intensity relies on an increased combustion of carbohydrate in muscle. Clearly, the exercising T1DM has a choice of fuels to use dependent on the amount of exercise, i.e., duration, intensity, and its type. Knowledge of how stores of liver and muscle of carbohydrate are used or preserved by preferential use of fat determines how blood glucose levels respond to exercise. Furthermore, different exercise models evoke different patterns of change in energy stores that also complicate an understanding of the blood glucose response to exercise. Understanding variation in metabolic changes in T1DM individuals is a first step towards understanding the efficacy of pre-exercise alterations in insulin and/or carbohydrate supplementation.

3.2   Exercise-Induced Hypoglycemia with Different Exercise Types

3.2.1   *Endurance Exercise*

Endurance exercise-induced hypoglycemia is a frequent occurrence in T1DM individuals and represents a challenge to good glycemic control [1–3] when compared with sprinting or intermittent exercise patterns mimicking games activities [4–6]. In response to a single bout of continuous endurance exercise, evidence has demonstrated patients with T1DM may develop a hypoglycemic episode [2, 3, 7]. For example, Campaigne et al. [2] investigated the effects of different diets and insulin adjustments prior to a 45-min bout of steady state cycling that was performed at 60% of VO_2 peak. Six out of the nine patients experienced hypoglycemic episodes within 5 h of completing the exercise which was independent of prior insulin dosage or post-exercise feeding. The authors suggested the findings might reflect an enhanced glucose uptake following the reduction in muscle glycogen stores due to exercise. Moreover, in a study by Tsalikian et al. [3] hypoglycemia developed overnight more frequently in T1DM children after performance of continuous exercise that day (four 15-min periods of walking at a heart rate of ~140 bpm) compared to nights when daily exercise was not performed. The results showed that plasma glucose concentrations decreased by at least 25% during or immediately after the exercise period in 41 subjects, with 11 demonstrating blood glucose concentrations of ≤60 mg/dL during or immediately after walking. Thus, it appears that the incidence of developing a post-exercise hypoglycemic episode following continuous endurance exercise is significant and ranges from 15% to 66% in T1DM patients across studies [1–3].

3.2.2 Sprint Exercise

The performance of a short sprint before or after continuous moderate-intensity exercise can reduce the degree of hypoglycemia following exercise in T1DM patients [4, 8]. In these two separate studies, 7 T1DM males were recruited to complete 20 min of cycle ergometry at an exercise intensity equivalent to 40% VO_2 peak with a 10-s sprint performed before [8] or after [4] the low-intensity cycling. The control trial in each study was 20-min cycling at 40% VO_2 peak with no sprinting. In both studies, the 20-min bout of cycling resulted in a significant fall in blood glucose values 2 h after exercise; however, the addition of a 10-s sprint placed before or after the endurance exercise significantly attenuated the drop in blood glucose concentration. The mechanisms explaining the improved post-exercise glycemia were not clear, but the authors suggested that there was an increased hepatic glucose release in response to the sprint due to greater counter-regulatory hormones and/or greater circulating lactate after exercise which may have contributed to liver gluconeogenesis and/or restoration of reduced muscle carbohydrate stores.

3.2.3 Intermittent Exercise

Sport and recreational activities vary greatly in terms of muscular recruitment, technical requirements, exercise intensity, and duration. In contrast to endurance-based activities (such as constant pace running, cycling, or swimming), where energy supply is more evenly matched to the energy demands of the activity, most sporting activities are intermittent in nature. Examples of this type of exercise pattern can be seen in field games (football, rugby, and hockey), racquet sports (tennis, squash, and badminton), and court games (basketball, volleyball, and netball). In recent years, there has been an increase in the number of studies employing exercise protocols that attempt to replicate typical patterns of intermittent activities, while remaining well controlled within a laboratory environment. Research has demonstrated that the performance of intermittent high-intensity sprints (INT; 11 × 4-s cycle sprints, every 2 min for 20 min) did not increase the risk of developing hypoglycemia during and for 60 min post-exercise, when compared to a resting control trial [5]. The researchers demonstrated blood glucose levels fell by 4 $mmol\cdot l^{-1}$ during INT compared to 2 $mmol\cdot l^{-1}$ during the control trial. Interestingly, blood glucose did not continue to fall following exercise resulting in similar glucose levels by 50 min in post-INT exercise and control trials. Moreover, intermittent high-intensity (INT) exercise has been shown to preserve blood glucose concentrations more than continuous (CON) exercise and reduce the risk of hypoglycemia during and after exercise [6, 9]. In a study by Guelfi et al. [6], blood glucose responses to both continuous and intermittent exercise were compared. Participants performed 30 min of cycling at 40% VO_2 peak (CON) or 30 min of cycling at 40% VO_2 peak, with 4 s maximal sprints interspersed every 2 min (INT). Blood glucose responses revealed a smaller decline during INT exercise, despite performing more work. Moreover, blood glucose remained stable for 60 min post-exercise, whereas they continued to decline under CON. The preserved blood glucose concentrations were suggested to be related to the stimulatory effects of catecholamines and growth hormone on liver glycogenolysis. It is interesting to note that none of the aforementioned research that utilized high-intensity exercise protocols employed pre-exercise rapid-acting insulin reductions unlike the apparent common practice in endurance exercise (see Sect. 3.4.1). This may be because of the greater likelihood of post-exercise hyperglycemia in INT exercise from the combined effects of a small amount of circulating insulin-reducing glucose uptake and an increased counter-regulatory hormone-stimulated effect on hepatic glucose release. On the other hand, the potential to avoid hypoglycemia, or at least improve the stability of post-exercise blood glucose concentrations, may be worthy of investigation.

At present, the literature examining different exercise factors affecting blood glucose responses within T1DM individuals has employed cycling exercise [2, 4–6, 8, 10–19]. Cycling is a primarily concentric form of exercise, i.e., the muscle shortens as it contracts. However, in many daily activity patterns including non-body-weight-supported exercises, such as walking, jogging, or running, there is a significant proportion of eccentric muscle action, where the muscle lengthens in the performance of the movement. Eccentric muscle actions have been demonstrated to hinder insulin action and glucose uptake for many hours following exercise [20, 21]. Such data suggest an additional layer of complexity to the understanding of post-exercise glycemia in response to different patterns of exercise in the T1DM individual.

From a practical point of view, although much more work is needed to explore glycemic responses to real-life sports and exercise patterns "in the field," the specificity of submaximal endurance exercise as the "exercise of choice" for some T1DM cohorts is clear. In research studies examining the glycemic responses to high-intensity exercise, participant mean age was young (i.e., 21–22 years old) [4, 6, 8]. It is less likely that older T1DM individuals are inclined to perform high-intensity intermittent exercise as a method to preserve blood glucose after exercise, as the risk of injury may be more significant [22]. Additionally, although high-intensity (90–100% VO_2 max) exercise will increase cardiovascular fitness more so than lower intensity exercise [23], research suggests that when lower intensity exercise exceeds 35 min, there are similar gains in cardiovascular fitness, when compared with short-duration high-intensity training [22]. For these reasons, methods to help preserve glycemia during and after submaximal endurance exercise should continue to be explored.

3.2.4   Resistance Exercise

Resistance exercise is important in the glycemic control of T2DM individuals [24, 25]; however, its effect on glycemic control within T1DM is unclear with research demonstrating no change in HbA_{1c} after a resistance training program [26, 27].

Additionally, data on the acute effects of a single session of resistance exercise on glycemia and metabolism are sparse.

A single resistance exercise session did not affect post-exercise insulin sensitivity in T1DM individuals [28]. In this study, 2 groups of 7 T1DM individuals were placed under a euglycemic-hyperinsulinemic clamp before resting (control) or performing 5 sets of 6 repetitions, at 80% of 1 repetition maximum, of a combined lower leg extension and flexion movement (i.e., quadriceps extension and hamstring curl). The clamp procedure was repeated at 12 and 36 h following the resistance and control protocol. After exercise, insulin sensitivity did not differ from baseline at 12 and 36 h post-exercise; moreover, there were no differences when compared to the control group. However, caution should be taken when interpreting this data. There is a large contribution from muscle glycogen during resistance exercise [29–31], and its depletion is a key factor in exercise-induced increases in insulin sensitivity [32–34]. Furthermore, there is a rapid-replenishment of muscle glycogen stores within the first 2 h of completing a resistance exercise session [30]. Potentially, within the study of Jiminez et al. [28] differences in insulin sensitivity (and blood glucose concentrations) may have been more likely to occur in a shorter time frame after completion of the resistance protocol. In addition, the exercise protocol consisted of concentric-only muscle contractions, whereas free or machine-assisted resistance exercises consist of both eccentric and concentric muscle contractions. As previously mentioned, eccentric contractions hinder insulin action and glucose uptake within skeletal muscle for many hours following exercise [20, 21].

Resistance exercise is a potent stimulator of counter-regulatory hormones such as catecholamines, growth hormone, and cortisol in people that do not have diabetes [35–38]. Blood glucose increases in response to a single resistance exercise session [36] with a ~1.8 mmol·l^{-1} increase in blood glucose after 6 sets of 10 repetition back squats, at 80% of 1 repetition maximum in nondiabetes participants. Increases in blood glucose were related to increases in adrenaline ($r=0.6$) and noradrenaline ($r=0.9$) concentrations, respectively. Thus, available data suggest potential for resistance exercise to promote hyperglycemia, but to date, there is limited data to demonstrate this in T1DM individuals. The limited literature on the acute metabolic responses to resistance exercise in T1DM individuals warrants future research to develop more comprehensive blood glucose management strategies across all types of exercise.

3.3 Strategies for Preventing and/or Minimizing Post-exercise Hypoglycemia

In light of the aforementioned potential for hypoglycemia following some forms of exercise, strategies that help combat hypoglycemia have received considerable attention within the literature [2, 6, 12, 13, 15, 18, 39–41]. An important aspect of the research focuses on reducing the pre-exercise rapid-acting insulin dose [2, 15, 18].

3.3.1   The Efficacy of Pre-exercise Insulin Dose Reduction on Post-exercise Glycemia

The type of insulin is important to consider when examining its consequent effects on blood glucose concentrations. Currently, many T1DM individuals are treated with modern insulin analogues in a basal-bolus regimen; these rDNA insulins (e.g., insulin glargine/detemir and aspart/lispro/glulisine) offer very different, more favorable, action-time profiles and less variability than longer established insulins, such as regular human insulin and NPH insulin [19, 42, 43]. In recent years, research that has begun to emerge that has examined the effectiveness of pre-exercise rapid-acting insulin reductions employed in a basal-bolus insulin routine [18, 44–47].

3.3.1.1   Basal Insulins

The choice of basal insulin may influence the potential for hypoglycemia. In a multinational, randomized, 3-year crossover trial, T1DM individuals managed with basal insulin detemir, glargine, or neutral protamine Hagedorn (NPH) performed 30 min of exercise and were monitored over 150 min of recovery [48]. During exercise, 18 (38%) of 51 participants on glargine developed hypoglycemia compared with 5 (11%) and 6 (12%) participants on detemir and NPH, respectively. Furthermore, incidence of hypoglycemia in those participants on glargine was greater than detemir and NPH (19% vs. 14% and 11%, $P<0.001$). Thus, insulin detemir was associated with less hypoglycemia than insulin glargine, but not NPH insulin during and after exercise. Interestingly, compared to rapid-acting insulin [49], the effect of exercise appears minimal on absorption kinetics of some basal insulins. In one study in T1DM individuals, cycling (30 min, 65% VO_2 max) did not influence glargine absorption rate and produced similar declines in plasma glucose and insulin compared to a noncycling condition [17]. So, reductions to modern long-lasting insulins in a basal-bolus routine have the potential to influence circulating glucose concentrations; however, its manipulation before acute exercise may be impractical given the need for dose alterations for many hours prior to the exercise session. Finally, there is little research that has examined the effects of manipulations of basal insulins in T1DM individuals that are engaged in regular exercise training.

3.3.1.2   Rapid-Acting Insulins

Within the existing literature examining pre-exercise rapid-acting insulin reductions, recommendations have varied from 10% to 40% [39], >50% [2], 10% to 50% [40], 50% to 90% [15], and 50% to 75% [18] (Table 3.1). Some of the variation in the recommended reduction can be accounted for by differences in the insulin type used by participants and the exercise model employed (Table 3.1).

Table 3.1 Summary of literature investigating the effects of reducing pre-exercise insulin dose on the maintenance of glycemia

Reference	Participants	Participant insulin regimen	Insulin reduction	Exercise	Findings
Campaigne et al. [2]	9 T1DM males	2 daily – premixed (NPH and soluble)	A – 50% ↓ of intermediate insulin, B – 50% ↓ of soluble insulin, C – No change	45 min, continuous cycling at 60% VO$_2$max	Hypoglycemia occurred despite reductions. ↑ Nocturnal hypoglycemia under C. Hypoglycemia occurred despite insulin reductions
Rabasa-Lhoret et al. [18]	8 T1DM males	Basal ultralente with prandial lispro	No change, 50% or 75% ↓ in all exercise protocols	Cycling at A – 25% VO$_2$max for 1 h, B – 50% VO$_2$max for 30 and 60 min, C – 75% VO$_2$max for 30 min	No insulin reduction ↑ chance of hypoglycemia at all intensities. Appropriate adjustments maintain glycemia during and after exercise
Mauvais-Jarvis et al. [15]	12 T1DM males	NPH and regular insulin twice (n = 6) or three times (n = 6) daily	50% ↓ for subjects on twice-daily regimen, 90% ↓ for three times daily	1-h continuous cycling at 70% VO$_2$max	No reduction ↑ chance of hypoglycemia. 50–90% reductions depending on insulin regimen can maintain glycemia during and after exercise
West et al. [45]	7 T1DM (6 males, 1 female)	Basal insulin glargine with prandial insulin lispro or aspart	Administered normal, 75%, 50%, or 25% of rapid-acting insulin dose 2 h prior to exercise	45-min continuous running at 70% VO$_2$max	25% dose preserved blood glucose the most for 24 h post-exercise, despite consuming fewer carbohydrates. Severe rapid-acting insulin reductions do not increase the risk of developing hyperketonemia or ketoacidosis

An early study by Campaigne et al. [2] (Table 3.1) examined blood glucose responses during and after 45 min of cycling at 60% VO_2 max in 9 T1DM males who were treated with a twice-daily, intermediate/short-acting insulin mix. Despite 50% reductions in the intermediate or the soluble insulin prior to exercise, hypoglycemia still occurred in 6 of the 9 subjects at some point during or after exercise, mainly during the night of the trial day. Additionally, Mauvais-Jarvis et al. [15] (Table 3.1) examined pre-exercise insulin reductions during and for 2 h after exercise, within 12 T1DM individuals. Six of the participants were treated with regular insulin in the morning and at noon and NPH before bed, while the other six participants were treated with bi-daily mixed insulin regimen of 30% regular insulin combined with 70% NPH insulin. Participants performed 60 min of cycling at 70% VO_2 max, 90 min after a set meal where participants administered an unaltered insulin dose or a 90% insulin reduction (participants on 3 daily injections)/50% insulin reduction (bi-daily mixed regimen). Eight participants had to receive an oral glucose solution during the no insulin reduction condition due to rapidly falling plasma glucose concentrations. Plasma glucose levels were consistently higher during and for 2 h after exercise within the insulin reduction trial. It was concluded that a 50–90% reduction in insulin dose, depending on their insulin regimen, allowed T1DM individuals to engage in endurance exercise without causing hypoglycemia [15].

A limitation of the research of Campaigne et al. [2] and Mauvais-Jarvis et al. [15] was the lack of specific guidelines for pre-exercise insulin dose adjustments taking into consideration exercise intensity and duration. In addition, the duration of monitoring blood glucose was just 2–12 h, but hypoglycemia may develop up to 24 h after exercise [1, 3]; so a larger window of examination would allow determination of the effectiveness of the degree of insulin reduction. Finally, with the increased prescription of a basal-bolus regimen to treat many T1DM individuals, dose adjustments specific to this kind of treatment, as opposed to the use of mixed insulins in the studies above is worthy of more exploration.

Research by Rabasa-Lhoret et al. [18] (Table 3.1) strengthened the area by addressing some of the above-mentioned issues by examining alterations in rapid-acting insulin as part of a basal-bolus regimen (Ultralente with prandial insulin lispro) while also taking into consideration exercise intensity and duration. Participants performed 60 min cycling at 25% VO_2 max, 30 and 60 min at 50% VO_2 max, and 30 min at 75% VO_2 max. Blood glucose concentrations were monitored during and for an hour after exercise. All trials were performed following administration of a full insulin dose (Full), a 50% reduction (50%), and after a 75% reduction (25%). The researchers demonstrated that the drop in blood glucose that occurs with exercise at 25% VO_2 max for 60 min did not differ between Full and 50%, but higher pre-exercise glucose concentrations resulted in a safer glycemic profile following exercise. Plasma glucose at the end of exercise was $\Delta - 2.9 \pm 1.1$ mmol·l^{-1} below baseline after Full, compared with $\Delta - 0.6 \pm 0.9$ mmol·l^{-1} after 50%. This trend followed during exercise at 50% VO_2 max for 30 min; the decrease in plasma glucose, relative to rest, at the end of exercise was less under 50% ($\Delta - 0.4 \pm 1.3$ mmol·l^{-1}) compared with Full ($\Delta - 2.1 \pm 0.7$ mmol·l^{-1}) and resulted in greater plasma glucose concentrations during and for 1 h after exercise. Plasma glucose responses revealed that the greatest preservation of post-exercise glycemia occurred after a 75% insulin reduction, when exercising at 50% VO_2 max for an hour and 75% VO_2 max for 30 min. The 75% reduction trial resulted in a better maintenance of glycemia during and after exercise (~7–10 mmol·l⁻¹), with less chance of developing hypoglycemia, compared to just a 50% reduced dose, which elicited post-exercise concentrations of ~4.5–7 mmol·l⁻¹.

Large reductions to pre-exercise insulin lispro or aspart resulted in better preservation of blood glucose, during and after running in T1DM individuals (Fig. 3.1) [45]. In this study, effects of pre-exercise insulin reductions on consequent metabolic and dietary patterns for 24 h after running were examined in individuals with type 1 diabetes. Participants administered their full rapid-acting insulin dose or 75%, 50%, or 25% of it, immediately before consuming a carbohydrate rich meal. After 2 h, participants completed 45 min of running at 70% VO_2 peak. Pre-exercise peak insulin concentrations were greatest with the Full dose and consequently elicited the lowest blood glucose concentrations. Blood glucose decreased under all conditions with exercise, with the fall in the full dose greater than with 25% insulin. Blood glucose at 3 h post-exercise was greatest with the 25% dose. Interestingly, over the next 21 h, self-recorded blood glucose area under the curve was greater with the 25% dose compared with all other trials despite consuming less energy and fewer carbohydrates. Thus, a 75% reduction to pre-exercise insulin resulted in the greatest preservation of blood glucose, and a reduced dietary intake, for 24 h after running in individuals with type 1 diabetes.

3.3.2 The Safety of Strategies Employing Reductions to Rapid-Acting Insulin Dose

Exogenous insulin treatment reduces blood glucose, which prevents hyperglycemia and risk of ketosis [50]. Under normal physiological conditions, ketones (acetoacetate, β(beta)-hydroxybutyrate, and acetone) are produced through hepatic fatty acid metabolism during periods of low carbohydrate availability. Ketogenesis allows fat-derived energy to be generated in the liver and used by other organs, such as the brain, heart, kidney cortex, and skeletal muscle [51]. However, reduction or omission in insulin dose is a significant factor in the development of diabetic ketoacidosis accounting for 13–45% of reported DKA cases [52]. The formation of ketone bodies above nonphysiological levels (>1 mmol·l⁻¹) has been shown to increase oxygen radical formation and cause lipid peroxidation [53–55] as well as induce metabolic acidosis [51]. Diabetic ketoacidosis is characterized by an absolute or relative deficiency of circulating insulin and combined increases in counter-regulatory hormones (catecholamines, glucagon, cortisol, growth hormone), particularly glucagon and adrenaline, hyperglycemia, and metabolic acidosis [52]. Furthermore, physical exercise increases ketone body formation [56], alters acid-base balance, and increases counter-regulatory hormones. Therefore, the potential for a combined effect of a pre-exercise insulin reduction strategy and performance of exercise

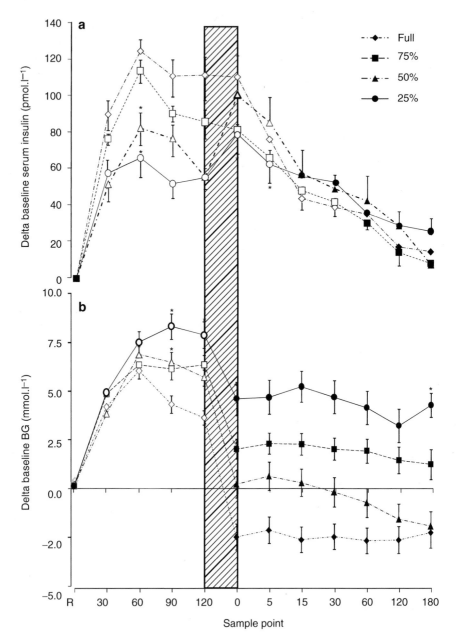

Fig. 3.1 Serum insulin and blood glucose responses to progressive reductions in rapid-acting insulin at rest and during and after 45 min of aerobic running (Reprinted with permission of the publisher from West et al. [45], Taylor & Francis)

might exacerbate ketogenesis and result in hyperketonemia (>1.0 mmol·l^{-1}) or development of ketoacidosis (>3.0 mmol·l^{-1}) [51]. However, reductions in pre-exercise rapid-acting insulin dose were not found to influence ketogenesis following running [44]. In this study, 7 T1DM participants attended the laboratory four times, each time consuming a 1.12 MJ wheat biscuit and peach meal (60 g carbohydrate, 2 g fat, 2 g protein), with Full (7.3 ± 0.2 units), 75% (5.4 ± 0.1 units), 50% (3.7 ± 0.1 units), or 25% (1.8 ± 0.1 units) of their rapid-acting insulin lispro or aspart. After a 2-h rest, participants completed 45-min running at $70 \pm 1\%$ VO$_2$ peak. Resting ketoacids (β-O-hydroxybutyrate) gradually decreased over 2-h rest with similar post-exercise peak β-OHB at 3 h. This preparatory strategy preserved blood glucose and posed no greater risk to exercising T1DM individuals in exercise-induced ketone body formation.

3.3.3 Current Recommendations for Carbohydrate Intake and Exercise in T1DM

The importance of carbohydrate for the exercising person with T1DM is in the provision of fuel for exercise as well as the avoidance of hypoglycemia during or after exercise. From a clinical exercise physiology perspective both are of utmost importance in ensuring the individual adapts safely to exercise. Carbohydrates come in a variety of forms with very different functional characteristics. The simplest forms of carbohydrates are the monosaccharides commonly referred to as "simple sugars" which include pentoses (e.g., arabinose, ribose, xylose) and hexoses (e.g., fructose, galactose, glucose, mannose). Disaccharides (e.g., lactose maltose, sucrose, isomaltulose) are comprised of pairs of monosaccharides linked together, while polysaccharides (e.g., glycogen or starches like amylin and amylopectin) are comprised of long chains of glucose molecules.

Important characteristics of carbohydrate, such as the amount and concentration, determine the rate of gastric emptying due to the resultant increase in volume and potential for intestinal feedback. The bolus temperature, pH, osmolality, viscosity, multiple carbohydrate content, and hypo- or hyperglycemic state also influence the rate of gastric emptying [57–59]. Thereafter, the entry of carbohydrate into the bloodstream from the small intestine is determined to a large degree by the type of carbohydrate. Glucose and galactose are transported into enterocytes in the small intestine by sodium/glucose co-transporter 1 (SGLT1), while fructose is transported into enterocytes by GLUT5 transporters. This has distinct implications for the resultant appearance of carbohydrate from ingestion to circulatory appearance. The transport of glucose by SGLT1 is saturable and somewhat independent of the ingested glucose load; so its entry into the bloodstream is rate-limited. However, the ingestion of multiple carbohydrates by involving more than one transport system can increase the carbohydrate transport rate into the bloodstream, e.g., by an increase in GLUT5-mediated transport of fructose. Therefore, the type of carbohydrate, i.e., mono-, di-, or polysaccharide can influence the rate of appearance in the circulation.

For example, hydrolysis of isomaltulose by a sucrose-isomaltase complex into glucose and fructose in the jejunum of the small intestine results in a slower carbohydrate transport rate into the portal vein circulation [60]. Indeed, reported values from several studies suggest exogenously ingested carbohydrates demonstrate a wide range in maximum circulatory appearance rates due to several of the above-mentioned factors [61]. However, an important observation from this research is a maximum appearance rate of carbohydrate into the bloodstream of ~1.0–1.1 $g \cdot min^{-1}$. This suggests a maximum of ~60–66 grams of ingested carbohydrate may contribute to the maintenance of blood glucose levels per hour of exercise.

There has been a wide range of recommendations for carbohydrate consumption before or during exercise in T1DM individuals that have condensed to three main strands, namely, (a) amounts based on pre-exercise blood glucose concentration (<5.6 or <6.7 mM, [39, 62]), (b) amounts based on exercise duration (20–60 g every 30 min [63], 60 $g \cdot h^{-1}$ [64]), or (c) amounts based on body mass (1–2 $g \cdot kg^{-1}$ BM [65, 66]). One criticism of blood glucose measurement before exercise is the lack of knowledge of blood glucose changes in the hours prior to measurement. Potentially, a single blood glucose reading may appear euglycemic but could be declining from previous values, in which case, exercise might accelerate the decline in circulating glucose to hypoglycemic levels.

Although there appears strong support for carbohydrate consumption before, during, and after exercise, the primary question for the T1DM individual is what amount of carbohydrate to consume. Hernandez et al. [13] (Table 3.2) suggested that 60–120 g of carbohydrates should be consumed in equal bolus before, during, and after exercise to prevent late-onset hypoglycemia. Iafusco recommended consumption of 15 g of "simple carbohydrates" immediately before exercise and consumption of a hypotonic sports drink (e.g., Gatorade®, 4% sucrose, 2% fructose) during exercise [41]. Dubé et al. [12] recommended a beverage containing 35 g of glucose should be consumed immediately before exercise to maintain blood glucose during 60 min of moderate-intensity exercise. During the exercise bout, 7 of 9 individuals required glucose infusion under a no-added carbohydrate trial; 0 g, 4 of 9 participants required glucose infusion under the 15 g trial, and 3 under the 30 g condition. Therefore, it appears glucose ingestion up to an upper limit of ~1 $g \cdot min^{-1}$ of exercise may facilitate optimal glucose appearance rates and preserve glycemia, reducing the occurrence of hypoglycemia.

Carbohydrate drink concentration is another important characteristic to consider in the avoidance of low blood glucose. Some research has recommended T1DM individuals consume a 10% carbohydrate solution before and during exercise to maintain glycemia (Table 3.2) [16]. Participants cycled at 55–60% VO_2 max for 60 min, consuming either an 8% or a 10% carbohydrate solution before and during exercise. Throughout the duration of the trial, blood glucose concentrations were lower under the 8% solution; and four individuals experienced hypoglycemia under this condition. Furthermore, blood glucose concentrations dropped ~1.8 $mmol \cdot l^{-1}$ in the hour post-exercise, whereas concentrations remained stable under the 10% condition. Additionally, to quickly correct falling blood glucose during exercise, Gallen [67] recommended consumption of a 15% carbohydrate solution. Drinks with a high carbohydrate concentration (ranging from 6% to 20%) have been shown to

Table 3.2 Summary of current literature examining carbohydrate consumption in order to prevent hypoglycemia during and after exercise

Reference	Participants	Participant insulin regimen	Protocol	Exercise	Findings
Hernandez et al. [13]	7 T1DM (6 males, 1 female)	Bovine/porcine ultralente with regular human insulin	Water (0 g CHO), whole milk (40 g), skim milk (66 g), sports drink A (121 g), and sports drink B (74 g) consumed in thirds immediately before, during, and after exercise. BG monitored 12 h post-exercise	60-min cycling at 60% VO_2 max. After 30 min, a 10-min rest period was carried out for fluid ingestion	No trial completely prevented hypoglycemia. Milk trials had ↓ pre-bed BG concentrations. During milk trials, no early morning incidents of hypoglycemia; there was 1 incident under sports drink B. Authors conclude CHO beverage must be consumed before, during, and after exercise. Amount may depend on level of glycogen depletion across participants
Dubé et al. [12]	9 T1DM (6 males, 3 females)	Bi-daily NPH and prandial insulin lispro	3 h after a standardized breakfast (8 kcal·kg⁻¹) participants consumed either 0, 15, or 30 g of glucose immediately before exercise	60-min continuous cycling at 50% VO_2 max	30 g delayed the time before glucose needed to be infused more than 15 g. 7 of 9 needed glucose infusion under 0 g, 4 of 9 under 15 g and 3 under 30 g. Authors estimate a beverage of 35 g of glucose is required to maintain BG for 60 min of moderate exercise
Perrone et al. [16]	16 T1DM (10 males, 6 females)	Intermediate or ultra-long insulin	Participants consumed an 8% (5.4 g glucose; 2.6 g fructose per 100 mL) or 10% (6.7 g glucose; 3.3 g fructose per 100 mL) before and during exercise	60-min continuous cycling at 55–60% VO_2 max	4 incidents of hypoglycemia during exercise under 8% and none under 10%. 60-min post-exercise BG ↓ under 8%, but ↔ under 10%. Authors recommend a 10% carbohydrate solution to avoid hypoglycemia during exercise
West et al. [47]	7 T1DM males	Basal insulin glargine with prandial insulin lispro or aspart	75 g of isomaltulose with a 75% reduced insulin dose, 120, 90, 60, and 30 min pre-exercise	45-min continuous running at 70% VO_2 max	5 out of 7 experienced post-exercise hypoglycemia after 120-min ingestion time. 30-min ingestion time completely prevented hypoglycemia and increased lipid oxidation during exercise

reduce gastric emptying rates in non-T1DM individuals [68–70]. Similarly, Schvarcz et al. [59] demonstrated a slowing of gastric emptying in T1DM individuals when blood glucose concentrations were clamped at 8 compared to 4 mmol·l^{-1}. In addition, gastric emptying rates are also negatively influenced by long-term poor glycemic control [71]. Conversely, low blood glucose concentrations increase gastric emptying rates in non-T1DM individuals [58]. Therefore, blood glucose concentrations and long-term glycemic control may be contributing factors to understanding the large inter-individual variability in blood glucose responses that exist after ingestion of carbohydrate.

None of the above-mentioned research in T1DM individuals employed a pre-exercise insulin reduction. Doing so could result in different carbohydrate requirements. Research is needed to examine the weight of insulin reduction against carbohydrate consumption on post-exercise glycemia.

3.3.4   Carbohydrate Type: The Glycemic Index

The glycemic index (GI) is a method of classifying carbohydrate-containing foods according to blood glucose responses following ingestion [72]. For example, carbohydrates with a high GI, such as white bread, will induce a rapid increase in blood glucose concentrations after ingestion [73]. Conversely, carbohydrates with a low GI, such as peaches, will induce more gradual increases with lower peaks in blood glucose [73].

From a diabetes management perspective, this classification of foodstuffs is useful as patients can include low GI (LGI) carbohydrates in their diet and, in doing so, benefit from greater feelings of satiety [73], improved insulin sensitivity and blood lipid profiles [74], lower daily mean blood glucose concentrations [75], and reduced incidence of hypoglycemia and reductions in HbA$_{1c}$ [76–78]. In one dietary study, consumption of LGI foodstuffs, such as peaches, kidney beans, or brown rice, resulted in continuously monitored glucose concentrations being within a target range of 3.9–9.9 mmol·l^{-1} more of the time than under a high GI (HGI) trial (67% vs. 47%). Furthermore, participants elicited a lower mean blood glucose concentration (LGI 7.6±2.0 vs. HGI 10.1±2.6 mmol·l^{-1}) and required less bolus insulin per 10 g of ingested CHO.

Based on the existing literature in nondiabetic individuals, consumption of LGI carbohydrates increases blood glucose concentration less than equivalent amounts of high glycemic carbohydrate [79, 80]. Additionally, LGI carbohydrates may suppress fat oxidation less during exercise, sparing both endogenous and exogenous carbohydrate use, resulting in better preservation of blood glucose during exercise and in the recovery period [81]. Only recently has research begun to emerge that has examined the metabolic responses to exercise after ingestion of different GI carbohydrates within T1DM in combination with insulin dose reductions. West et al. (Fig. 3.2) compared the alterations in metabolism and fuel oxidation in 8 T1DM individuals after pre-exercise ingestion of 75 g (10% solution) of either LGI

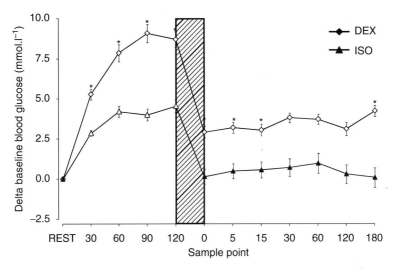

Fig. 3.2 Blood glucose responses to ingestion of high and low glycemic index carbohydrates at rest and during and after 45 min of aerobic running [46]. Hollow symbols indicate significant change from rest with each CHO condition. * indicates significant difference between CHO conditions at this time point (Reprinted with permission of the publisher from West et al. [46], Wolters Kluwer Health)

carbohydrate isomaltulose (ISO, GI = 32) or dextrose (DEX, GI = 96) 2 h before a 45-min treadmill run [46]. Blood glucose increased half as much in the isomaltulose trial compared to dextrose over the rest period ($\Delta + 4.5 \pm 0.4$ vs. $\Delta + 9.1 \pm 0.6$ mmol·l^{-1}, $P < 0.01$) and remained 21% lower for 3-h recovery. Additionally, during the later stages of exercise, there was a lower carbohydrate (ISO 2.85 ± 0.07 vs. DEX 3.18 ± 0.08 g·min^{-1}, $P < 0.05$) and greater lipid (ISO 0.33 ± 0.03 vs. DEX 0.20 ± 0.03 g·min^{-1}, $P < 0.05$) oxidation rate under the isomaltulose trial. Thus, consumption of a low GI carbohydrate improved blood glucose responses and supported continued use of lipid in spite of carbohydrate ingestion.

3.3.5 Pre-exercise Timing of Carbohydrate Consumption and Insulin Administration

The advice regarding timing of pre-exercise carbohydrate consumption and insulin administration is largely dependent upon the insulin type and the altered uptake kinetics that are associated with exercise [11, 19, 82]. Research has demonstrated that exercise can result in greater peaks in insulin as well as increasing absorption rates and ultimately increasing the risk of hypoglycemia [11, 19]. The altered rates of absorption are likely due to a combination of increases in exercise-induced blood flow [83–85] and temperature [86, 87].

Regular human insulin and animal preparations interact differently with exercise. Fernqvist et al. [82] demonstrated that the exercise-induced peak in insulin concentrations was less with regular human insulin as opposed to porcine insulin. Moreover, Tuominen et al. [19] demonstrated that rDNA insulins, human insulin, and the analogue insulin lispro also interact differently with exercise, with consideration of pre-exercise timing particularly important in subsequent insulin and blood glucose responses. Tuominen and colleagues identified that when exercise was performed 40 min after insulin administration, insulin lispro induced an earlier and 56% greater peak in insulin concentrations, resulting in a greater drop in blood glucose with exercise, when compared to regular human insulin. Moreover, when exercising this close to administration, the exercise bout was associated with a 2.2-fold greater risk of hypoglycemia. However, when exercising 3 h after insulin administration, the drop in blood glucose was less under insulin lispro and the risk of hypoglycemia was reduced by 46%, compared to regular human insulin. This research highlights pre-exercise timing as an important factor to consider, as the intense rise and peak in insulin that is elicited soon after administration of rapid-acting insulin, results in marked increases in the risk of hypoglycemia during exercise.

The lower variability and more favorable action-time profiles of the rapid-acting insulins [19, 42] make these analogues of insulin ideal for prandial use and have been shown to improve glycemic control within T1DM individuals, without increasing the risk of hypoglycemia [88]. However, the rapid rise in insulin concentrations (peaking 45–60 min after administration) [89] means that it is currently recommended to avoid administration of rapid-acting insulin within 90–120 min of exercise due to the risk of over-insulinization of the active musculature during exercise [39, 90], as demonstrated by the early work of Tuominen et al. [19]. Thus, at present, it is recommended that insulin dose should be reduced before performing exercise, regardless of the insulin type or time before exercise [2, 15, 18]. However, there is limited literature that examined pre-exercise timing as a factor to consider in subsequent blood glucose responses. Specifically, there are limited data available on the absorption kinetics of the insulin analogues when administered in reduced doses with the carbohydrate meal at different times prior to exercise. Within the study of Tuominen et al. [19], participants administered ~6.3 IU of insulin; however, if employing a heavy insulin reduction, as recommended by Rabasa-Lhoret et al. [18], pre-exercise insulin dose could be as little as ~3 IU. Therefore, there is potential that administering such small doses of insulin closer to exercise may not increase the risk of hypoglycemia. The study of West et al. [47] aimed to examine the influence of alterations in the timing of a 75% reduction in insulin administration and ingestion of a 10% low GI carbohydrate solution on glycemic and fuel oxidation responses prior to endurance running in T1DM individuals. Participants rested for 30 (30MIN), 60 (60MIN), 90 (90MIN), or 120 min (120MIN) before completing 45 min of running at 70% VO_2 peak. Pre-exercise blood glucose concentrations were lower for 30MIN compared with 120MIN ($P<0.05$). Exercising carbohydrate and lipid oxidation rates were lower and greater, respectively, for 30MIN compared with 120MIN ($P<0.05$). The drop in blood glucose during exercise was less for 30MIN (-3.7 ± 0.4 mmol·l^{-1}) compared with 120MIN (-6.4 ± 0.3 mmol·l^{-1}). During the first 60 min of the 3-h recovery, blood glucose concentrations were higher for 30MIN compared with 120MIN ($P<0.05$). In addition, there were no cases of hypoglycemia in 30MIN, one case in 60MIN, two in 90MIN, and five in the

120MIN condition. Therefore, a strategy involving heavy reductions to rapid-acting insulin and use of a low glycemic index carbohydrate administered 30 min before running improves pre- and post-exercise blood glucose responses in type 1 diabetes through subtle alterations in fuel metabolism promoting lipid combustion.

3.3.6 Preparatory Insulin and Carbohydrate Strategies and Exercise Performance

Carbohydrate consumption has the potential to alter endurance exercise performance in T1DM individuals. In a study by Ramires et al. [65] withholding neutral protamine Hagedorn porcine insulin for 12 h prior to exercise followed by administration of 1 g·kg^{-1} BM of dextrose 30 min before cycling at 55–60% VO_2 max to exhaustion resulted in a 12% improvement in cycling performance compared to a carbohydrate-free solution in participants with well-controlled T1DM. Preservation of carbohydrate stores through combustion of endogenous lipid use is conducive to an improvement in endurance capacity. However, although studies have demonstrated the importance of a carbohydrates glycemic index in influencing exercise capacity in nondiabetic individuals by such mechanisms [91], results have been equivocal [92]. Furthermore, scant research has addressed the relationship between carbohydrate type and endurance performance in T1DM individuals. This is surprising since the functional capacity of T1DM individuals is often lower than in matched individuals without diabetes, and, as an example, in the above-mentioned study by Ramires et al. [65], cycling performance to exhaustion was 62% lower (77 ± 6 vs. 125 ± 7 min, $P < 0.05$).

However, it may be inappropriate to employ an endurance "exercise to exhaustion" model to determine functional capacity in T1DM individuals given the risk of progressively lowering blood glucose concentrations to potentially hypoglycemic levels. Alternative exercise models in cycling ergometry advocating completion of an amount of work have been shown to reduce intra-subject variation compared to endurance capacity models [93]. Thus, the use of time or distance trials using a nonmotorized treadmill or cycling-based protocols to retain ecological validity of "real-life" movement patterns under controlled laboratory conditions might facilitate a deeper insight into the metabolic and performance effects of insulin reduction/carbohydrate administration strategies that avoid placing the T1DM individual at risk of hypoglycemia. In one study, seven T1DM individuals consumed isomaltulose or dextrose alongside a 50% reduction in rapid-acting insulin 2 h before an incremental run test followed by a 10-min distance trial where the objective was to cover as much distance as possible. There was a 50% lower peak blood glucose concentration before running after consumption of isomaltulose compared with dextrose. However, running performance was maintained during the high-intensity run performance in T1DM individuals [94]. Thus, consumption of a low GI carbohydrate improved glycemia and maintained run performance similar to that elicited using high GI carbohydrates. Some preliminary findings from our laboratory suggest some carbohydrates may confer a positive impact on exercise performance. We examined the influence of ingestion of a high molecular mass carbohydrate waxy barley starch (WBS; GI=98) on glycemia and endurance performance in T1DM compared with dextrose. WBS carbohydrates have been shown to improve high-intensity exercise performance capacity in individuals without diabetes [95]. In a similar protocol to that employed by Bracken et al. [94], preliminary data from our laboratory demonstrated similar glycemic responses to ingestion of high (WBS) and low (DEX) molecular weight carbohydrates in T1DM individuals; however, distance in the last quarter of a 10-min performance run was significantly greater after ingestion of WBS compared with DEX (WBS 323 ± 21 vs. dextrose 301 ± 20 m, $P=0.001$ [96] (*unpublished data*). Thus, it appears more research is warranted into the functional characteristics of carbohydrates and exercise performance.

3.4 Practical Advice

The principles of rapid-acting insulin reduction and carbohydrate ingestion form an important strategy in the daily glycemic management of those with T1DM wishing to be physically active. A schematic to improve blood glucose responses to exercise that takes into account these and other factors is graphically illustrated in Fig. 3.3. Many of these factors are already supported by the ADA/ACSM or IDF guidelines for those T1DM individuals wishing to exercise safely. It is important to state that there is no one strategy that fits all T1DM individuals and a degree of trial and error (at least initially) is involved to minimize the risk of hypoglycemia before or after beginning regular physical activity. Internet websites like www.runsweet.com or those of diabetes charities support the contributions from physically active or athletic individuals and allow more confidence to refine generic components of strategies to preserve blood glucose concentrations.

The main factors involved in safe participation of T1DM individuals in exercise are comprised of:

3.4.1 *Monitoring of Blood Glucose Before Physical Activity*

Use caution if blood glucose concentrations are >17 mM (300 mg·dL^{-1}) and no ketones are present. However, avoid exercising if blood glucose levels are >14 mM (250 mg·dL^{-1}) and ketosis is present. If glucose levels are <5.5 mM (100 mg·dL^{-1}), carbohydrate ingestion will be required before exercise begins.

3.4.2 *Ingestion of Carbohydrate*

Carbohydrate ingestion is dependent on the pre-exercise blood glucose concentrations and knowledge of the volume and type of exercise. Aim to consume carbohydrates based on a maximum intake of 60 g·h^{-1} of exercise. Low glycemic index carbohydrates

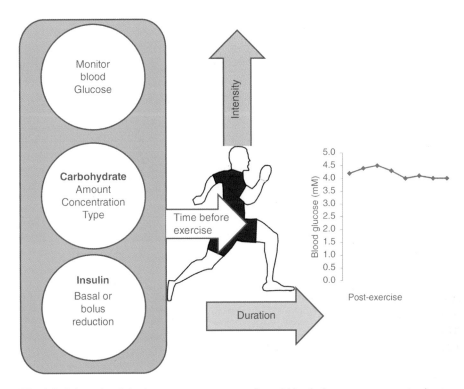

Fig. 3.3 Schematic of the important components of good blood glucose management prior to physical activity

may be recommended before exercise with the aim of stabilizing glucose during and after physical activity. If glucose levels are low, consumption of high GI carbohydrates like dextrose tablets may help restore glucose to euglycemic levels.

3.4.3 Reduction of Rapid-Acting Insulin

Research is available to support the use of rapid-acting insulin reduction with extended exercise sessions. Through trial and error, more knowledge of the exercise type and volume will allow refinement of the exact degree of the rapid-acting insulin reduction in each individual.

3.4.4 Awareness of Time of Insulin Reduction: Carbohydrate Ingestion Before Exercise

Although research suggests not administering insulin 1–2 h before exercise, more recent research suggests reduced rapid-acting insulin dose in conjunction with low

GI carbohydrate consumption allows a shorter period of time before exercise (i.e., 30 min) with better maintenance of post-exercise glycemia.

3.4.5 Knowledge of Exercise Volume and Type

A single sprint has very different metabolic responses to prolonged aerobic exercise. Therefore, knowledge of the athlete's individual responses to these forms of exercise alongside an understanding of the metabolic effects of increased intensity or volume in one specific exercise will aid in combative strategies to counter low blood glucose.

3.4.6 Blood Glucose Monitoring Post-exercise

Low blood glucose has the potential to occur many hours after exercise. Therefore, regular post-exercise monitoring of glucose may prevent late-onset hypoglycemia.

3.5 Future Research

Although it has been shown to be beneficial to reduce pre-exercise rapid-acting insulin and/or consume carbohydrates in response to certain exercise types, much work remains in optimizing these and other factors to safely preserve blood glucose during and after different volumes of one exercise (e.g., aerobic exercise) or specific to different forms of exercise (e.g., sprint or resistance exercise). From an aerobic-endurance exercise point of view, research to examine "fat-burning" strategies to preserve limited carbohydrate stores in an attempt to improve glycemic control and increase performance is an attractive area to pursue. At the other end of the exercise spectrum, more knowledge of the metabolic effects of resistance exercise in T1DM individuals is needed. Continued examination of the metabolic effects of modification of exogenous insulin and/or carbohydrate consumption has two modest but important aims, namely, to improve performances of T1DM individuals in their chosen sport and increase the numbers of those with T1DM safely participating in physical activity.

3.6 Conclusions

Pre-exercise reductions in exogenous insulin and/or carbohydrate consumption improve glycemia and may improve performance during some forms of exercise. However, the exact weighting of the determinants of the insulin reduction – carbohydrate consumption strategy – specific to the type and volume of exercise, remains to be determined. Additionally, due to the complexity of the interrelated components of physical exercise, i.e., duration, intensity, mode, and frequency, the strategy may be specific to the model of exercise employed, e.g., endurance vs. sprint exercise. Nonetheless, the existing research examining manipulation of pre-exercise insulin and carbohydrates offers some suggestions to the physically active T1DM individual, the majority of whom use basal-bolus routines and many of whom have better knowledge of "carbohydrate counting." With continued research, development of exercise-specific strategies with a little trial and error may allow each T1DM individual to safely engage in all forms of physical activity.

References

1. MacDonald MJ. Postexercise late-onset hypoglycaemia in insulin-dependent diabetic patients. Diabetes Care. 1987;10:584–8.
2. Campaigne BN, Wallberg-Henriksson H, Gunnarsson R. Glucose and insulin responses in relation to insulin dose and caloric intake 12 h after acute physical exercise in men with IDDM. Diabetes Care. 1987;10:716–21.
3. Tsalikian E, Maurus N, Beck RW, Janz KF, Chase HP, et al. Impact of exercise on overnight glycemic control in children with type 1 diabetes mellitus. J Paediatr. 2005;147:528–34.
4. Bussau VA, Ferreira LD, Jones TW, Fournier PA. The 10-s maximal sprint: a novel approach to counter an exercise-mediated fall in glycemia in individuals with type 1 diabetes. Diabetes Care. 2006;29:601–6.
5. Guelfi KJ, Jones TW, Fournier PA. Intermittent high-intensity exercise does not increase the risk of early post-exercise hypoglycaemia in individuals with type 1 diabetes. Diabetes Care. 2005;28(2):416–8.
6. Guelfi KJ, Jones TW, Fournier PA. The decline in blood glucose levels is less with intermittent high-intensity compared with moderate exercise in individuals with type 1 diabetes. Diabetes Care. 2005;28(6):1289–94.
7. Iscoe KR, Riddell MC. Continuous moderate-intensity exercise with or without intermittent high-intensity work: effects on acute and late glycaemia in athletes with type 1 diabetes mellitus. Diabet Med. 2011;28(7):824–32.
8. Bussau VA, Ferreira LD, Jones TW, Fournier PA. A 10-s sprint performed prior to moderate-intensity exercise prevents early post-exercise fall in glycaemia in individuals with type 1 diabetes. Diabetologia. 2007;50(9):1815–8.
9. Maran A, Pavan P, Bonsembiante B, Brugin E, Ermolao A, Avogaro A, Zaccaria M. Continuous glucose monitoring reveals delayed nocturnal hypoglycaemia after intermittent high-intensity exercise in nontrained patients with type 1 diabetes. Diabetes Technol Ther. 2010. doi:10.1089/dia.2010.0038.
10. Chokkalingam K, Tsintzas K, Norton L, Jewell K, Macdonald IA, Mansell PI. Exercise under hyperinsulinaemic conditions increases whole-body glucose disposal without affecting muscle glycogen utilisation in type 1 diabetes. Diabetologia. 2007;50:414–21.
11. Dandona P, Hooke D, Bell J. Exercise and insulin absorption from subcutaneous injection site. Br Med J. 1980;280:479–80.
12. Dubé MC, Weisnagel J, Homme DP, Lavoie C. Exercise and newer insulins: how much glucose supplement to avoid hypoglycemia. Med Sci Sports Exerc. 2005;37:1276–82.
13. Hernandez JM, Moccia T, Fluckey JD, Ulbrecht JS, Farrell PA. Fluid snacks to help persons with type 1 diabetes avoid late onset post-exercise hypoglycemia. Med Sci Sports Exerc. 2000;32:904–10.

14. Jenni S, Oetliker S, Allemann M. Fuel metabolism during exercise in euglycaemia and hyperglycaemia in patients with type 1 diabetes mellitus – a prospective single-blinded randomised crossover trial. Diabetologia. 2008;51:1457–65.

15. Mauvais-Jarvis F, Sobngwi E, Porcher R, Garnier JP, Vexiau P, Duvallet A, Gautier JF. Glucose response to intense aerobic exercise in type 1 diabetes. Diabetes Care. 2003;26:1316–7.

16. Perrone C, Laitano O, Mayer F. Effect of carbohydrate ingestion on the glycemic response to type 1 diabetic adolescents during exercise. Diabetes Care. 2005;28:2537–8.

17. Peter R, Luzio SD, Dunseath G, Miles A, Hare B, Backx K, Pauvaday V, Owens DR. Effects of exercise on the absorption of insulin glargine in patients with type 1 diabetes. Diabetes Care. 2005;28:560–5.

18. Rabasa-Lhoret R, Bourque J, Ducros F, Chiasson J. Guidelines for premeal insulin dose reduction for postprandial exercise of different intensities and durations in type 1 diabetic subjects treated intensively with a basal-bolus insulin regimen (ultralente-lispro). Diabetes Care. 2001;24:625–30.

19. Tuominen JA, Karonen SL, Melamies L, Bolli G, Koivisto VA. Exercise-induced hypoglycaemia in IDDM patients treated with a short-acting insulin analogue. Diabetologia. 1995; 38:106–11.

20. Asp S, Daugaard JR, Richter EA. Eccentric exercise decreases glucose transporter GLUT4 protein in human skeletal muscle. J Physiol. 1995;482:705–12.

21. Asp S, Daugaard JR, Kristiansen S, Kiens B, Richter EA. Eccentric exercise decreases maximal insulin action in humans. J Physiol. 1996;494:891–8.

22. Wenger HW, Bell GJ. The interactions of intensity, frequency and duration of exercise training in alerting cardiorespiratory fitness. Sports Med. 1986;3:345–56.

23. Tabata I, Nishimura K, Kouzaki M, Hirai Y, Ogita F, Miyachi M, Yamamoto K. Effects of moderate-intensity endurance and high-intensity intermittent training on anaerobic capacity and VO₂max. Med Sci Sports Exerc. 1996;28:1327–30.

24. Sigal RJ, Kenny GP, Boule NG, Wells GA, Prudhomme D, Fortier M, Reid RD, Tulloch H, Coyle D, Phillips P, Jennings A, Faffey J. Effects of aerobic training, resistance training, or both on glycemic control in type 2 diabetes: a randomized trial. Ann Intern Med. 2007; 147:357–69.

25. Jorge ML, de Oliveira VN, Resende NM, Paraiso LF, Calixto A, Diniz AL, Resende ES, Ropelle ER, Carvalheira JB, Espindola FS, Jorge PT, Geloneze B. The effects of aerobic, resistance, and combined exercise on metabolic control, inflammatroy markers, adipocytokines, and muscle insulin signalling in patients with type 2 diabetes mellitus. Metabolism. 2011;60(9):1244–52. doi:10.1016/j.metabol.2011.01.006.

26. Durak EP, Jovanovic-Peterson L, Peterson CM. Randomized crossover study of effect of resistance training on glycemic control, muscular strength, and cholesterol in type 1 diabetic men. Diabetes Care. 1990;13:1039–43.

27. Ramalho AC, de Lourdes Lima M, Nunes F, Cambuí Z, Barbosa C, Andrade A, Viana A, Martins M, Abrantes V, Aragão C, Temístocles M. The effect of resistance versus aerobic training on metabolic control in patients with type-1 diabetes mellitus. Diabetes Res Clin Pract. 2006;72:271–6.

28. Jiminez C, Santiago M, Sitler M, Boden G, Homko C. Insulin-sensitivity responses to a single bout of resistive exercise in type 1 diabetes mellitus. J Sport Rehabil. 2009;18:564–71.

29. Essen-Gustavsson B, Tesch PA. Glycogen and triglyceride utilization in relation to muscle metabolic characteristics in men performing heavy-resistance exercise. Eur J Appl Physiol Occup Physiol. 1990;61:5–10.

30. Robergs RA, Pearson DR, Costill DL, Pascoe DD, Benedict MA, Lambert CP, Zachwieja JJ. Muscle glycogenolysis during differing intensities of weight-resistance exercise. J Appl Physiol. 1991;70:1700–6.

31. Tesch PA, Ploutz-Snyder LL, Ystrom L, Castro MJ, Dudley GA. Skeletal muscle glycogen loss evoked by resistance exercise. J Strength Cond Res. 1998;12:67–73.

32. Bogardus C, Thuillez P, Ravussin E, Vasquez B, Narimiga M, Azhar S. Effect of muscle glycogen depletion in vivo in insulin action in man. J Clin Invest. 1983;72:1605–10.

33. Munger R, Temler E, Jallut D, Haesler E, Felber JP. Correlations of glycogen synthase and phosphorylase activities with glycogen concentration in human musclebiopsies. Evidence for a double-feedback mechanism regulating glycogen synthesis and breakdown. Metabolism. 1993;42:36–43.
34. Zachwieja JJ, Costill DL, Beard GC, Robergs RA, Pascoe DD, Anderson DE. The effects of a carbonated carbohydrate drink on gastric emptying gastro-intestinal distress, and exercise performance. Int J Sports Nutr. 1992;2:229–38.
35. Fry AC, Kraemer WJ, Stone MH, Warren BJ, Fleck SJ, Kearney JT, Gordon SE. Endocrine responses to overreaching before and after 1 year of weightlifting. Can J Appl Physiol. 1994;19:400–10.
36. French DN, Kraemer WJ, Volek JS, Spiering BA, Judelson DA, Hoffman JR, Maresh CM. Anticipatory responses of catecholamines on muscle force production. J Appl Physiol. 2007;102(1):94–102.
37. Matsuse H, Nago T, Takano Y, Shiba N. Plasma growth hormone is elevated immediately after resistance exercise with electrical stimulation and voluntary muscle contraction. Tohoku J Exp Med. 2010;222:69–75.
38. Leite RD, Prestes J, Rosa C, De Salles BF, Major A, Miranda H, Simao R. Acute effect of resistance training volume on hormonal responses in trained men. J Sports Med Phys Fitness. 2011;51:322–8.
39. De Feo P, Di Loreto C, Ranchelli A, Fatone C, Gam-belunghe G, Lucidi P, Santeusanio F. Exercise and diabetes. Acta Biomedica. 2006;77:14–7.
40. Grimm JJ. Exercise in type 1 diabetes. In: Nagi D, editor. Exercise and sport in diabetes. Hoboken: Wiley; 2005. p. 25–43.
41. Iafusco D. Diet and physical activity in patients with type 1 diabetes. Acta Biomedica. 2006;77:41–6.
42. Brange J, Vølund A. Insulin analogs with improved pharmacokinetic profiles. Adv Drug Deliv Rev. 1999;35:307–35.
43. Leopore M, Pampanelli S, Fanelli C, Porcellatim F, Bartocci L, Di Vincenzo A. Pharmacokinetics and pharmacodynamics of subcutaneous injection of long-acting human insulin analogue glargine, NPH insulin, and ultralente human insulin and continuous subcutaneous infusion of insulin lispro. Diabetes. 2000;49:2142–8.
44. Bracken RM, West D, Stephens JW, Kilduff L, Luzio S, Bain SC. Impact of pre-exercise rapid-acting insulin reductions on ketogenesis following running in type 1 diabetes. Diabet Med. 2011;28(2):218–22.
45. West DJ, Morton RD, Bain SC, Stephens JW, Bracken RM. Blood glucose responses to reductions in pre-exercise rapid-acting insulin for 24 h after running in individuals with type 1 diabetes. J Sports Sci. 2010;28(7):781–8.
46. West DJ, Morton RD, Stephens JW, Bain SC, Kilduff LP, Luzio S, Still R, Bracken RM. Isomaltulose improves post-exercise glycemia by reducing CHO oxidation in T1DM. Med Sci Sports Exerc. 2011;43(2):204–10.
47. West DJ, Stephens JW, Bain SC, Kilduff LP, Luzio S, Still R, Bracken RM. A combined insulin reduction and carbohydrate feeding strategy 30 min before running best preserves blood glucose concentration after exercise through improved fuel oxidation in type 1 diabetes mellitus. J Sports Sci. 2011;29(3):279–89.
48. Arutchelvam V, Heise T, Dellweg S, Elbroend B, Minns I, Home PD. Plasma glucose and hypoglycaemia following exercise in people with type 1 diabetes: a comparison of three basal insulins. Diabet Med. 2009;26(10):1027–32.
49. Koivisto VA, Felig P. Alterations in insulin absorption and in blood glucose control associated with varying insulin injection sites in diabetic patients. Ann Intern Med. 1980;92(1):59–61.
50. Cryer PE. The prevention and correction of hypoglycaemia. In: Jefferson LS, Cherrington AD, editors. The endocrine pancreas and regulation of metabolism. New York: Oxford University Press; 2001. p. 45–56.
51. Laffel L. Ketone bodies: a review of physiology, pathophysiology and application of monitoring to diabetes. Diabetes Metab Res Rev. 1999;15:412–26.

52. Wallace TM, Matthews DR. Recent advances in the monitoring and management of diabetic ketoacidosis. Q J Med. 2004;97:773–80.
53. Jain SK, McVie R, Jaramillo JJ, Chen Y. Hyperketonemia (acetoacetate) increases oxidizability of LDL + VLDL in type-1 diabetic patients. Free Radic Biol Med. 1998;24:175–81.
54. Jain SK, McVie R. Hyperketonemia can increase lipid peroxidation and lower glutathione levels in human erythrocytes in vitro and in type 1 diabetic patients. Diabetes. 1999;48:1850–5.
55. Jain SK, McVie R, Jackson R, Levine SN, Lim G. Effect of hyperketonemia on plasma lipid peroxidation levels in diabetic patients. Diabetes Care. 1999;22:1171–5.
56. Køeslag JH, Noakes TD, Sloan AW. Post-exercise ketosis. J Physiol (Lond). 1980;301: 79–90.
57. Leiper JB, Aulin KP, Söderlund K. Improved gastric emptying rate in humans of a unique glucose polymer with gel-forming properties. Scand J Gastroenterol. 2000;35(11):1143–9.
58. Schvarcz E, Palmer M, Aman J, Lindkvist B, Beckman KW. Hypoglycaemia increases the gastric emptying rate in patients with type 1 diabetes mellitus. Diabet Med. 1993;10:660–3.
59. Schvarcz E, Palmer M, Aman J, Horowitz M, Stridsberg M, Berne C. Physiological hyperglycaemia slows gastric emptying in normal subjects and patients with insulin-dependent diabetes mellitus. Gastroenterology. 1997;113:60–6.
60. Lina BAR, Jonker D, Kozianowski G. Isomaltulose (Palatinose®): a review of biological and toxicological studies. Food Chem Toxicol. 2002;40:1375–81.
61. Jeukendrup AE, Jentjens RL. Oxidation of carbohydrate feedings during prolonged exercise: current thoughts, guidelines and directions for future research. Sports Med. 2000;29(6):407–24.
62. Steppel JH, Horton ES. Exercise in the management of type 1 diabetes mellitus. Rev Endocr Metab Disord. 2003;4:355–60.
63. Diabetes mellitus and exercise. American Diabetes Association. Diabetes Care. 1997;20(12): 1908–12.
64. Gallen I. Exercise in type 1 diabetes. Diabet Med. 2003;20:1–17.
65. Ramires PR, Forjaz CL, Strunz CM, Silva ME, Diament J, Nicolau W, Liberman B, Negrão CE. Oral glucose ingestion increases endurance capacity in normal and diabetic (type I) humans. J Appl Physiol. 1997;83(2):608–14.
66. Riddell MC, Iscoe K. Physical activity, sport and pediatric diabetes. Pediatr Diabetes. 2006;7(1):60–70.
67. Gallen I. The management of insulin treated diabetes and sport. Pract Diab Int. 2005; 22:307–12.
68. Davis JM, Burgess WA, Slentz CA, Bartoli WP. Fluid availability and sports drinks differing in carbohydrate type and concentration. Am J Clin Nutr. 1990;51:1054–7.
69. Maughan RJ, Leiper JB. Limitations to fluid replacement during exercise. Can J Appl Physiol. 1999;24:173–87.
70. Murray R, Bartoli WP, Eddy DE, Horn MK. Gastric emptying and plasma deuterium accumulation following ingestion of water and two carbohydrate-electrolyte beverages. Int J Sports Nutr. 1997;7:144–53.
71. Jing M, Rayner CK, Jones KL, Horowitz M. Diabetic gastroparesis: diagnosis and management. Drugs. 2009;69:971–86.
72. Wolever TM, Jenkins DJ, Jenkins AL, Josse RG. The glycemic index: methodology and clinical implications. Am Soc Clin Nutr. 1991;54:846–54.
73. Foster-Powell K, Holt SHA, Brand-Miller JC. International table of glycaemic index and glycemic load values. Am J Clin Nutr. 2002;76:5–56.
74. Jenkins DJ, Wolever TM, Kalmusky J, Giudici S, Giordano C, Wong GS, Bird JN, Patten R, Hall M, Buckley G. Low glycemic index carbohydrate foods in the management of hyperlipidemia. Am J Clin Nutr. 1985;42:604–17.
75. Nansel TR, Gellar L, McGill A. Effect of varying glycemic index meals on blood glucose control assessed with continuous glucose monitoring in youth with type 1 diabetes on basal-bolus insulin regimens. Diabetes Care. 2008;31:695–7.

76. Brand JC, Colagiuri S, Crossman S, Allen A, Truswell AS. Low glycaemic index carbohydrate foods improve glucose control in non-insulin dependent diabetes mellitus (NIDDM). Diabetes Care. 1991;14:95–101.
77. Gilbertson HR, Brand-Miller JC, Thorburn AW, Evans S, Chondros P, Wether GA. The effect of flexible low glycemic index dietary advice versus measured carbohydrate diets on glycemic control in children with type 1 diabetes. Diabetes Care. 2001;34:1137–43.
78. Thomas DE, Elliott EJ, Baur L. Low glycemic index or low glycemic load diets for overweight and obesity. Cochrane Database Syst Rev. 2007;18:1–38.
79. DeMarco H, Sucher KP, Cisar CJ, Butterfield GE. Pre-exercise carbohydrate meals: application of glycemic index. Med Sci Sports Exerc. 1999;31:164–70.
80. Achten J, Jentjens RL, Brouns F, Jeukendrup AE. Exogenous oxidation of isomaltulose is lower than that of sucrose during exercise in men. J Nutr. 2007;137:1143–8.
81. Stevenson EJ, Williams C, Mash LE, Phillips B, Nute ML. Influence of high-carbohydrate mixed meals with different glycemic indexes on substrate utilisation during subsequent exercise in women. Am J Clin Nutr. 2006;84:354–60.
82. Fernqvist E, Linde B, Ostman J, Gunnarsson R. Effects of physical exercise on insulin absorption in insulin-dependent diabetics. A comparison between human and porcine insulin. Clin Physiol. 1986;6:489–97.
83. Lauritzen T, Binder C, Faber OK. Importance of insulin absorption, subcutaneous blood flow, and residual beta-cell function in insulin therapy. Acta Paediatr Scand. 1980;283:81–5.
84. Linde B, Gunnarsson R. Influence of aprotinin on insulin absorption and subcutaneous blood flow in type 1 (insulin-dependent) diabetes. Diabetologia. 1985;28:645–8.
85. Vora JP, Burch A, Peters JR, Owens DR. Absorption of radiolabelled soluble insulin in type 1 (insulin dependent) diabetes: influence of subcutaneous blood flow and anthropometry. Diabet Med. 1993;10:736–43.
86. Koivisto VA. Sauna-induced acceleration in insulin absorption from subcutaneous injection site. Br Med J. 1980;280:1411–3.
87. Koivisto VA, Fortney S, Hendler R, Felig P. A rise in ambient temperature augments insulin absorption in diabetic patients. Metabolism. 1981;30:402–5.
88. Tamás GY, Marre M, Astorga R, Dedov I, Jacobsen J, Lindholm A. Glycaemic control in type 1 diabetic patients using optimised insulin aspart or human insulin in a randomised multinational study. Diabetes Res Clin Pract. 2001;54:105–14.
89. Plank J, Wutte A, Brunner G, Siebenhofer A, Semlitsch B, Sommer R, Hirschberger S, Pieber T. A direct comparison of insulin aspart and insulin lispro in patients with type 1 diabetes. Diabetes Care. 2002;25:2053–7.
90. Perry E, Gallen IW. Guidelines on the current best practice for the management of type 1 diabetes, sport and exercise. Pract Diab Int. 2009;26:116–23.
91. Moore LJ, Midgley AW, Thomas G, Thurlow S, McNaughton LR. The effects of low- and high-glycemic index meals on time trial performance. Int J Sports Physiol Perform. 2009;4(3):331–44.
92. Wong SH, Chen YJ, Fung WM, Morris JG. Effect of glycemic index meals on recovery and subsequent endurance capacity. Int J Sports Med. 2009;30(12):898–905.
93. Jeukendrup A, Saris WH, Brouns F, Kester AD. A new validated endurance performance test. Med Sci Sports Exerc. 1996;28(2):266–70.
94. Bracken RM, Page R, Gray B, Kilduff LP, West DJ, Stephens JW, Bain SC. Isomaltulose improves glycaemia and maintains run performance in type 1 diabetes. Med Sci Sports Exerc. 2011; [Epub ahead of print] doi: 10.1249/MSS.0b013e31823f6557.
95. Stephens FB, Roig M, Armstrong G, Greenhaff PL. Post-exercise ingestion of a unique, high molecular weight glucose polymer solution improves performance during a subsequent bout of cycling exercise. J Sports Sci. 2008;26(2):149–54.
96. Bracken RM, Page R, Gray B, West D, Kilduff L, Stephens JW, Bain SC. Waxy barley starch improves high intensity run performance in type 1 diabetes. 2012. Paper in preparation.

Chapter 4
Physical Activity in Childhood Diabetes

Krystyna A. Matyka and S. Francesca Annan

4.1 Introduction

Physical activity is an important part of childhood. It is important for normal childhood development, to maintain healthy bones and body composition, and is useful in developing and maintaining social contacts. Physical activity is no less important for children and young people with diabetes. It is actively encouraged but presents significant challenges for diabetes management for the child, family, and the diabetes team. Physical activity can lead to fluctuations in blood glucose levels that can be difficult to manage or to avoid. In this chapter, we will provide some background to the developmental aspects of physical activity in children and young people and suggest some strategies for managing type I diabetes during periods of physical activity.

4.2 Definitions

Physical activity is defined as any force exerted by skeletal muscle that results in energy expenditure above resting level. Exercise is defined as a subset of physical activity that is volitional, planned, structured, repetitive, and aimed at improvement or maintenance of any aspect of fitness or health. Sport is a subset of physical

K.A. Matyka, M.B.B.S., M.D., M.R.C.P.C.H. (✉)
Division of Metabolic and Vascular Health, Warwick Medical School,
Clinical Sciences Research Laboratories, University Hospital,
Clifford Bridge Road, Coventry CV2 2DX, UK
e-mail: k.a.matyka@warwick.ac.uk

S.F. Annan, B.Sc. (Hons), PGCert
Department of Nutrition and Dietetics, Alder Hey Children's NHS Foundation Trust,
Eaton Road, West Derby, Liverpool, Merseyside L12 2AP, UK
e-mail: francesca.annan@nhs.net

I. Gallen (ed.), *Type 1 Diabetes*,
DOI 10.1007/978-0-85729-754-9_4, © Springer-Verlag London Limited 2012

activity that involves structured competitive situations governed by rules. Physical fitness is a set of attributes that people have or achieve that relates to the ability to perform physical activity [1].

4.3 Developmental Changes and Physical Activity

There are quite marked variations in patterns of physical activity throughout childhood as a result of childhood development. These changes will be a reflection of the dramatic changes in stature, body composition, and neuromuscular development that occur. There will be improvements in strength and coordination and hence physical ability, and these will change constantly throughout childhood and into young adult life [1]. Changes in cognitive ability of children will allow them to participate in more structured and organized events involving either exercise or sporting activities. There are also significant differences between boys and girls throughout the period of development, with boys being more active than girls even in the early years.

This period of development will depend not only on the physical attributes of the child but also on the opportunities provided both within the environment and also by adult carers: data suggest that children are more likely to be active if their parents are active and encourage physical activity [2]. It is beyond the scope of this chapter to go into the developmental changes which will influence physical activity in childhood in any detail. However, there are changes in muscle strength, pulmonary function, cardiovascular function, and aerobic fitness throughout childhood and into early adult life [1]. Some of these changes occur as a result of developmental changes in stature and body composition: it is well described that boys will develop more muscle mass going through puberty and girls will predominantly accrue more fat mass [1]. Yet some of these changes will also be mediated by physical activity itself which will influence body composition. Thus, some of the differences between children of similar age and developmental stage may be explained by their access to opportunities to be physically active [3].

Infants less than 1 year of age will be doing little in the form of vigorous movement as they are yet to develop the necessary skills to be active with any degree of confidence. This changes quickly over the first few years of life as the young child learns to crawl, shuffle, walk, run, climb stairs, and so on. As the skills increase, the intensity of the activity is likely to increase along with the complexity. Preschool children are likely to be active through play involving a mixture of activity and social interaction [4]. Primary school children will start to participate in more structured activity, or exercise, within PE lessons, although it is likely that they will participate in unstructured activity in the playground at break times. Once young people go to secondary school, the nature of physical activity may change again and become more structured and potentially become restricted to organized events or sports.

Data suggest that along with these changes in type of activity, there are also changes in the amount of physical activity that is performed. It is well described that activity levels decrease as children get older and become adolescents [5]. The reasons for this are likely to be multifactorial and include both physiological (rapid growth and pubertal changes) as well as environmental and societal factors. The increased emphasis on academic achievement is likely to be a significant barrier to regular physical activity for a number of teenage pupils. As already mentioned, data also highlight gender differences throughout the life course with girls performing significantly less physical activity than boys. Again, the reason for this is likely to be complex. It is plausible that there are physiological factors which mediate the decrease in physical activity which is particularly pronounced in teenage girls. However, it is also well described that boys use physical activity as a method of socializing with their peer group, while girls are more likely to have other methods for social interactions which do not include physical activity [6].

These developmental changes will have significant implications to the management of diabetes in children of different ages. Physical activity improves physical fitness which in turn improves insulin sensitivity: those children who are most physically active are likely to need lower doses of insulin compared to those who are more sedentary [7]. Assessing both the quantity and intensity of physical activity performed by children and young people with diabetes is likely to be as important as assessing nutritional intake; yet in the clinical setting, it is a hugely challenging exercise.

4.4 Assessing Physical Activity in Childhood

There are significant difficulties in the accurate, objective measurement or assessment of physical activity particularly in childhood. There are a number of different methods of assessment ranging from questionnaires to more objective measures involving monitoring of movement or heart rate [8, 9]. Questionnaires create the greatest concern. Data can be recorded either prospectively or retrospectively, and both methods have significant flaws. Retrospective data collection may be imprecise and challenging with children who lack the cognitive ability to accurately recall details of activity patterns and report them without bias [10]. Studies suggest that children younger than 9 years old will have problems reliably reporting physical activity patterns [11]. On the other hand, prospective data collection is labor intensive as it requires detailed documentation of all physical activity performed in predefined time blocks sometimes as short as 15 min. Again, this can be very difficult for young children but is also a challenge for older children and young people who will easily tire of the intensity of this procedure [10]. Questionnaires are often used as part of research studies where large number of subjects are to be studied; yet they are likely to have significant limitations within a clinical context [8, 9].

More objective measures of assessing physical activity using either heart rate or activity monitors are likely to provide better quality data with respect to the amount of activity performed [8, 9]. However, they do not provide information on the type of activity performed. Activity monitors can measure either heart rate or physical activity or a combination of the two. Measurement of heart rate only has limitations in that a number of other physiological variables can lead to an increase in heart rate other than physical activity. For example, stress, excitement, or an increased temperature can all lead to an increase in heart rate. On the other hand, measurement of activity with a movement sensor such as an accelerometer also causes problems particularly with movement artifacts, leading to erroneously high levels of activity. In addition, some types of physical activity are not captured very well with an accelerometer worn on the waistband; activities such as cycling are examples of this. Many activity monitors are also not waterproof, and so water-based activities are not included as part of the assessment. More recent activity monitors provide a combination of both heart rate measurement and accelerometry and are thought to be a more robust assessment of patterns of physical activity in both children and adults [12]. Using standardized metabolic equations, many of these monitors can provide estimates of energy expenditure, although some of the physiological assumptions used in these calculations have not been validated in studies of children [13]. Many of these monitors are reasonably expensive; so their use in large community-based studies can be unfeasible. Familiarity with their use is necessary if they are to be valuable within a clinical setting.

A combination of an objective measurement of physical activity using an activity monitor in combination with an activity diary is likely to provide the best information with respect to both type and frequency of physical activity [8, 9]. Most countries will have national recommendations for levels of physical activity in children and young people. It does appear that the majority of these recommendations suggest at least 60 min of moderate to vigorous physical activity (activity which leads to an increase in heart rate or feelings of sweatiness) per day [14].

4.5   Patterns of Physical Activity in Children with Diabetes

A number of studies have been performed to examine patterns of physical activity in children with diabetes [15–19]. These studies on the whole have used questionnaires to collect data on levels of activity. The results from these studies have been rather variable with studies suggesting both increased and decreased levels of activity when compared to children who are otherwise healthy. A study in 2010 from North America has examined physical activity and electronic media use in young people with both type I and type II diabetes [15]. The study examined compliance with the physical activity recommendations for children and young people which was either 30 min per day of vigorous physical activity or 60 min per day of moderate to vigorous physical activity for adolescents. The study found that 81% of adolescents with type I diabetes met these target criteria compared to 80% of healthy controls. Only 68% of adolescents with type II diabetes met these national guidelines [15]. Another study from Italy examined computer use, free time activities, and metabolic control in 115 patients aged 10–35 years [16]. The authors found that in the group as a whole, the mean time spent playing sports was 2 ½ h per week, with a range from 0 to 8 h. Twenty five subjects, i.e., 29%, did not practice any kind of physical activity at all [16]. A much larger study from Norway evaluated physical activity patterns of 723 children with type I diabetes aged from 6 to 19 years using a questionnaire that could estimate total amount of time spent on inactivity and light, moderate, and vigorous activity [17]. The study found that 54% of the participants did not fulfill the international recommendations of 60 min of moderate to vigorous activity per day. Not surprisingly, girls were less active than boys in childhood and in adolescents. Worryingly, 43% of the participants watched TV for more than 2 h a day: TV viewing was found to be related to overweight in children and adolescents with type I diabetes. The study found no statistical differences in physical activity between the different intensified insulin regimens, and pump patients were not less active than other patients with diabetes [17]. A study of heart rate monitoring in 127 children with diabetes and 200 controls in France showed that schoolchildren with diabetes were significantly more active than healthy peers when considering moderate activity [18]. In addition, teenagers with diabetes were also significantly more active when considering moderate and vigorous activity. Furthermore, there was a negative correlation between the most recent glycated hemoglobin and the time spent in light activities in schoolchildren [18]. Another study from Sweden of 26 adolescent girls with type I diabetes and 49 controls using accelerometers showed that there was a tendency toward a lower total amount of physical activity in the diabetes group, but the difference between the study groups did not reach statistical significance [19].

4.6 Beneficial Effects of Physical Activity

4.6.1 Well-being

In the nondiabetic population, there is now fairly strong evidence of a positive association between physical activity and psychological well-being. A Cochrane review from 2004 found that physical activity is associated with reduction in depression, anxiety, and stress and with increased self-esteem, although it was felt there were few data available on which to make this assumption [20]. Physical activity is encouraged in the majority of patients with chronic illnesses who are able to be physically active in a safe and pain-free manner.

There are a number of reasons why physical activity may be important for psychological well-being in patients with type I diabetes. The incidence of depression is significantly higher in patients with diabetes than in the healthy population: children with type I diabetes have a two- to threefold increased incidence of depression compared to healthy controls [21].

There have been few studies which have specifically examined psychological well-being and physical activity in children with type I diabetes. A study by Edmunds at al from the United Kingdom studied 36 participants aged between 9 and 15 years with a mean duration of type I diabetes of almost 6 years [22]. The participants filled in a number of questionnaires including the Quality of Life for

Youths questionnaire, the Self-Efficacy for Diabetes scale, and the Physical Self-Perception Profile for Children. Physical activity was assessed using heart rate monitoring for 2 weeks and 2 weekend days. This small study found that 16 (47%) of children participated in at least 60 min per day of moderate to vigorous physical activity. Twenty-six (76%) engaged in at least 30 min of moderate to vigorous physical activity per day. Again, boys reported higher levels of both moderate to vigorous physical activity and vigorous physical activity compared to girls. Boys reported higher self-esteem than females, but self-efficacy with respect to diabetes management was higher in females than males. Self-reported quality of life was above the median value for this scale, and males reported better quality of life than females in all subscales. Correlation analysis revealed no significant associations between moderate to vigorous physical activity and self-esteem, self-efficacy, quality of life, or glycemic control [22]. The authors concluded that the role of physical activity as part of disease management may reduce the extent to which physical activity is seen as fun. They also felt that there might be a significant element of worry involved that blood glucose levels will be affected by physical activity both in the short term and later on that night which would impact on the psychological benefits of physical activity [22]. Emotional concerns have also been described by parents who have been asked about their experiences of learning to cope with a diagnosis of diabetes in one of their offspring. Feelings of sadness and guilt resurfaced at times when their child's diabetes is brought to the forefront: for example, at times of physical activity when a child may have to stop playing a sport because they start to feel low [23]. Studies have shown that parental support is essential to promote physical activity in healthy populations of children [2]. Studies of families of children with diabetes have shown that parental conflict around physical activity was related to decreased activity in children with type I diabetes. The authors suggested that nagging and criticism as well as arguing about physical activity make a child less likely to engage [24]. However, other parents report the importance of fostering normality by allowing their children to be physically active with other children [25]. In this study, parents reported that they did what they had to do so that their child with diabetes could do anything they wanted to do. Planning and vigilance was especially evident for parents of children with diabetes, reflecting the difficult negotiations necessary to maintain good blood glucose control around periods of activity [25]. Schools also play an important role in encouraging children to be active. In a qualitative study of how children with chronic disease and their parents manage physical activity, one child with asthma reported "one of the PE teachers used to treat me as if I was about to die, that's so annoying!" [25].

In a report from the Hvidoere Study Group on childhood diabetes, a large group of just over 2,000 adolescents with an average age of 14 ½ years were asked to complete three questionnaires: the Diabetes Quality of Life – Short Form, questions on psychological well-being and health perception from the Health Behaviour in School Children WHO project (HBSC), and five questions on physical activity and sedentary lifestyle from the HBSC survey 2001 [26]. Questions on physical activity focused on the number of days during the last week being moderately physically active for more than 60 min per day. The average HbA1c of the whole sample was $8.2 \pm 1.4\%$. Boys reported not only being more physically active but also doing less school homework and spending more time on the computer than girls. Older respondents were less physically active but did more school homework and spent more time on the computer. Physical activity was also positively correlated with nearly all markers of psychological health with more activity associated with greater well-being, fewer symptoms, less worry, greater perception of health, and general quality of life [26].

4.6.2   Cardiovascular Benefits

Regular physical activity which leads to improvement in physical fitness has significant cardiovascular and metabolic benefits in both children and adults [27]. Type I diabetes is associated with a significantly increased risk of cardiovascular disease, and so physical activity is important to this group of patients [28]. There have been few studies examining cardiovascular risk factors with respect to physical activity in children with type I diabetes.

Reduced heart rate variability is an independent predictor of heart disease and risk of heart disease in healthy populations of adults [29, 30].

Heart rate variability in 93 children with type I diabetes aged 8–12 years was compared to 107 matched healthy control children [31]. Level of physical activity was assessed using a questionnaire which could divide activity levels into low, moderate, or high. This study showed that children with type I diabetes who had low levels of activity had significantly lower heart rate variability at rest when compared to healthy controls [31]. Aerobic fitness has also been examined in some studies. One study has examined physical activity levels using an accelerometer and cardiorespiratory fitness by a treadmill test in children with three different chronic diseases and compared them to healthy controls [32]. Forty-five obese children, 31 children with juvenile idiopathic arthritis, 48 children with type I diabetes, and 85 healthy children took part in the study. This study showed that 60% of healthy controls met the recommended daily 60 min of moderate to vigorous physical activity, but only 39% of children with type I diabetes met these criteria. In the group as a whole, lower cardiorespiratory fitness was associated with female gender and low daily physical activity. This study did not find any significant differences in cardiorespiratory fitness in children with diabetes [32]. Other studies confirm these findings: using an incremental exercise test on a bicycle ergometer in late pubertal adolescent girls with diabetes, there were no differences in aerobic power compared to healthy siblings [33]. In another study, significant differences in aerobic capacity were found between in people with type I diabetes and healthy controls [34]. The study also used an incremental treadmill test and found that subjects with type I diabetes had lower maximal heart rates and lower time to exhaustion compared to healthy controls; however, there was a wide variation in the age range (and probably pubertal status) of both cohorts, and it is difficult to assess the robustness of the data [34].

The beneficial effects of physical activity on cardiovascular risk profiles have been examined in young people with diabetes. A multicenter study of over

23,000 patients attending 209 centers in Germany and Austria examined lipid profiles, blood pressure, glycated hemoglobin, and body mass index and compared them to levels of physical activity, as assessed by questionnaire [35]. The group was divided into 10,392 patients who performed no physical activity outside of school per week, 8,607 who performed 1–2 episodes of at least 30 min per week, and 4,252 who performed at least 30 min of physical activity more than three times a week. With increasing frequency of physical activity, the percentage of patients with dyslipidemia decreased from 41% in the physically inactive group to 34% in the most active group. There was no difference in systolic or diastolic blood pressure among the groups, but there was a lower glycated hemoglobin in patients with a higher frequency of physical activity ($p < 0.00001$), and this effect was found in both sexes and in all age groups [35]. A study examining noninvasive markers of atherosclerosis using flow-mediated dilation and intima-media thickness with high-resolution ultrasonography found that patients ($n = 32$) with type I diabetes had higher intima-media thickness and reduced flow-mediated dilation compared to control subjects ($n = 42$) [36]. When children with diabetes were assessed based on their level of daily physical activity, those children who did 60 or more minutes of moderate to vigorous physical activity were found to have higher flow-mediated dilation compared to the inactive group, and similar differences were found when comparing inactive and active healthy subjects. Again, the group studied was of a wide age range from 6 to 17 years, and it does not appear that pubertal status was controlled for, although it was assessed [36].

4.7 Effects on Glucose and Glycemic Control

Exercise increases the risk of hypoglycemia in type I diabetes, and this risk is both acute and delayed. A very elegant study has examined glucose requirements during moderate-intensity afternoon exercise in adolescents with type I diabetes [37]. Nine adolescents with a mean age of 16 years and duration of diabetes of approximately 8 years were studied using exercise clamp studies. The aim of the study was to maintain glucose levels in the euglycemic range using an infusion of a fixed dose of insulin but variable doses of intravenous dextrose. A standardized "dose" of exercise was performed at 16:00 hours with 45 min of cycling on a cycle ergometer at an intensity of approximately 55% of their peak aerobic capacity. A second euglycemic clamp study was performed at rest with no periods of exercise. This study shows that glucose infusion rates to maintain stable glucose levels were increased during and shortly after exercise and again from 7 to 11 h after exercise. Counterregulatory hormone levels were measured and were similar between exercise and rest days, although there was a peak immediately after exercise [37]. This study suggests that patients are risk of hypoglycemia during and shortly after exercise and again from 7 to 11 h after exercise. If exercise is performed late in the day, this risk of delayed hypoglycemia will occur during sleep. In addition, the peak in counterregulatory hormone responses immediately after exercise can cause blood glucose levels to rise for a while after exercise. This means that patients need less insulin during activity but then may need extra insulin straight after exercise which is often when they are checking their blood glucose level [37]. This response to physical activity does appear to be reproducible within patients. Nine adolescent boys with type I diabetes were tested, using six 10-min cycling bouts at moderate intensity separated by a 5-min rest period, on two separate occasions 5–17 days apart. Plasma glucose levels for each time period from the beginning of exercise to the end of the recovery period were unchanged between the two sessions [38]. Carbohydrate intake, insulin injections, exercise bouts, and their timing were identical in both sessions. This does suggest that patients who can monitor themselves intensively around periods of activity can learn a great deal with respect to making adjustments to their diabetes regimen to keep glucose levels at acceptable values during exercise [38].

Another study has examined the effect of physical activity in 50 subjects with type I diabetes aged 11–17 years. Blood glucose was frequently sampled on a day of physical activity (a standardized afternoon exercise session on a treadmill) compared to a day of inactivity [39]. Current guidelines from the American Diabetes Association for the management of exercise for patients with type I diabetes were used to try to avoid hypoglycemia during exercise [40]. Despite this, 11 (22%) of patients developed hypoglycemia during exercise. In addition, the mean glucose concentration overnight was lower on the exercise day than on a rest day. Hypoglycemia was more frequent on exercise nights occurring in 13 (26%) of nights [39].

Studies have also examined the effects of physical activity on long-term glycemic control. Two large epidemiological studies have found rather conflicting results. The Hvidoere Study Group found that physical activity, as assessed by questionnaires based on retrospective reporting of amounts of physical activity, has shown no link with glycemic control, as judged by glycated hemoglobin levels [26]. Furthermore, there were also no associations with reported frequency of severe hypoglycemia or diabetic ketoacidosis [26]. In contrast, a study using cross-sectional analysis of data from 19,000 patients with type I diabetes aged 3–20 years showed that regular physical activity is a major factor influencing glycemic control [41]. Again, physical activity data were collected using questionnaires and subjects were divided based on the frequency of physical activity bouts of greater than 30 min per week. No association was noted between the frequency of physical activity and episodes of severe hypoglycemia. Data on episodes of mild hypoglycemia were not collected [41]. Neither of these studies was designed to look at a link between physical activity and glycemic control. One study of 81 youth with type I diabetes aged 11–16 years who were randomized either to usual care or personal trainer intervention found that glycated hemoglobin levels increased in the control group by 0.3%, whereas there was a decrease in the intervention group of 0.39% over a 2-year period [42]. Another study examined the impact of preexisting glycemic control on the beneficial effects of physical activity on glycated hemoglobin. Twenty-four adolescents with type I diabetes with glycated hemoglobin levels either higher or lower than 9% participated in 12 weeks of supervised exercise followed by 12 weeks of unsupervised training [43]. The study found no improvements in HbA1c in those who are either poorly controlled or well controlled [43].

4.8 Managing Diabetes During Physical Activity

4.8.1 Insulin Adjustment

Management of type I diabetes around the times of physical activity is fraught with problems particularly among children and young people. However, it is also a significant concern to adults in whom fear of hypoglycemia is the most significant barrier to physical activity [44]. There has been surprisingly little research into the management of activity in childhood diabetes.

The American Diabetes Association has provided guidelines to the management of diabetes and exercise; however, this is very much a consensus statement rather than an evidence-based document [40]. ISPAD has also produced some guidelines [45]. These guidelines assume that episodes of activity are planned and that the level of physical activity can be reasonably well predicted. This may be possible in young people and adults but becomes more problematic when considering young children and toddlers. As mentioned earlier, young children are less likely to have planned episodes of physical activity or exercise, and data suggest that they are more likely to have multiple short bouts of potentially intense activity [46]. Planning for this kind of physical activity is almost impossible to do with any degree of accuracy. If parents are aware that their child may have opportunity for physical activity during the day at school, they may plan to make reductions in insulin doses during the day or a range for extra snacks, but the weather or whim of the child could turn these plans upside down.

A few studies have examined the management of physical activity with particular emphasis on hypoglycemia avoidance. The DirecNet study group has studied a group of 49 children with type I diabetes aged 8–17 years of age [47]. All children were on insulin pump therapy and were studied on 2 days during which time they had structured exercise sessions. On one day, basal insulin was stopped during exercise, and on the second day, basal insulin was continued. The standardized exercise sessions consisted of four 15-min treadmill cycles at a target heart rate of 140 beats per minute. The study found that hypoglycemia during exercise occurred less frequently when the basal insulin was discontinued ($p < 0.003$). Post-exercise hyperglycemia was more frequent when basal insulin had been discontinued [47]. Another study of ten adolescents using a similar study design found no difference between having a pump off and the pump on during exercise [48]. This study did find that delayed hypoglycemia was more common than hypoglycemia during exercise, suggesting that even though it may be possible to avoid hypoglycemia during planned exercise, delayed hypoglycemia, which often occurs at night time, is more problematic to avoid [48].

In an attempt to avoid post-exercise nocturnal hypoglycemia, Taplin et al. studied 16 adolescents on insulin pump therapy using a 60-min exercise session followed by an overnight reduction in basal rates by 20% for 6 h or oral terbutaline at a dose of 2.5 mg [49]. Terbutaline did result in an avoidance of hypoglycemia overnight; however, there were significantly more episodes of hyperglycemia compared to basal rate reduction (blood glucose greater than 13.8 mmol/l). Blood glucose profiles were better overnight with a basal rate reduction, but there was still more hyperglycemia than was clinically acceptable [49].

There are pragmatic adjustments that have been suggested in terms of insulin dosing around the time of planned episodes of physical activity [50]. If exercise is to be taken within 2 h of a mealtime bolus of rapid-acting insulin, the dose needs to be reduced to avoid exercise-induced hypoglycemia. If the exercise is of moderate to high intensity, a premeal reduction of 50% is recommended. If exercise is to be taken greater than 2 h after a mealtime bolus, there does not need to be a reduction in insulin dose. If the exercise is anaerobic or in hot conditions or at a time of competition stress, then an increase in insulin dose may be needed. Those patients on insulin pump therapy will be able to make reductions in their basal rates both during and after physical activity. It is likely that different types of physical activity as well as different intensities of activity are likely to need varying adjustments to basal rates at these times. It would be very useful for children, young people, and their parents to do much more rigorous monitoring of physical activity, nutrition, and blood glucose levels around the time of physical activity. It may then be possible for the diabetes team to work closely with families to develop plans for diabetes management that are personalized.

4.9 Nutrition and Exercise

Nutrition advice is another strategy that can be used to achieve glycemic control during exercise. Nutritional aspects of glycemic control and prevention of long-term complications are summarized in the 2009 International Society for Pediatric and Adolescent Diabetes (ISPAD) consensus guidelines [51]. Where nutrition is used to manage blood glucose levels, it should not compromise the diets of young people with diabetes. Information about what young people with type 1 diabetes eat demonstrates that often they fail to achieve the recommendations made for health [52, 53]. Management of exercise and physical activity needs to balance health benefits with hypoglycemia risk.

4.10 Unplanned or Spontaneous Physical Activity

Nutrition advice for unplanned and spontaneous physical activity usually focuses on hypoglycemia prevention. Where exercise is unplanned, the usual nutritional advice is to consume additional carbohydrate to prevent hypoglycemia. This carbohydrate should not contribute to an increased intake of saturated fats or disrupt

Table 4.1 Estimated average energy requirements for children 7–18 years in the UK

Sex and age (years)	Estimated average requirement for energy[a] (kcal/day)
Boys	
7–10	1,970
11–14	2,220
15–18	2,750
Girls	
7–10	1,740
11–14	1,845
15–18	2,110

[a]Values taken from UK dietary reference values, 1991 [62]

energy balance and encourage weight gain. Children and families will benefit from guidance on the suitable carbohydrate-containing foods to use in these situations.

4.11 Management of Regular Physical Activity and Exercise

Regular and planned activities such as games lessons in schools, attendance at sports clubs, and activity trips require nutrition advice appropriate to the level of participation in the sport/activity. Advice for individual children needs to consider energy balance, glycemic control, and insulin adjustment strategies. Nutritional advice for hypoglycemia prevention should not increase overall energy intake and contribute to weight gain.

Individual advice plans will depend on insulin treatment regimens. Conventional twice-daily biphasic insulin regimens provide fewer options for insulin adjustment to manage blood glucose levels during activity especially activities performed in the afternoon in schools/clubs. The use of intensive therapy increases the options available, insulin doses can be adjusted at meals before and after activity, and background/basal insulin adjustments can also be made. For many, this may be a more appropriate strategy to prevent excess energy intake and weight gain.

Children and young people with diabetes have the same energy requirements as their peers. Dietary reference values (DRVs) for populations usually summarize energy recommendations across population groups; estimated average requirements (EAR) meet the needs of 50% of a population group. In the UK, DRVs published by the Department of Health in 1991 give a summary of EAR for energy across age groups, based on weight and average activity levels (Table 4.1). By contrast, the 2006 Australia and New Zealand nutrient reference values give estimated energy expenditure values based on average weight, age, and physical activity factors (Table 4.2) and do not present this data averaged across age ranges.

Advice to manage the hypoglycemia risks associated with exercise should not increase energy intake beyond expenditure, and care is needed when interpreting energy requirements from DRV to ensure that estimated average values apply to the individual.

Energy expenditure and carbohydrate needs to prevent hypoglycemia will vary with age and weight. For most young people undertaking regular physical activity of moderate intensity lasting up to 60 min per day, broad guidelines on exercise

Table 4.2 Calculated energy requirement for age and physical activity level in Australia and NZ

Sex and age (years)	Calculated average energy requirements		
	Light activity PAL 1.6	Moderate activity PAL 1.8	Vigorous activity PAL 2.2
Boys			
7	1,670	1,866	2,272
11	2,105	2,368	2,870
15	2,679	3,014	3,684
Girls			
7	1,555	1,746	2,129
11	1,913	2,153	2,631
15	2,248	2,535	3,086

Values for energy requirements for light, moderate, and vigorous activity levels taken from nutrient reference values for Australia and New Zealand [61]

Table 4.3 Summary of exercise management strategies for regular planned activity

	Management advice
Exercise within peak insulin action	Consider decreasing pre-exercise insulin food bolus by up to 50%
	If exercise is aerobic or duration greater than 45 min, consume carbohydrate (1 g/kg/h) at 20-min intervals to maintain blood glucose levels
	Check blood glucose levels before, during, and after activity. If blood glucose is below 4 mmol/l, delay exercise until blood glucose level is normal
	If blood glucose level is >10 mmol/l, delay carbohydrate intake until 20 min into activity
	If blood glucose level is >15 mmol/l, check for ketones and manage high blood glucose levels before exercise commences
	Consume adequate fluids
Anaerobic activities, e.g., basketball, athletic field events, sprint events	Check blood glucose levels to assess responses to exercise
	If activity last longer than 45 min, consume carbohydrate during exercise for fuel
	Consume meal or snack within 1 h of finishing exercise to reduce risk of post-exercise hypoglycemia
Aerobic activities	Consume additional carbohydrate and/or adjust insulin when exercise lasts 45 min or longer
Team sports	Monitor blood glucose levels during and after activity
	If within peak action of insulin, consider reducing insulin doses
	Consume snack and fluid at half time; if competition stress increases blood glucose levels, consider small corrective dose of insulin
Post-exercise	Consume carbohydrate snack or meal with fluids after exercise
	If blood glucose levels raised post-exercise, treat with caution
	Consume pre-bed snack whenever exercise duration is 60 min or longer

management can be used and adapted according to blood glucose responses. These broad guidelines should cover blood glucose level, type and duration of activity, timing of activity, appropriate amounts and type of carbohydrate needed, and post-exercise hypoglycemia prevention [45].

Key characteristics of advice for regular activity are summarized in Table 4.3.

If more detailed advice about nutrition and sport is needed, then the information and guidance for training and competition nutrition can be adapted to meet the needs of the individual based on estimation of energy and carbohydrate needs.

4.12   Management of Training/Competitive Sports

Young athletes require adequate nutrition to grow, to develop, and to fuel performance [54, 55]. A healthy diet is an essential part of training for sports performance. As with diabetes, most recommendations are extrapolated from adult guidelines. Nutritional considerations for young athletes include growth and development as well as health and performance. Meyer in 2007 [56] and Jeukendrup and Cronin in 2011 [57] summarize an appropriate nutritional intake as one that will support training and recovery as well as limiting problems that may occur due to nutritional deficiency and injury. While diabetes disrupts glucose homeostasis, it does not alter the nutritional requirements associated with sport. Managing diabetes and achieving an appropriate nutritional intake can present the athlete, family, and health-care professionals with a number of challenges. This section will discuss how best to advise young athletes to maximize performance ability through good nutrition.

Education and counseling of young athletes with type 1 diabetes needs to consider all the factors that influence food choice and the impact of diabetes management. Neumark-Sztainer et al. summarize the influencing factors as hunger, food cravings, appeal of food, time considerations, convenience, food availability, peer influence, parental influence, health beliefs, mood, body image, habit, cost, and media [58].

4.12.1   Practice Tips

- In clinical practice, a diet history is the usual method of assessing dietary intake; food intake checklists and 24-h recalls of food intake are useful tools in young athletes.
- Asking young athletes about goals for their sport helps to provide effective behavioral strategies for each individual.

4.13   Energy Balance

Energy requirements vary with age, growth, and activity levels. Achieving an appropriate energy intake is of paramount importance to ensure that the demands of training do not have a negative impact on growth and maturation. In the general population, energy requirements based on age and average activity levels and weight are available through dietary reference values. Energy requirements given in dietary reference tables are unlikely to meet the needs of young athletes undertaking regular training, and daily energy needs will be influenced by the volume of training being undertaken.

4.14   Assessment of Energy Requirements

Energy requirements can be calculated using predictive equations and energy costs of particular exercise types. Predictive formulas include Schofield's age-, mass-, and gender-specific equation; Harrell's age-, gender-, and pubertal-specific equation; and WHO/FAO/UNU equation [59]. Within pediatric population subgroups, each predictive equation has varying agreement with calorimetry dependent on the population characteristics. A comparison by Rodriguez et al. in 2000 recommends the use of Schofield's height and weight equation for estimation of resting energy expenditure (REE) [60]. The Schofield height and weight equation is used in the Australian dietary reference values, whereas UK DRVs use the WHO/FAO/UNU equation [61, 62].

Once REE is calculated, information about the energy costs of exercise or activity is required to estimate total daily energy expenditure (TEE). Estimation of TEE can be made using either physical activity factors to estimate daily energy requirements or use of activity diaries to calculate the energy expenditure associated with sports. Data on the energy costs of activity in young athletes are limited; use of adapted tables of metabolic equivalents (METs) allows some attempt to quantify energy costs of exercise [63]. Use of adult physical activity data to estimate energy costs of exercise may underestimate the actual energy requirements due to the decrease in energy cost per unit of body weight with age. Recent work to develop a compendium of energy expenditures in youth has been published by Ridley et al. [64, 65]. The MET data from these compendium tables can be used to assess energy expenditure during exercise (see Box 1).

Anthropometric assessment including monitoring of height and weight on centile charts, skinfold, and circumferences should be used to assess body composition and growth. In practice, assessment of energy requirements is a key first step in providing sports nutrition advice as the recommendations for protein, carbohydrate, and fat intake are all based on the energy needs of the athlete.

4.14.1   Practice Tips

• A detailed history of activity and training is needed to calculate energy requirements.

Box 1: Example Use of MET Data to Calculate Energy Expenditure
Example
A boy who weighs 45 kg and is 150 cm tall doing 60 min basketball has a REE of 1,452 kcal/24 h using Schofield HW equation.
Energy expenditure per min = 1.0 kcal/min
Basketball light effort has a MET of 7.2
Energy expenditure for 60 min basketball = $(1.0 \times 7.2 \times 60)$ 435 kcal/h

- Activity diaries can be used but may not be completed accurately; adequate time is needed in the consultation to take a detailed activity history.
- Energy requirements should be calculated for each individual.

4.15 Carbohydrate

Energy metabolism in young athletes differs through the ages and stages of development; younger prepubertal athletes generally have a greater dependence on fat rather than carbohydrate as fuel source compared to postpubertal and adult athletes. However, despite these differences in energy metabolism, carbohydrate remains the main dietary fuel source for young people. Carbohydrate intake in adults has been well studied, and the benefits of ingestion of carbohydrate pre- and post-exercise are well documented [66].

4.15.1 Type of Exercise

Adult recommendations consider the carbohydrate needs of athletes according to the type of sport being undertaken. Detailed information about the carbohydrate needs of endurance versus strength/power sports is available. There is little information available about specific sports types and the younger competitor. For all sports types, the key consideration is achieving the appropriate intake for growth and maturation. The type of exercise will impact on blood glucose responses as strength and power sports are predominantly anaerobic and therefore likely to raise blood glucose levels. Appropriate adjustments in insulin should be made to achieve blood glucose targets rather than adjustments in food intake which may be detrimental to overall energy balance.

4.15.2 Timing of Carbohydrate Ingestion with Exercise

Studies on the ingestion of carbohydrate before and during exercise in children have shown equivocal results. In adults, it is accepted practice that carbohydrate should be consumed 1–3 h prior to exercise bouts, during exercise bouts of greater than 60–90 min duration, and within 1–2 h of completing exercise to maximize muscle recovery. Despite the limited body of available evidence about performance benefits of carbohydrate ingestion for younger athletes, it is appropriate to recommend that carbohydrate is ingested before and after exercise, and for the young athlete with diabetes, carbohydrate should be consumed during any exercise where the duration of the activity is 60 min or longer.

4.15.3   Pre-exercise Meal/Snack Suggestions

Fruit and low fat milk or yogurt	Sandwich with low fat filling
Low fat cereal bars	Jacket potato with filling
Breakfast cereals with low fat milk	Pasta with tomato based sauce
Dried fruit	Breakfast cereal with milk and fruit
Homemade cakes/muffins/scones	Soup and bread

4.15.4   Amount of Carbohydrate

Reviews looking at the carbohydrate requirements in younger athletes conclude that intakes should be in the order of 50–60% of energy intake. The age-related differences in glycolytic capacity, which appear to relate to stage of development rather than chronological age, mean that it is difficult to set age-specific requirements. Work by Riddell and colleagues has shown that carbohydrate utilization during exercise shows age- and sex-related differences [67–70]. Consideration of carbohydrate intake in young athletes with type 1 diabetes needs to account for both performance and hypoglycemia prevention particularly during endurance sports. In a review of physical activity and pediatric diabetes, Riddell and Iscoe [50] suggest that carbohydrate requirements for youth with diabetes are of the magnitude of 1.0–1.5 g/kg body weight/h of exercise during peak insulin action. The amount of carbohydrate required to maintain blood glucose levels will fall with diminishing insulin levels. An alternative method of estimating carbohydrate requirement is the amount which supports the energy cost of the activity. If the energy cost of the exercise is known, using the assumption that 60% of total energy is provided by carbohydrate allows the calculation of carbohydrate requirements.

Example: Energy expenditure of 435 kcal/h for a 45-kg boy doing basketball would equate to 65-g carbohydrate per hour of basketball.

When exercise is performed during peak insulin action, reductions in insulin can be used as an alternative to consuming additional carbohydrate. This strategy should be used within a management plan that ensures total daily energy intake is adequate for the volume of training being undertaken.

For anaerobic sports, adjustment in insulin doses may be needed to maintain blood glucose levels and enable appropriate amounts of carbohydrate to be consumed for fuel.

4.15.5   Type of Carbohydrate

Nutritional recommendations for diabetes promote healthy low-fat, low glycemic index (GI) carbohydrate choices. The glycemic index describes the rate at which a carbohydrate food produces glucose in the blood. At present, there is no evidence to support advising particular carbohydrate types during exercise in children and adolescents. Diets should be based on the same healthy carbohydrate choices recommended in diabetes management. However, where higher carbohydrate requirements are difficult to achieve, the addition of high GI carbohydrate foods may make the diet more palatable. The use of medium to high GI carbohydrate foods in the recovery period may be of particular importance in achieving recommended amounts of carbohydrate immediately post-exercise.

4.15.6 Practical Carbohydrate Management

- Young athletes should be advised to consume a diet that provides 50–60% of their total energy requirements as carbohydrate. Carbohydrate sources should be spread across the day to ensure that there are opportunities to maximize both muscle and liver glycogen both before and after exercise. For exercise performed during peak insulin activity, 1–1.5 g carbohydrate/kg/h of activity is recommended.
- The amount of carbohydrate intake during exercise will depend on the duration and type of exercise to be performed and the timing of the exercise in relation to the peak action of the insulin.
- For all exercise, it is recommended that the energy cost of the activity is used to guide carbohydrate requirements during exercise.
- Carbohydrate needs during exercise will change and should be reviewed on a regular basis.
- Carbohydrate advice should include guidance on the amount and type of carbohydrate to be consumed before and after exercise to maximize muscle glycogen stores.
- Insulin management needs to be adjusted according to food intake and blood glucose responses.
- Carbohydrate consumed during exercise should be distributed throughout the activity wherever possible, consuming carbohydrate every 10–20 min throughout exercise rather than all at the beginning of a training bout.

4.16   Protein

Children and adolescents have higher protein requirements than adults to support growth. Protein requirements in athletes will be higher than their peers. Protein recommendations in diabetes management decrease to 0.8–1 g protein/kg body weight in later adolescence. This level of protein intake will not be high enough for competitive athletes. However, protein intakes are often higher than the recommended intakes given in national Recommended Daily Allowances (RDAs). Aiming for a protein intake of 10–15% of total energy requirements will usually meet protein needs associated with training and development [71]. Protein requirements in adult athletes vary with type of sport with endurance athletes having lower protein requirements than strength/power athletes [72]. The range of protein requirements in adults is 1.2–1.7 g/kg/day [66]. Adolescent athletes are unlikely to need more than 2 g protein/kg/day [73]. Provided a varied diet is consumed, protein intakes will be adequate, but additional advice may be needed for vegetarian athletes and those with poor dietary choices [74]. Consuming protein mixed with carbohydrate (recovery snacks) post-exercise may be beneficial in the prevention of late-onset hypoglycemia. Recovery snack ideas include fruit smoothie, low-fat milk shake, yogurt drinks, mini pancakes, fruit, and yogurt.

4.16.1 Practice Tips

- Most young athletes will achieve adequate protein intakes if they consume 10–15% of total energy as protein.
- Vegetarian athletes may need additional advice about quality of protein intake.
- The addition of low-fat dairy products to the post-exercise recovery meal/snack will provide a mix of protein and carbohydrate that may be beneficial in preventing late-onset hypoglycemia.

4.17 Fat

There is no difference in recommendations for fat intake from those made for the general population. While younger athletes may use fat in preference to carbohydrate as a fuel source during exercise, they do not need to consume fat as a fuel source. Fat should provide no more than 30% of dietary energy and with no more than 10% from saturated fat. Food choices should be as low fat as possible in most situations. Careful advice about snack choices used to increase carbohydrate intake will prevent increases in saturated fat intake.

4.18 Fluid, Hydration, and Thermoregulation

Excess heat produced during exercise is lost through evaporation of sweat and convection of heat from the surface of the skin. The ability to perform exercise is affected by hydration status. Dehydration of 1–2% in adults has been demonstrated to compromise function and performance. Studies comparing adults and children have shown similar effects of dehydration on performance. Exertional heat illness, e.g., cramps, exhaustion, and heat stroke, will occur with losses of 3% body weight. Dehydration can be elicited during exercise due to the environment, prior state of hydration, and duration of exercise. Thirst is recognized as a poor indicator of hydration and fluid needs; so young athletes need guidance and drinking plans to achieve adequate fluid intakes.

Clear guidelines exist for adults about voluntary fluid intake during activity; a review by Rowland has suggested that fluid requirements in child athletes (aged 8–13 years) are 13 ml/kg/h of exercise and 4 ml/kg in the post-exercise recovery period [75]. The American Academy of Pediatrics [76] also provides guidance on fluid and climatic heat stress in child and adolescent athletes. This statement provides additional advice about exercise in conditions that increase heat stress, i.e., high temperatures and humidity. Recommendations include reduction in intensity in exercise when relative humidity and air temperature are above critical levels. Heat stress in the young athlete with diabetes may exacerbate hyperglycemia particularly during competition, anaerobic activity, and when hyperglycemia exists due to lack of insulin. Fluid advice needs to be practical and achieve an appropriate daily fluid intake. Fluid requirements can be assessed by pre- and post-exercise weights. If weight is lost through an exercise bout, this is due to inadequate fluid intake during exercise. As a general guide, weight loss × 1.5 will replace fluid losses, e.g., 500 g of weight loss requires at least 750 ml of additional fluid. Regular monitoring of weight changes during training in different climatic conditions will provide information about individual sweat losses and fluid needs.

4.19 Practical Fluid Management

- Before exercise, sufficient fluid should be consumed through the day to ensure adequate levels of hydration. A drink should be consumed with each meal and snack. Drinking plans should encourage intake of around 500 ml of fluid 1–2 h before activity. Drinking additional fluid 15 min before exercise will help to ensure adequate hydration at the start of training/competition. Sipping 150–200 ml fluid is advised. Water is the most appropriate drink choice before exercise. Beverages with high concentrations of sugar empty slowly from the stomach, and for this reason, glucose/energy drinks are not recommended as pre-exercise beverages.
- During exercise, fluid should be consumed every 15–20 min; for exercise that lasts 60 min or longer or is of high intensity, a sports drink is recommended. This may also help prevent problems with low blood glucose levels. Commercial sports drinks also provide sodium and electrolytes. These encourage drinking as they improve taste. Water is an appropriate fluid choice for exercise lasting less than 60 min; however, flavoring the water with sugar squashes may improve intake due to the improved taste.
- Post-exercise fluid is needed as part of the muscle recovery process. Ideally, a drink should be consumed within 15 min of completing a bout of exercise. This can be a carbohydrate-containing fluid. Young athletes should be encouraged to drink as much as possible after exercise. Consuming food and fluid post-exercise helps rehydration as well reducing post-exercise hypoglycemia risks.

4.20 Vitamins and Minerals

Vitamins and minerals have key roles in metabolism; for athletes, these roles include immune function, antioxidant supply, and energy metabolism. If food intakes meet energy requirements from a varied balanced diet, then it is likely that vitamin and mineral intakes will be adequate. RDAs can be used to assess adequacy of vitamin and mineral intakes; however, it is not known if these are appropriate for higher activity levels. In the general population, calcium and iron intakes are often below recommended levels. Calcium requirements are greater during childhood and adolescence. Restriction of dairy products can occur particularly as a method of reducing fat and calorie intake. Iron intakes are also affected by energy restriction as well as increased losses associated with endurance and high-intensity training. Female athletes are at particular risk of iron depletion/deficiency due the combined effects of higher requirements due to growth and menstrual losses. Iron depletion in young athletes is common. Particular attention to vitamin and mineral intakes will be needed for sports where a lower energy intake is required to maintain lower body weights, e.g., gymnastics and dance, wrestling, and boxing.

4.20.1 Practice Tips

- Nutrition advice should include assessment and monitoring of vitamin and mineral intakes.
- Use of low-fat dairy products as recovery foods will help ensure adequate calcium intakes.
- Achieving the recommended "5 a day" will help to ensure adequate vitamin intakes.

4.21 Supplements and Ergogenic Aids

Adolescent athletes are likely to use supplements. This supplement use ranges from multivitamin and mineral supplements to products marketed to improve performance. Supplement use in a group of junior athletes at World Junior Championships was as high as 62%. Popular supplements include whey protein and creatine, as well as caffeine. Most sporting authorities recommend that these supplements are not used in athletes aged under 18 years. Athletes with diabetes need the same guidance as their peers about supplement use, including counseling about the risk of contamination and lack of evidence for performance benefits. Additional counseling should be provided about antidoping and insulin use. In some sports, Therapeutic Use Exemption is required under the age of 18 years. Advice should be sort from individual sporting bodies.

4.22   Sport-Specific Considerations

4.22.1   Endurance Sports

Training programs for endurance sports generally increase energy and macronutrient requirements significantly. Iron and calcium intakes may be of particular concern in younger endurance athletes. Requirements for energy, protein, carbohydrate, iron, and calcium should be reviewed regularly.

4.22.2   Power/Strength Sports

Strength and power sports are predominantly anaerobic activities, and therefore glycolytic in nature, which can present very specific challenges for the young athlete with diabetes. The expected blood glucose response to this type of activity is increasing blood glucose profile during the sport. Achieving an adequate energy intake during the training or competition necessitates counseling about appropriate insulin adjustment strategies to maintain blood glucose levels. This may include advice to increase insulin delivery to allow fuel utilization. Anaerobic exercise usually depletes glycogen stores so can have profound effects on blood glucose levels 1–2 h post-exercise. Using recovery snacks in the immediate post-exercise period can prevent this.

Many of these sports will have weight categories, and young athletes may use inappropriate strategies including fluid, calorie, and carbohydrate restriction to achieve target weights. These athletes are likely to benefit from the support of a sports dietitian to allow them to achieve weight targets with an appropriate nutritional intake.

4.22.3   Team Sports

Team sports are often characterized by intermittent high-intensity exercise which moderates blood glucose effects. Nutritional needs include adequate fluid replacement as well as sufficient energy intake to promote muscle recovery and maintenance of lean body mass.

4.22.4   Competition and Travel

All athletes need advice and support about what to eat and drink during competition particularly when travel is involved. The need to adjust insulin, monitor blood glucose levels, and achieve an appropriate nutritional intake needs planning. It is likely due to the hormonal responses to competition stress that additional insulin or adjustments in timing of insulin delivery will be needed. High blood glucose levels will impair performance ability. To ensure adequate fuel supply to exercising muscles, meals, snacks, and insulin need to be timed to achieve target blood glucose levels during events.

When competition involves travel to different venues, availability of suitable food choices may be an issue. Fussy eating will compromise both nutritional intake and blood glucose management if food refusal results in inadequate intake. It may be necessary to provide additional support and plan with team managers who have a pastoral role about how they will ensure the athlete with diabetes consumes an adequate amount of food and fluid. The principles of management of food, fluid, and travel include ensuring adequate fluid is consumed during travel, researching food availability at the destination, and taking supplies to ensure that energy and carbohydrate needs are met, as well as the usual considerations for travel and type 1 diabetes.

4.22.5   Practical Tips for Travel and Competition

- Stick to familiar foods and drinks, find out what food will be available, and pack suitable kit bag snacks to maintain energy and carbohydrate intake.
- Have small regular snacks during tournaments and matches, where possible consume carbohydrate and fluid at half time, check blood glucose levels, and adjust insulin according to responses to exercise and competition.

4.23   Summary

Nutrition is a key component of the management of diabetes and sports performance. For all young people, advice based on healthy food choices with appropriate use of carbohydrate to prevent exercise-induced hypoglycemia is needed. Individual energy requirements will dictate food and fluid needs, and wherever possible, individual management strategies should be devised based on nutritional requirements, type of sport, and blood glucose responses.

4.24   Conclusion

In recent years, there has been an increasing focus on rigorous diabetes management with the use of intensive diabetes regimens and nutritional interventions. Physical activity is important for both physical and mental health and should be recommended for all children and young people with type 1 diabetes. However, much more work needs to be done if we are going to be able to support our young patients in being active without the added risks of marked glycemic variability or increased treatment burden.

References

1. Armstrong N, van Mechelen W. Paediatric exercise science and medicine. Oxford: Oxford University Press; 2008.
2. Mulvihill C, Rivers K, Aggleton P. Physical activity 'at our time': qualitative research among young people aged 5 to 15 years and parents. Health Education Authority 2000. ISBN 0 7521 1748 3.
3. Williams HG, Pfeiffer KA, O'Neill JR, Dowda M, McIver KL, Brown WH, Patel R. Motor skill performance and physical activity in preschool children. Obesity. 2008;16:1421–6.
4. McKenzie TL, Sallis JF, Nader PR, Broyles SL, Nelson JA. Anglo- and Mexican-American preschoolers at home and at recess: activity patterns and environmental influences. J Dev Behav Pediatr. 1992;13:173–80.
5. Health Survey for England 2002. Joint Health Surveys Unit: National Centre for Social Research Department of Epidemiology and Public Health at the Royal Free and University College Medical School. In: Sproston K, Primatesta P, editors. http://www.archive2.official-documents.co.uk/document/deps/doh/survey02/hcyp/hcyp01.htm
6. Cockburn C, Clarke G. "Everybody's looking at you!": girls negotiating the 'femininity deficit' they incur in physical education. Women's Studies Int Forum. 2002;25:651–65.
7. Bunt JC, Salbe AD, Harper IT, Hanson RL, Tataranni PA. Weight, adiposity, and physical activity as determinants of an insulin sensitivity index in Pima Indian children. Diabetes Care. 2003;26:2524–30.
8. Adamo KB, Prince SA, Tricco AC, Connor-Gorber S, Tremblay M. A comparison of indirect versus direct measures for assessing physical activity in the pediatric population: a systematic review. Int J Pediatr Obes. 2009;4:2–27.
9. Reilly JJ, Penpraze IV, Hislop I, Davies G, Grant S, Paton JY. Objective measurement of physical activity and sedentary behaviour: review with new data. Arch Dis Child. 2008;93:614–9.
10. Baranowski T, Dworkin R, Cieslik CJ, et al. Reliability and validity of self-report of aerobic activity: Family Health Project. Res Q Exerc Sport. 1984;55:308–17.
11. Sallis JF. Self-report measures of children's physical activity. J Sch Health. 1991;61:215–9.
12. Brage S, Brage N, Franks PW, Ekelund U, Wareham NJ. Reliability and validity of the combined heart rate and movement sensor Actiheart. Eur J Clin Nutr. 2005;59:561–70.
13. Brage S, Brage N, Franks P, Ekelund U, Wong M, Andersen L, Froberg K, Wareham N. Branched equation modelling of simultaneous accelerometry and heart rate monitoring improves estimate of directly measured physical activity energy expenditure. J Appl Physiol. 2004;96:343–51.
14. WHO. Global recommendations on physical activity for health. WHO Press, Geneva, Switzerland. 2010.
15. Lobelo F, Liese AD, Liu J, Mayer-Davis EJ, D'Agostino Jr RB, Pate RR, Hamman RF, Dabelea D. Physical activity and electronic media use in the SEARCH for diabetes in youth case-control study. Pediatrics. 2010;125:e1364–71.
16. Benevento D, Bizzarri C, Pitocco D, Crino A, Moretti C, Spera S, Tubili C, Costanza F, Maurizi A, Cipolloni L, Cappa M, Pozzilli P, IMDIAB Group. Computer use, free time activities and metabolic control in patients with type 1 diabetes. Diabetes Res Clin Pract. 2010;88:e32–4.
17. Overby NC, Margeirsdottir HD, Brunborg C, Anderssen SA, Andersen LF, Dahl-Jorgensen K, Norwegian Study Group for Childhood Diabetes. Physical activity and overweight in children and adolescents using intensified insulin treatment. Pediatr Diabetes. 2009;10:135–41.
18. Massin MM, Lebrethon MC, Rocour D, Gerard P, Bourguignon JP. Patterns of physical activity determined by heart rate monitoring among diabetic children. Arch Dis Child. 2005;90:1223–6.
19. Sarnblad S, Ekelund U, Aman J. Physical activity and energy intake in adolescent girls with Type 1 diabetes. Diabet Med. 2005;22:893–9.

20. Ekeland E, Heian F, Hagen KB, Abbott J. Nordheim L. Exercise to improve self esteem in children and young people. Cochrane Database Syst Rev. 2004.
21. Hood KK, Huestis S, Maher A, Butler D, Volkening L, Laffel LMB. Depressive symptoms in children and adolescents with type 1 diabetes: association with diabetes-specific characteristics. Diabetes Care. 2006;29:1389–91.
22. Edmunds S, Roche D, Stratton G, Wallymahmed K, Glenn SM. Physical activity and psychological well-being in children with Type 1 diabetes. Psychol Health Med. 2007;12:353–63.
23. Bowes S, Lowes L, Warner J, Gregory JW. Chronic sorrow in parents of children with Type 1 diabetes. J Adv Nurs. 2009;65:992–1000.
24. Mackey ER, Streisand R. Brief report: the relationship of parental support and conflict to physical activity in preadolescents with type 1 diabetes. J Pediatr Psychol. 2008;33: 1137–41.
25. Fereday J, MacDougall C, Spizzo M, Darbyshire P, Schiller W. "There's nothing I can't do–I just put my mind to anything and I can do it": a qualitative analysis of how children with chronic disease and their parents account for and manage physical activity. BMC Pediatr. 2009;9:1.
26. Aman J, Skinner TC, de Beaufort CE, Swift PG, Aanstoot HJ, Cameron F, Hvidoere Study Group on Childhood Diabetes. Associations between physical activity, sedentary behavior, and glycemic control in a large cohort of adolescents with type 1 diabetes: the Hvidoere Study Group on Childhood Diabetes. Pediatr Diabetes. 2009;10:234–9.
27. Janssen I, LeBlanc AG. Systematic review of the health benefits of physical activity and fitness in school aged children and youth. Int J Behav Nutr Phys Activity. 2010;7:40.
28. Grundy SM, Benjamin IJ, Burke GL, Chait A, Eckel RH, Howard BV, Mitch W, Smith Jr SC, Sowers JR. Diabetes and cardiovascular disease. A statement for healthcare professionals from the American Heart Association. Circulation. 1999;100:1134–46.
29. Tsuji H, Venditti Jr FJ, Manders ES, Evans JC, Larson MG, Feldman CL, Levy D. Reduced heart rate variability and mortality risk in an elderly cohort. The Framingham heart study. Circulation. 1994;90:878–83.
30. Dekker JM, Crow RS, Folsom AR, Hannan PJ, Liao D, Swenne CA, Schouten EG. Low heart rate variability in a 2-minute rhythm strip predicts risk of coronary heart disease and mortality from several causes: the ARIC study. Circulation. 2000;102:1239–44.
31. Chen SR, Lee YJ, Chiu HW, Jeng C. Impact of physical activity on heart rate variability in children with type 1 diabetes. Childs Nervous System. 2008;24:741–7.
32. Maggio AB, Hofer MF, Martin XE, Marchand LM, Beghetti M, Farpour-Lambert NJ. Reduced physical activity level and cardiorespiratory fitness in children with chronic diseases. Eur J Pediatr. 2010;169:1187–93.
33. Heyman E, Delamarche P, Berthon P, Meeusen R, Briard D, Vincent S, DeKerdanet M, Delamarche A. Alteration in sympathoadrenergic activity at rest and during intense exercise despite normal aerobic fitness in late pubertal adolescent girls with type 1 diabetes. Diabetes Metab. 2007;33:422–9.
34. Komatsu WR, Gabbay MAL, Castro ML, Saraiva GL, Chacra AR, De Barros Neto TL, Dib SA. Aerobic exercise capacity in normal adolescents and those with type 1 diabetes mellitus. Pediatr Diabetes. 2005;6:145–9.
35. Herbst A, Kordonouri O, Schwab KO, Schmidt F, Holl RW. DPV Initiative of the German Working Group for Pediatric Diabetology Germany. Impact of physical activity on cardiovascular risk factors in children with type 1 diabetes: a multicenter study of 23,251 patients. Diabetes Care. 2007;30:2098–100.
36. Trigona B, Aggoun Y, Maggio A, Martin XE, Marchand LM, Beghetti M, Farpour-Lambert NJ. Preclinical noninvasive markers of atherosclerosis in children and adolescents with type 1 diabetes are influenced by physical activity. J Pediatr. 2010;157:533–9.
37. McMahon SK, Ferreira LD, Ratnam N, Davey RJ, Youngs LM, Davis EA, Fournier PA, Jones TW. Glucose requirements to maintain euglycemia after moderate-intensity afternoon exercise in adolescents with type 1 diabetes are increased in a biphasic manner. J Clin Endocrinol Metabol. 2007;92:963–8.

38. Temple MY, Bar-Or O, Riddell MC. The reliability and repeatability of the blood glucose response to prolonged exercise in adolescent boys with IDDM. Diabetes Care. 1995; 18:326–32.
39. Tsalikian E, Mauras N, Beck RW, Tamborlane WV, Janz KF, Chase HP, Wysocki T, Weinzimer SA, Buckingham BA, Kollman C, Xing D, Ruedy KJ, Diabetes Research in Children Network Direcnet Study Group. Impact of exercise on overnight glycemic control in children with type 1 diabetes mellitus. J Pediatrics. 2005;147:528–34.
40. American Diabetes Association. Diabetes mellitus and exercise. Diabetes Care. 2000;23:s50–4.
41. Herbst A, Bachran R, Kapellen T, Holl RW. Effects of regular physical activity on control of glycemia in pediatric patients with type 1 diabetes mellitus. Arch Pediatr Adolesc Med. 2006;160:573–7.
42. Nansel TR, Iannotti RJ, Simons-Morton BG, Plotnick LP, Clark LM, Zeitzoff L. Long-term maintenance of treatment outcomes: diabetes personal trainer intervention for youth with type 1 diabetes. Diabetes Care. 2009;32:807–9.
43. Roberts L, Jones TW, Fournier PA. Exercise training and glycemic control in adolescents with poorly controlled type 1 diabetes mellitus. J Pediatr Endocrinol. 2002;15:621–7.
44. Brazeau A, Rabasa-Lhoret R, Strychar I, Mircescu H. Barriers to physical activity among patients with type 1 diabetes. Diabetes Care. 2008;31:2108–9.
45. Robertson K, Adolfsson P, Scheiner G, Hanas R, Riddell MC. Exercise in children and adolescents with diabetes. Pediatr Diabetes. 2009;10:154–68.
46. Berman N, Bailey R, Barstow TJ, Cooper DM. Spectral and bout detection analysis of physical activity patterns in healthy, prepubertal boys and girls. Am J Hum Biol. 1998;10:289–97.
47. Tsalikian E, Kollman C, Tamborlane WB, Beck RW, Fiallo-Scharer R, Fox L, Janz KF, Ruedy KJ, Wilson D, Xing D, Weinzimer SA, Diabetes Research in Children Network (DirecNet) Study Group. Prevention of hypoglycemia during exercise in children with type 1 diabetes by suspending basal insulin. Diabetes Care. 2006;29:2200–4.
48. Admon G, Weinstein Y, Falk B, Weintrob N, Benzaquen H, Ofan R, Fayman G, Zigel L, Constantini N, Phillip M. Exercise with and without an insulin pump among children and adolescents with type 1 diabetes mellitus. Pediatrics. 2005;116:e348–55.
49. Taplin CE, Cobry E, Messer L, McFann K, Chase HP, Fiallo-Scharer R. Preventing post-exercise nocturnal hypoglycemia in children with type 1 diabetes. J Pediatrics. 2010;157:784–8.
50. Riddell MC, Iscoe KE. Physical activity, sport, and pediatric diabetes. Pediatr Diabetes. 2006;7:60–70.
51. Smart C, Aslander-van Vliet E, Waldron S. Nutritional management in children and adolescents with diabetes. Pediatric Diabetes. 2009;10 Suppl 12:100–17.
52. Rovner AJ, Nansel TR. Are children with type 1 diabetes consuming a healthful diet?: a review of the current evidence and strategies for dietary change. Diabetes Educ. 2009;35:97–107.
53. Mehta SN, Haynie DL, Higgins LA, Bucey NN, Rovner AJ, Volkening LK, et al. Emphasis on carbohydrates may negatively influence dietary patterns in youth with type 1 diabetes. Diabetes Care. 2009;32:2174–6.
54. Steen SN. Timely statement of The American Dietetic Association: nutrition guidance for adolescent. J Am Diet Assoc. 1996;96:611.
55. Steen SN. Timely statement of The American Dietetic Association: nutrition guidance for child athletes. J Am Diet Assoc. 1996;96:610.
56. Meyer F, O'Connor H, Shirreffs SM. Nutrition for the young athlete. J Sports Sci. 2007;25:73–82.
57. Jeukendrup A, Cronin L. Nutrition and elite young athletes. Med Sports Sci. 2011;56:47–58.
58. Neumark-Sztainer D, Story M. Factors influencing food choices of adolescents: findings from focus-group discussions. J Am Diet Assoc. 1999;99:929.
59. Schofield WN. Predicting basal metabolic rate, new standards and review of previous work. Hum Nutr Clin Nutr. 1985;39 Suppl 1:5–41.

60. Rodríguez G, Moreno LA, Sarría A, Fleta J, Bueno M. Resting energy expenditure in children and adolescents: agreement between calorimetry and prediction equations. Clin Nutr. 2002;21:255–60.
61. National Health and Medical Research Council. Nutrient reference values for Australia and New Zealand. 2006.
62. Department of Health. Report on health and social subjects 41: dietary reference values for food energy and nutrients for the United Kingdom. London: HMSO; 1991.
63. Ainsworth BE, Haskell WL, Whitt MC, Irwin ML, Swartz AM, Strath SJ, et al. Compendium of physical activities: an update of activity codes and MET intensities. Med Sci Sports Exerc. 2000;32:S498–504.
64. Ridley K, Ainsworth BE, Olds TS. Development of a compendium of energy expenditures for youth. Int J Behav Nutr Phys Act. 2008;5:1–8.
65. Ridley K, Olds TS. Assigning energy costs to activities in children: a review and synthesis. Med Sci Sports Exerc. 2008;40:1439–46.
66. Position of the American Dietetic Association. Dietitians of Canada, and the American College of Sports Medicine: nutrition and athletic performance. J Am Diet Assoc. 2009;109:509–27.
67. Riddell MC. The endocrine response and substrate utilization during exercise in children and adolescents. J Appl Physiol. 2008;105:725–33.
68. Timmons BW, Bar-Or O, Riddell MC. Energy substrate utilization during prolonged exercise with and without carbohydrate intake in preadolescent and adolescent girls. J Appl Physiol. 2007;103:995–1000.
69. Timmons BW, Bar-Or O, Riddell MC. Influence of age and pubertal status on substrate utilization during exercise with and without carbohydrate intake in healthy boys. Appl Physiol Nutr Metab. 2007;32:416–25.
70. Timmons BW, Bar-Or O, Riddell MC. Oxidation rate of exogenous carbohydrate during exercise is higher in boys than in men. J Appl Physiol. 2003;94:278–84.
71. Phillips SM, Moore DR, Tang JE. A critical examination of dietary protein requirements, benefits, and excesses in athletes. Int J Sport Nutr Exerc Metab. 2007;17:S58–76.
72. Tipton KD, Witard OC. Protein requirements and recommendations for athletes: relevance of ivory tower arguments for practical recommendations. Clin Sports Med. 2007;26:17–36.
73. Petrie HJ, Stover EA, Horswill CA. Nutritional concerns for the child and adolescent competitor. Nutrition. 2004;20:620–31.
74. Barr SI, Rideout CA. Nutritional considerations for vegetarian athletes. Nutrition. 2004;20:696–703.
75. Rowland T. Fluid replacement requirements for child athletes. Sports Med. 2011;41:279–88.
76. American Academy of Pediatrics. Committee on Sports Medicine and Fitness. Climatic heat stress and the exercising child and adolescent. Pediatrics. 2000;106:158–9.

Chapter 5
The Role of Newer Technologies (CSII and CGM) and Novel Strategies in the Management of Type 1 Diabetes for Sport and Exercise

Alistair N. Lumb

5.1 Introduction

Long-acting insulin analogues (insulin glargine (Lantus), sanofi-aventis; insulin detemir (Levemir), Novo Nordisk) are now used to provide basal insulin therapy for the majority of people using multiple daily injection (MDI) treatment regimens for type 1 diabetes. These insulins have provided significant benefit in terms of greater stability of circulating insulin levels [1, 2], which in turn has led to more stable blood glucose levels and a reduction in rates of hypoglycemia, particularly nocturnal hypoglycemia [3, 4]. However, as has been explained elsewhere in this volume, circulating insulin levels can vary considerably during sport and exercise in those without diabetes. An unfortunate consequence of stabilizing insulin levels in those with type 1 diabetes is, therefore, a significant risk of dysglycemia during exercise. For example, during endurance exercise in those without diabetes, such as prolonged running or cycling, insulin levels fall [5] to allow the mobilization of carbohydrate and lipid fuel sources [6], with insulin secretion falling to below fasting levels [7]. These fuel sources provide the energy required by exercising muscle and allow blood glucose levels to be maintained within a tight range. In people with diabetes using MDI therapy, insulin levels remain reasonably stable during exercise [5]. This limits the body's ability to mobilize the required fuel sources and therefore results in a significant risk of hypoglycemia. The (somewhat inelegant) solution to this problem is usually the ingestion of carbohydrate, which can be problematic to maintain in some sports and also reduces the benefit of exercise if weight control is one of the intended outcomes.

In spite of the option to ingest more carbohydrate, it is well recognized that the major limiting factor preventing adults with type 1 diabetes from taking on a more

A.N. Lumb, B.A., Ph.D., M.B.B.S., M.R.C.P.
Diabetes Centre, Wycombe Hospital, Buckinghamshire Healthcare NHS Trust,
Queen Alexandra Road, High Wycombe, Buckinghamshire HP11 2TT, UK
e-mail: alilumb@hotmail.com

I. Gallen (ed.), *Type 1 Diabetes*,
DOI 10.1007/978-0-85729-754-9_5, © Springer-Verlag London Limited 2012

active lifestyle is the fear of hypoglycemia [8], and some experts suggest that this may also be the case for children [9]. The aim of this chapter is to discuss how technologies such as continuous subcutaneous insulin infusion (CSII or "insulin pump" therapy) and continuous glucose monitoring (CGM) can be used to help overcome the particular challenges presented by sport and exercise in the context of type 1 diabetes. Some novel strategies to avoid hypoglycemia will also be considered, which at least offer an alternative to the requirement for carbohydrate ingestion.

5.2 Continuous Subcutaneous Insulin Infusion and Hypoglycemia During Exercise

CSII has become an increasingly important option in the therapy of type 1 diabetes over recent years. Treatment involves the insertion of a temporary cannula into the subcutaneous tissue through which rapid-acting insulin is infused continuously using an electronically controlled pump. CSII therapy permits numerous bolus insulin doses to be given without the need for a physical injection each time and also means that background insulin levels can be adjusted much more easily than with MDI therapy as they are provided by a variable infusion of rapid-acting analogue insulin rather than a subcutaneous bolus of longer-acting insulin. This gives much greater flexibility in insulin delivery than MDI therapy.

It is recognized in people without diabetes that aerobic exercise is associated with a fall in insulin concentrations [5]. In view of this, the strategies for adjustment of CSII therapy during exercise have focused on the reduction or cessation of insulin infusion during exercise, based on the reasonable theory that this should approximate more closely to the physiological situation and therefore reduce rates of hypoglycemia. Early studies carried out in adults using CSII therapy in the 1980s (and therefore in the era predating rapid-acting analogue insulins) showed mixed results [10, 11]. As expected, continuing basal insulin infusion at the usual rate was demonstrated to result in hypoglycemia. A 50% reduction in the prandial insulin bolus with a meal taken 90 min prior to exercise was shown to reduce rates of hypoglycemia, and a reduction in insulin basal rate between 50% and 100% was also shown to be beneficial in reducing rates of hypoglycemia [11].

In contrast, cessation of basal infusion 30 min prior to 45 min of exercise at 60% VO_2 max, with basal infusion stopped for a total of 3 h (and hence restarted at the usual rate 105 min following exercise), resulted in the avoidance of hypoglycemia during postprandial exercise in the morning but not in the afternoon [10]. Three out of seven participants performing postprandial exercise in the afternoon suffered hypoglycemia, and comparison with previous results suggested little benefit of the strategy of cessation of basal insulin infusion over leaving the infusion running at the usual rate. Interestingly, in the three participants who did suffer hypoglycemia, insulin levels did not decline during exercise. This failure to achieve the expected reduction in circulating insulin by reducing infused insulin likely explains why the strategy failed to produce the anticipated results.

Avoiding hypoglycemia during exercise is a particular focus for children, adolescents, and their parents as children's play tends to be very active. Strategies to allow children to play safely while avoiding significant hypoglycemia are clearly important for children to live as normally as possible with diabetes, and therefore, the majority of the more recent evidence regarding the management of CSII therapy for sport and exercise therefore comes from work with younger people with type 1 diabetes.

Studies in children using CSII with analogue insulins have yielded clearer evidence of the benefits of reducing basal insulin infusion rate during exercise. One such study, designed to simulate unplanned postprandial exercise in children and adolescents aged between 10 and 19 years, compared the effect of reducing basal rate to 50% of normal during exercise with that of removing the insulin pump altogether for the exercise period [12]. Exercise occurred on average just under 2 h following the most recent meal, which was accompanied by the usual insulin bolus in order to simulate the unplanned exercise, and consisted of 40–45 min exercise on a cycle ergometer at 60% VO_2 max. Little difference was found in the physiological response to exercise between the two groups, and two of ten participants suffered hypoglycemia (defined as blood glucose <70 mg/dl, equivalent to <3.9 mmol/l) in each group. Interestingly, the exercise sessions with a hypoglycemic event began at lower glucose levels and higher insulin levels (for three subjects, 10–50% higher) than the other sessions performed by the same participants, again suggesting that the problem for these individuals was a failure to achieve the intended reduction in circulating insulin by the reduction in insulin being infused. This is consistent with the notion that the strategy of reducing insulin delivery is the correct one, but that if doing so does not result in a reduction in circulating insulin levels, then problems with hypoglycemia may persist. It also demonstrates that insulin levels at the start of exercise are important, and therefore reducing infused insulin some time before exercise may be more useful than making the reduction at the start of exercise. We shall return to this later.

A study in children and adolescents aged between 8 and 17 investigated whether stopping basal insulin at the start of exercise could reduce the frequency of hypoglycemia compared to when basal insulin infusion is continued at its usual rate [13]. Exercise occurred approximately 4 h following the most recent meal and consisted of four sessions of 15 min walking on a treadmill to a target heart rate of 140 bpm with a 5-min rest between each session. The two conditions were presented in a crossover design. In the condition where the basal insulin infusion was suspended, this was done at the start of exercise with the basal infusion restarted after 2 h (and thus 45 min after the exercise period). Exercise started with blood glucose between 120 and 200 mg/dl (6.7 and 11.1 mmol/l). There was a significant reduction in the fall in blood glucose during exercise when basal insulin was suspended, leading to a reduction in rates of hypoglycemia from 43% to 16%. Only 9% of the children who suspended basal insulin and started exercise with a blood glucose >130 mg/dl (7.2 mmol/l) suffered hypoglycemia. The beneficial effect of suspending basal insulin was consistent in subgroups based on HbA1c, age, gender, and usual frequency of exercise. However, a consequence of stopping basal insulin was a significant increase in the rates of hyperglycemia. No abnormal ketone levels were recorded during the exercise period, although it should be noted that ketone readings were not recorded in the 45 min after exercise finished.

Taken together, the results of these studies suggest how CSII therapy might be adjusted for exercise, although the optimal strategy has not been identified and will likely vary from person to person. With CSII therapy using rapid-acting insulin analogues, it has been demonstrated that a reduction in basal insulin infusion at the start of a relatively short period of moderate exercise will help avoid hypoglycemia both during the period of exercise and also immediately afterward. The optimal reduction is not clear, but for most people basal insulin infusion should be reduced by somewhere between 50% and 100% (i.e., suspension of basal insulin). Whether there is a benefit of an earlier reduction in basal rate has not yet been investigated. The available evidence suggests that circulating insulin levels at the start of exercise are important, and the time-action profile of the available rapid-acting analogue insulins suggests that the earliest effect of a reduction in basal rate will occur at around 10–15 min [14, 15]. In order to reduce circulating insulin levels at the start of exercise, therefore, it might seem sensible to suggest that a reduction in basal infusion rate should be made some time prior to starting exercise. Unfortunately, there is as yet no experimental evidence to support this view or guide when such a reduction should be made. An extension of this reasoning would be to consider whether basal rate should be increased again before exercise finishes, as insulin levels in those without diabetes would increase at the end of exercise. Again, while this strategy makes physiological sense and has been used with some success in individual athletes, there are as yet no data to support whether this might be beneficial in general.

As one might suspect, suspending basal insulin at the start of exercise does increase the risk of hyperglycemia, although it was not observed to increase the risk of ketosis during a short period of exercise and may therefore be the ideal option in groups (e.g., very young children) where significant hypoglycemia may have long-term consequences. It should be noted, however, that the avoidance of hypoglycemia may not be the only focus of attention for athletes of any age with type 1 diabetes. Many report that hyperglycemia has a deleterious effect on performance, and there are also obvious implications for overall glycemic control. Furthermore, it is important to note that while significant ketosis was not observed during 45 min of exercise following the suspension of basal insulin, the theoretical risk of ketosis remains for longer suspension of basal infusion, and this has also not been investigated in detail.

5.3   Continuous Glucose Monitoring and Exercise

Continuous glucose monitoring (CGM) has been increasingly available since the late 1990s. This technology employs a sensor to measure glucose concentrations in the subcutaneous tissue using a glucose oxidase reaction or microdialysis method, and circulating glucose is then estimated from this concentration using an algorithm and some assumptions about the equilibrium in glucose levels between the two regions [6]. Earlier systems recorded glucose data which could only be accessed once the sensor had been removed, but "real-time" CGM systems have become available which allow users to access glucose readings and information about their rate and direction of change while the sensor is being worn. Many experts feel that CGM will prove to be a useful technology to help people with type 1 diabetes improve metabolic control around exercise – both through the ability to react to changes detected at the time of exercise and also through the provision of information which will allow individuals to plan more accurately how to adjust carbohydrate intake and insulin doses for exercise in the future [6].

The use of real-time continuous glucose monitoring systems in general has been shown to reduce hypoglycemia in well-controlled adults and children with type 1 diabetes while also allowing for an improvement in overall glycemic control [16, 17]. Data looking at the accuracy of CGM during exercise have been encouraging. CGM accurately determines interstitial glucose levels during 1 h of intensive cycling exercise (spinning) and also accurately reflects the direction of change of blood glucose levels [18]. In a separate study, the FreeStyle Navigator CGM system was found to accurately reflect the magnitude of the fall in blood glucose levels seen with moderate treadmill exercise in a group of children, albeit with a 10-min delay [19].

This delay, however, represents one of the major challenges with using CGM to prevent hypoglycemia during exercise. There is a recognized time lag between changes in blood glucose and changes in glucose levels in the interstitial compartment at rest [20], which is similar to the 10-min time lag reported above. As a result, in both of the above studies, the CGM was unable to keep up with the rapidly falling glucose levels seen during intense aerobic exercise and, therefore, tended to overestimate the actual blood glucose reading when compared with capillary blood samples [18, 19]. In one study designed to examine the factors affecting CGM system calibration, CGM accurately detected only 65% of hypoglycemic events during exercise when three calibrations per day were used and only 69% when four calibrations per day were used [21].

Strategies are now being developed to overcome this limitation. Using real-time CGM with an alarm, people with uncomplicated type 1 diabetes and no evidence of hypoglycemia unawareness suffered significantly fewer episodes of hypoglycemia during exercise (30 min at 40% VO$_2$ max) when a low-glucose warning alarm was set to 5.5 mmol/l compared to when the alarm was set to 4 mmol/l or no alarm was used [22]. The alarm was used to trigger carbohydrate intake to avoid incipient hypoglycemia. Interestingly, the CGM still overestimated capillary glucose by an average of 1.6 mmol/l, meaning that even using the higher alarm threshold did not completely eliminate hypoglycemia. Based on their results, the authors therefore recommend this strategy in situations where glucose levels can be expected to fall rapidly, such as during moderate exercise similar to that used in their experimental protocol.

An extension of this strategy has been piloted during a sports camp for adolescents with diabetes [9]. Participants aged between 9 and 17 wore real-time CGM during a variety of different exercise situations. An algorithm was used in which carbohydrate intake was advised based both on real-time CGM readings and also the sensor's indication of their rate of change. Blood glucose levels were maintained within target to a great extent, with a reduction in hypoglycemia compared to expected levels and no hyperglycemia. The authors recognize that this is a pilot study in which there was no control group, and variables such as exercise intensity, age, and body weight were not taken into account. Also of concern was that no results were obtained from 6 of 25 participants recruited because of sensor data loss or the sensor falling out. However, the algorithm was surprisingly successful in spite of these limitations, and this certainly suggests a possible important future role for CGM in the management of diabetes in the context of sport and exercise.

5.4   CSII, CGM, and Nocturnal Hypoglycemia

Nocturnal hypoglycemia following exercise is a well-recognized problem in type 1 diabetes and has been observed following both aerobic [23, 24] and mixed forms [25] of exercise. The exact mechanism for this is not clear, although it is certainly possible that the exercise-induced recruitment of GLUT-4 receptors to the surface of the muscle cell may be involved. Another contributing factor is likely to be that exercise blunts the counterregulatory response to subsequent hypoglycemia [26]. One strategy which has been used to combat the risk of nocturnal hypoglycemia following exercise is to reduce basal insulin doses on the night after an exercise bout. This can be problematic when done in the context of an MDI regimen as it increases the risk of subsequent hyperglycemia.

   In those using CSII, it would be reasonable to suspect that reducing basal insulin for some of the nights following exercise might be able to reduce the risk of nocturnal hypoglycemia without significant hyperglycemia resulting. As with many other aspects of the management of CSII for exercise, this hypothesis has been tested in children [27]. Children and adolescents with type 1 diabetes treated with CSII underwent 4×15 min bursts of treadmill exercise at around 4 p.m. with 5-min rest periods in between. For the night after the exercise, they either reduced their basal insulin by 20% from 9 p.m. to 3 a.m., took 2.5 mg orally of terbutaline (a β-adrenoceptor agonist), or received no intervention. Both ingestion of terbutaline and reduction in basal insulin infusion resulted in a reduction of nocturnal hypoglycemia, but ingestion of terbutaline did result in an increase in morning hyperglycemia as had previously been found with adults [28]. While further studies may permit a more appropriate dose of terbutaline to be selected in future, being able to reduce nocturnal basal insulin infusion for a limited period of time offers a means to reduce nocturnal hypoglycemia without the need for additional pharmacological therapy. In those treated with CSII, this represents a successful solution to the problem of nocturnal hypoglycemia following exercise. As the authors themselves say, "The flexibility to adjust basal rates by the hour remains one of the most attractive features of an insulin pump and is … particularly useful for the active person with T1DM."

   An attractive strategy, combining CSII and CGM, may be of particular benefit in those experiencing nocturnal hypoglycemia following exercise. There is a commercially available insulin pump (Paradigm® Veo™, Medtronic Inc., Northridge, CA) which can be set to cease insulin infusion for a period of 2 h in response to CGM glucose readings below a certain threshold, referred to as the low-glucose suspend (LGS) function. In a six-center trial, 31 adults with type 1 diabetes were studied during a period of standard CSII therapy compared with a 3-week period using CSII with LGS [29]. In those with the highest frequency of nocturnal hypoglycemia, there was a significant reduction in the duration of nocturnal hypoglycemia (defined as CGM glucose <2.2 mmol/l or 40 mg/dl) from 46.2 min/day for conventional CSII to 1.8 min/day for CSII with LGS. Clearly this strategy could be beneficial in avoiding hypoglycemia following exercise. Furthermore, knowing that hypoglycemia can affect the counterregulatory hormone response to subsequent exercise and that this effect increases with increasing severity of hypoglycemia [30], it is possible that preventing nocturnal hypoglycemia in this way could also help prevent hypoglycemia and maintain performance during exercise the following day.

5.5   Novel Strategies for Preventing Hypoglycemia During Exercise

The majority of strategies designed to reduce dysglycemia (primarily hypoglycemia) during exercise involve adjustments to carbohydrate intake or insulin dosing. More recently, consideration has been given to trying to prevent exercise-induced hypoglycemia through augmentation of the counterregulatory response to exercise. One very inventive way is the use of a 10-s maximal effort sprint either before [31] or after [32] exercise. When such a sprint was performed at the beginning of a recovery period after 20 min of moderate exercise at 40% VO_2 max, there was no further fall in blood glucose levels, whereas a further significant fall in glucose levels was seen in the control condition when no sprint was performed [32]. Performing the sprint was associated with an increase in catecholamine, cortisol, growth hormone, and lactate levels, although it is not clear which of these were important for attenuating the fall in blood glucose. Interestingly, performing a 10-s sprint prior to similar exercise did not attenuate the drop in blood glucose levels seen during the exercise, but it did again attenuate the drop in blood glucose levels seen after exercise in the control group where no sprint was performed [31]. This was in spite of a significant rise in circulating catecholamine and lactate levels immediately following the sprint.

Both of these studies therefore demonstrate the benefit of the 10-s maximal sprint performed either before or after exercise in preventing a postexercise fall in blood glucose. This is particularly useful in that it provides a strategy which does not require preplanning and ingestion of significant amounts of carbohydrate. Interestingly, it is also possible that the benefit of performing a 10-s sprint prior to exercise was underestimated. The augmented catecholamine response was not shown to affect the fall in blood glucose levels during exercise, but this was with blood glucose levels well above hypoglycemia. Glucose fell on average by 3 mmol/l during the exercise period, and given that exercise commenced at around

11 mmol/l, this suggests a fall from 11 to 8 mmol/l. It has been demonstrated that carbohydrate oxidation is favored over fat oxidation as the source of energy for exercising muscle at a blood glucose level of 11 mmol/l when compared with 7 mmol/l [33], so participants in the trial would have been predisposed to preferential use of carbohydrate and hence a fall in blood glucose. This may have masked any benefit of the higher levels of catecholamines during the exercise period and may explain why the benefit was only seen when glucose levels fell into the normal range during the period of recovery. It would be useful to see whether the 10-s sprint might attenuate the fall in blood glucose during moderate exercise if blood glucose at the start of exercise was closer to the normal range.

Caffeine is of benefit in hypoglycemia, particularly nocturnal hypoglycemia, in type 1 diabetes, when the hypoglycemia is not specifically related to exercise [34, 35]. In particular, caffeine enhances the counterregulatory hormone response to hypoglycemia as well as increases symptoms accompanying hypoglycemia which allow earlier treatment of hypoglycemia and therefore reduce the chance of neuroglycopenia developing [36]. With exercise, we have found that caffeine in doses of 5 mg/kg taken 30 min prior to exercise reduces the need for carbohydrate treatment to prevent hypoglycemia during exercise in people with type 1 diabetes [37]. This is a preliminary study but offers another strategy for the prevention of hypoglycemia during exercise in type 1 diabetes which does not require much planning and does not involve the ingestion of extra carbohydrate.

5.6   Practical Aspects of CSII and Exercise

While CSII appears to provide an excellent solution to many of the problems posed by managing type 1 diabetes for sport and exercise, there are important practical considerations which need to be taken into account. Insulin pump therapy is expensive to provide relative to MDI, with a significant initial outlay for the pump and then ongoing costs for consumables. Improving athletic performance may not be seen as an appropriate justification for the extra cost, although a reduction in hypoglycemia and improvement in metabolic control could be. While the pumps are robust, it may not be practical to wear them for some contact sports because of the risk of damage even if they are carried in a protective case. There are some reports that newer patch pumps can be placed in locations on the body where they are protected from damage (e.g., the inner thigh), but these may not always be ideal locations for insulin delivery. Participation in sport may also increase the risk of cannula displacement, which carries the risk of ketoacidosis if not detected early enough. Not all pumps are adequately waterproof for swimming, and increased exposure to treated swimming pool water or seawater may reduce the useful life of any waterproof seals. The risk to the pump can be reduced by keeping it in a waterproof container while in the water, but this reduces access to the pump and may result in excessive bulkiness.

5.7   Summary and Practical Advice

The importance of insulin in the regulation of fuel production during exercise means that there is a significant risk of dysglycemia during exercise in type 1 diabetes where insulin is exogenously administered. The flexibility in basal insulin infusion afforded by CSII is an attractive solution to the problem of hypoglycemia with aerobic exercise, in theory at least allowing the person with diabetes to approximate more closely the metabolic state during exercise which is seen in those without diabetes. In doing this, it is hoped that performance will be optimized.

It seems likely that insulin infusion rates should be reduced prior to exercise, as circulating insulin levels at the start of exercise are a predictor of hypoglycemia during exercise. Exactly when such a reduction should be made is not clear. For practical purposes, based on the pharmacokinetics of the rapid-acting analogue insulins used in CSII therapy, the reduction should probably be made 30–45 min prior to the start of exercise. The exact amount by which basal infusion should be reduced is also not clear, but based on available evidence, it is likely to be somewhere between 50% and 100% (i.e., cessation of basal insulin infusion). It is not clear when a normal basal rate should be restarted, but doing so at the end of exercise may reduce the risk of postexercise hyperglycemia (although, as detailed below, later reductions may be required for the avoidance of nocturnal hypoglycemia). Complete removal of the insulin pump at the start of aerobic exercise is a strategy that will help avoid hypoglycemia, but at the expense of hyperglycemia. It is possible that this will result in an impairment of athletic performance and, therefore, may be the best strategy for those in whom the avoidance of hypoglycemia is the paramount consideration, but not for those in whom performance is of greater importance.

CGM can provide useful information regarding the direction of change of blood glucose levels during exercise, although when using standard real-time CGM, there is still a significant risk of hypoglycemia in aerobic exercise when blood glucose levels fall rapidly. Strategies are being developed to help mitigate this risk. Low-glucose thresholds need to be set significantly higher than the minimum glucose level hoped for, with benefit seen for alarms used to trigger carbohydrate replacement and checking of capillary glucose when glucose falls to 5.5 mmol/l. An algorithm used to guide carbohydrate replacement taking into account both the level of interstitial glucose and its rate of change may point the way to how CGM technology could best be employed in the future to help avoid hypoglycemia during exercise.

Nocturnal hypoglycemia following exercise is a well-recognized phenomenon in type 1 diabetes. Reducing the CSII basal rate by 20% between 9 p.m. and 3 a.m. has been shown to reduce the risk of this in children without increasing the risk of morning hyperglycemia. This result may well transfer to adults, although the timing of the reduction may need to be altered due to adults going to sleep later in the day. Low-glucose suspend insulin pumps have been shown to be useful in reducing nocturnal hypoglycemia in those most at risk of this, and this may also be a useful technique to avoid nocturnal hypoglycemia following exercise.

Augmenting the counterregulatory hormone response to exercise offers an alternative means of avoiding hypoglycemia which can help avoid the significant planning often required for the adjustment of insulin doses. It may also help avoid, or at least reduce, the need for extra carbohydrate supplementation which can be problematic if one of the aims of exercise is weight control. A 10-s maximal effort sprint either immediately before or after exercise attenuates a postexercise fall in blood glucose. While it has not been shown to attenuate the fall in glucose during exercise, this was tested during exercise in conditions of hyperglycemia when carbohydrate oxidation is favored. High doses of caffeine have also been shown to reduce the need for carbohydrate supplementation to avoid hypoglycemia during exercise.

5.8   Areas for Future Research

Further research is needed to identify the optimal way to manage CSII for exercise. A clearer understanding of the pharmacokinetics and pharmacodynamics of rapid-acting insulin analogues when used for CSII will be useful to underpin this. Further research is required to identify both the optimal time to alter basal insulin rate prior to exercise and also to identify exactly what this alteration should be to permit athletes with diabetes to optimize their performance. It would also be helpful to test whether restarting the normal basal rate prior to finishing an exercise session would avoid postexercise hyperglycemia and may permit greater reductions to (or even cessation of) basal insulin infusion to be made prior to exercise without subsequent hyperglycemia. It may well be that the alterations to basal rate which provide the best approximation to normal physiology will provide the optimum means of managing CSII for exercise, but this also requires further testing.

More detailed analysis of strategies using CGM to guide carbohydrate replacement during exercise is required to see whether the early promise shown by these strategies can be fulfilled. The use of low-glucose suspend technology to avoid nocturnal hypoglycemia following exercise should also be assessed, as well as the effect this has on the counterregulatory response to any subsequent exercise. Assessment of the effect of the 10-s maximal sprint during euglycemic exercise would be interesting, to see whether such a strategy might be able to protect against the fall in blood glucose in these conditions. Similarly, using other means to augment the counterregulatory hormone response to exercise might also offer further strategies to help avoid hypoglycemia during exercise without the requirement for significant carbohydrate ingestion.

5.9   Conclusions

The ability to adjust basal insulin infusion rates in CSII therapy means that, in our clinic, we now class CSII therapy as the gold standard in athletes with diabetes where it is practical. It is difficult to assess blood glucose levels accurately with

CGM during a period of rapid change (such as during exercise), meaning that closed-loop insulin delivery is likely to remain difficult in this context for some time. However, current knowledge permits individuals to develop extremely successful strategies for the management of diabetes for sport and exercise using CSII. Real-time CGM is likely to play an increasingly important role in this, permitting accurate carbohydrate replacement based on individual requirements. Managing diabetes for sport and exercise is not easy, but improvements in the available technology and our understanding of how best to use it can only help to increase the numbers of successful athletes with diabetes.

References

1. Heise T, Nosek L, Ronn BB, Endahl L, Heinemann L, Kapitza C, et al. Lower within-subject variability of insulin detemir in comparison to NPH insulin and insulin glargine in people with type 1 diabetes. Diabetes. 2004;53(6):1614–20.
2. Lepore M, Pampanelli S, Fanelli C, Porcellati F, Bartocci L, Di VA, et al. Pharmacokinetics and pharmacodynamics of subcutaneous injection of long-acting human insulin analog glargine, NPH insulin, and ultralente human insulin and continuous subcutaneous infusion of insulin lispro. Diabetes. 2000;49(12):2142–8.
3. Ratner RE, Hirsch IB, Neifing JL, Garg SK, Mecca TE, Wilson CA. Less hypoglycemia with insulin glargine in intensive insulin therapy for type 1 diabetes. U.S. Study Group of Insulin Glargine in Type 1 Diabetes. Diabetes Care. 2000;23(5):639–43.
4. Hermansen K, Fontaine P, Kukolja KK, Peterkova V, Leth G, Gall MA. Insulin analogues (insulin detemir and insulin aspart) versus traditional human insulins (NPH insulin and regular human insulin) in basal-bolus therapy for patients with type 1 diabetes. Diabetologia. 2004;47(4):622–9.
5. Petersen KF, Price TB, Bergeron R. Regulation of net hepatic glycogenolysis and gluconeogenesis during exercise: impact of type 1 diabetes. J Clin Endocrinol Metab. 2004;89(9):4656–64.
6. Riddell M, Perkins BA. Exercise and glucose metabolism in persons with diabetes mellitus: perspectives on the role for continuous glucose monitoring. J Diabetes Sci Technol. 2009;3(4):914–23.
7. Marliss EB, Vranic M. Intense exercise has unique effects on both insulin release and its roles in glucoregulation: implications for diabetes. Diabetes. 2002;51 Suppl 1:S271–83.
8. Brazeau AS, Rabasa-Lhoret R, Strychar I, Mircescu H. Barriers to physical activity among patients with type 1 diabetes. Diabetes Care. 2008;31(11):2108–9.
9. Riddell MC, Milliken J. Preventing exercise-induced hypoglycemia in type 1 diabetes using real-time continuous glucose monitoring and a new carbohydrate intake algorithm: an observational field study. Diabetes Technol Ther. 2011;13(8):819–25.
10. Edelmann E, Staudner V, Bachmann W, Walter H, Haas W, Mehnert H. Exercise-induced hypoglycaemia and subcutaneous insulin infusion. Diabet Med. 1986;3(6):526–31.
11. Sonnenberg GE, Kemmer FW, Berger M. Exercise in type 1 (insulin-dependent) diabetic patients treated with continuous subcutaneous insulin infusion. Prevention of exercise induced hypoglycaemia. Diabetologia. 1990;33(11):696–703.
12. Admon G, Weinstein Y, Falk B, Weintrob N, Benzaquen H, Ofan R, et al. Exercise with and without an insulin pump among children and adolescents with type 1 diabetes mellitus. Pediatrics. 2005;116(3):e348–55.
13. Tsalikian E, Kollman C, Tamborlane WB, Beck RW, Fiallo-Scharer R, Fox L, et al. Prevention of hypoglycemia during exercise in children with type 1 diabetes by suspending basal insulin. Diabetes Care. 2006;29(10):2200–4.

14. Heise T, Nosek L, Spitzer H, Heinemann L, Niemoller E, Frick AD, et al. Insulin glulisine: a faster onset of action compared with insulin lispro. Diabetes Obes Metab. 2007;9(5):746–53.

15. Arnolds S, Rave K, Hovelmann U, Fischer A, Sert-Langeron C, Heise T. Insulin glulisine has a faster onset of action compared with insulin aspart in healthy volunteers. Exp Clin Endocrinol Diabetes. 2010;118(9):662–4.

16. Battelino T, Phillip M, Bratina N, Nimri R, Oskarsson P, Bolinder J. Effect of continuous glucose monitoring on hypoglycemia in type 1 diabetes. Diabetes Care. 2011;34(4):795–800.

17. Juvenile Diabetes Research Foundation Continuous Glucose Monitoring Study Group. Effectiveness of continuous glucose monitoring in a clinical care environment: evidence from the Juvenile Diabetes Research Foundation continuous glucose monitoring (JDRF-CGM) trial. Diabetes Care. 2010;33(1):17–22.

18. Iscoe KE, Campbell JE, Jamnik V, Perkins BA, Riddell MC. Efficacy of continuous real-time blood glucose monitoring during and after prolonged high-intensity cycling exercise: spinning with a continuous glucose monitoring system. Diabetes Technol Ther. 2006;8(6):627–35.

19. Wilson DM, Beck RW, Tamborlane WV, Dontchev MJ, Kollman C, Chase P, et al. The accuracy of the FreeStyle Navigator continuous glucose monitoring system in children with type 1 diabetes. Diabetes Care. 2007;30(1):59–64.

20. Boyne MS, Silver DM, Kaplan J, Saudek CD. Timing of changes in interstitial and venous blood glucose measured with a continuous subcutaneous glucose sensor. Diabetes. 2003;52(11):2790–4.

21. Buckingham BA, Kollman C, Beck R, Kalajian A, Fiallo-Scharer R, Tansey MJ, et al. Evaluation of factors affecting CGMS calibration. Diabetes Technol Ther. 2006;8(3):318–25.

22. Iscoe KE, Davey RJ, Fournier PA. Increasing the low-glucose alarm of a continuous glucose monitoring system prevents exercise-induced hypoglycemia without triggering any false alarms. Diabetes Care. 2011;34(6):e109.

23. McMahon SK, Ferreira LD, Ratnam N, Davey RJ, Youngs LM, Davis EA, et al. Glucose requirements to maintain euglycemia after moderate-intensity afternoon exercise in adolescents with type 1 diabetes are increased in a biphasic manner. J Clin Endocrinol Metab. 2007;92(3):963–8.

24. Tsalikian E, Mauras N, Beck RW, Tamborlane WV, Janz KF, Chase HP, et al. Impact of exercise on overnight glycemic control in children with type 1 diabetes mellitus. J Pediatr. 2005;147(4):528–34.

25. Maran A, Pavan P, Bonsembiante B, Brugin E, Ermolao A, Avogaro A, et al. Continuous glucose monitoring reveals delayed nocturnal hypoglycemia after intermittent high-intensity exercise in nontrained patients with type 1 diabetes. Diabetes Technol Ther. 2010;12(10): 763–8.

26. Sandoval DA, Guy DL, Richardson MA, Ertl AC, Davis SN. Effects of low and moderate antecedent exercise on counterregulatory responses to subsequent hypoglycemia in type 1 diabetes. Diabetes. 2004;53(7):1798–806.

27. Taplin CE, Cobry E, Messer L, McFann K, Chase HP, Fiallo-Scharer R. Preventing post-exercise nocturnal hypoglycemia in children with type 1 diabetes. J Pediatr. 2010;157(5): 784–8.

28. Raju B, Arbelaez AM, Breckenridge SM, Cryer PE. Nocturnal hypoglycemia in type 1 diabetes: an assessment of preventive bedtime treatments. J Clin Endocrinol Metab. 2006;91(6): 2087–92.

29. Choudhary P, Shin J, Wang Y, Evans ML, Hammond PJ, Kerr D, et al. Insulin pump therapy with automated insulin suspension in response to hypoglycemia: reduction in nocturnal hypoglycemia in those at greatest risk. Diabetes Care. 2011;34(9):2023–5.

30. Galassetti P, Tate D, Neill RA, Richardson A, Leu SY, Davis SN. Effect of differing antecedent hypoglycemia on counterregulatory responses to exercise in type 1 diabetes. Am J Physiol Endocrinol Metab. 2006;290(6):E1109–17.

31. Bussau VA, Ferreira LD, Jones TW, Fournier PA. A 10-s sprint performed prior to moderate-intensity exercise prevents early post-exercise fall in glycaemia in individuals with type 1 diabetes. Diabetologia. 2007;50(9):1815–8.

32. Bussau VA, Ferreira LD, Jones TW, Fournier PA. The 10-s maximal sprint: a novel approach to counter an exercise-mediated fall in glycemia in individuals with type 1 diabetes. Diabetes Care. 2006;29(3):601–6.

33. Jenni S, Oetliker C, Allemann S, Ith M, Tappy L, Wuerth S, et al. Fuel metabolism during exercise in euglycaemia and hyperglycaemia in patients with type 1 diabetes mellitus–a prospective single-blinded randomised crossover trial. Diabetologia. 2008;51(8):1457–65.

34. Watson J, Kerr D. The best defense against hypoglycemia is to recognize it: is caffeine useful? Diabetes Technol Ther. 1999;1(2):193–200.

35. Richardson T, Thomas P, Ryder J, Kerr D. Influence of caffeine on frequency of hypoglycemia detected by continuous interstitial glucose monitoring system in patients with long-standing type 1 diabetes. Diabetes Care. 2005;28(6):1316–20.

36. Debrah K, Sherwin RS, Murphy J, Kerr D. Effect of caffeine on recognition of and physiological responses to hypoglycaemia in insulin-dependent diabetes. Lancet. 1996;347(8993): 19–24.

37. Gallen IW, Ballav C, Lumb AN, Carr J. Caffeine supplementation reduces exercise induced decline in blood glucose and subsequent hypoglycaemia in adults with type 1 diabetes (T1DM) treated with multiple daily insulin injection (MDI). Poster 1184-P presented at the 70th Scientific Sessions of the American Diabetes Association, Orlando, Florida: 25–29 June 2010.

Chapter 6
Hypoglycemia and Hypoglycemia Unawareness During and Following Exercise

Lisa M. Younk and Stephen N. Davis

6.1 Introduction

Attention to diet, including meal composition and timing, is integral to all athletes' training programs. Athletes with type 1 diabetes mellitus (type 1 DM) face the added task of administering insulin to carefully match energy availability and requirements. Avoiding both hyper- and hypoglycemia is a continual challenge for all patients with type 1 DM but is even more difficult for athletes who experience extreme changes in fuel utilization between periods of rest and exercise.

Hyperglycemia during exercise can be detrimental to performance. Insulin-induced hypoglycemia, however, not only hinders performance but also can render (uncommonly) seizure, coma, and/or death; and (more commonly) decreased quality of life and/or increased anxiety with regard to glycemic control.

Counterregulation is the term used to describe the systemic response to a blood glucose that falls below the body's normal postabsorptive level. The primary goal of counterregulation is to maintain an adequate supply of blood glucose to the brain. While this priority does not change during exercise, it is also important that the exercising muscle continues to receive enough substrate to maintain performance level. Counterregulation occurs in healthy individuals generally only during periods of fasting and exercise. Patients with type 1 DM rely on this response much more frequently, both during rest (regardless of absorptive state) and exercise, as hyperinsulinization

L.M. Younk, B.S.
Department of Medicine, University of Maryland School of Medicine,
10-055 Bressler Research Building, 655 W. Baltimore St., Baltimore, MD 21201, USA
e-mail: lyounk@medicine.umaryland.edu

S.N. Davis, M.B.B.S., FRCP, FACP (✉)
Department of Medicine, University of Maryland School of Medicine,
22 S. Greene Street, Room N3W42, Baltimore, MD 21201, USA
e-mail: sdavis@medicine.umaryland.edu

I. Gallen (ed.), *Type 1 Diabetes*,
DOI 10.1007/978-0-85729-754-9_6, © Springer-Verlag London Limited 2012

occurs as a result of the need to administer exogenous insulin that, to this day, does not adequately mimic physiological fluctuations in endogenous insulin secretion.

This chapter will describe and compare the counterregulatory responses that occur during hypoglycemia and exercise in healthy individuals and in individuals with type 1 DM. Factors that increase the risk for hypoglycemia will also be discussed with special attention to the risk associated with blunted counterregulation and hypoglycemia unawareness. A general overview of the current state of research regarding the causes of and treatments for these syndromes is provided. The chapter will conclude with clinical approaches to preventing and responding to an acute hypoglycemic event.

6.2 Normal (Nondiabetic) Cascade of Events During Hypoglycemia

Unlike muscle cells, which can modulate fuel selection among blood glucose, fatty acid, triglyceride, and/or glycogen metabolism, neurons rely, acutely, almost entirely on glucose transported from the bloodstream across the blood-brain barrier. Normal brain function is supported only within a narrow range of glucose levels. Thus, when blood glucose begins to fall, numerous changes occur throughout the body to maintain an adequate supply of substrate to the brain. Glucose uptake is inhibited peripherally, blood flow is shunted away from the splenic bed and skeletal muscle, and hepatic glucose production increases.

The counterregulatory response to acute hypoglycemia in healthy individuals primarily involves a decrease in insulin secretion, followed by increases in glucagon and epinephrine. Cortisol and growth hormone also increase during hypoglycemia but generally only gain importance during prolonged glucose deprivation. Stepped hyperinsulinemic hypoglycemic clamps (of decreasing glucose levels) have been used to investigate thresholds for the onset of counterregulatory hormones in healthy individuals [1–4]. Under resting conditions, insulin secretion decreases at ~4.5 mmol/l [1, 2]. Glucagon, epinephrine, growth hormone, cortisol, and pancreatic polypeptide (an indirect marker of parasympathetic activation) all increase ~3.6–3.9 mmol/l [1–5]. Muscle sympathetic nerve activity (MSNA; a direct, real-time measurement of sympathetic activation) increases between ~3.3 and 3.8 mmol/l [5]. These responses occur at similar thresholds between men and women albeit with lower levels of counterregulatory hormones generated in women [2, 5, 6]. The reason for these differences is not well understood, but increased levels of estrogen appear to play an important role [7].

Although the secretion of counterregulatory hormones is critical for the protection against hypoglycemia, it is ultimately an individual's symptoms – his or her perception of the physiological changes associated with hypoglycemia – that prompts ingestion of food and consequent cessation of counterregulation. Symptoms can be classified according to origin (see Table 6.1). Autonomic symptoms, also known as neurogenic symptoms, are adrenergic and cholinergic symptoms generated as a result of increased neural sympathetic activity and catecholamine release from the adrenal medulla. From studies in adrenalectomized patients, it appears that these symptoms arise primarily

Table 6.1 Symptoms of hypoglycemia

Autonomic/neurogenic	Neuroglycopenic	Unspecified
Sweaty	Confused, difficulty thinking/ concentrating	General malaise
Shaky, tremor, trembling	Blurry vision	Headache
Palpitations, pounding heart	Tired, drowsy	Nausea
Anxious, nervous	Difficulty speaking	
Tingling	Uncoordinated	
Hungry	Odd behavior	
	Weak	
	Dizzy	
	Warm	

from the sympathetic neural response [8], although in another study, adrenergic symptoms were correlated primarily with epinephrine levels [9]. Work from our laboratory has determined that during euglycemic conditions, epinephrine levels simulating those found during moderate hypoglycemia are responsible for ~20% of autonomic symptoms [10]. Sweating, shakiness/tremor/trembling, palpitations/pounding heart, anxiousness/nervousness, tingling, and hunger are typical autonomic symptoms experienced during hypoglycemia [8, 11]. Neuroglycopenic symptoms arise from the effects of low blood glucose in the brain per se and cannot be reduced by pharmacologic adrenergic or panautonomic blockade [12]. Included in this group are confusion/difficulty thinking or concentrating, blurred vision, tiredness/drowsiness, difficulty speaking, discoordination, odd behavior, weakness, dizziness, and warmness [11]. Neuroglycopenic symptoms intensify as blood glucose continues to fall, progressing to severe cognitive dysfunction if hypoglycemia is not treated. In addition to the autonomic and neuroglycopenic symptoms described above, patients may also detect a feeling of general malaise, which could include headache and/or nausea [13]. Emotional responses may also increase [14] along with a shift in general mood states during hypoglycemia.

In healthy people, the threshold for autonomic and neuroglycopenic symptoms can be slightly variable [15] but is generally ~3.0 mmol/l. Cognitive dysfunction arises ~2.6 mmol/l [1–4]. Although men tend to have a more robust counterregulatory response to hypoglycemia, symptoms do not appear to follow a pattern of sexual dimorphism, with similar symptom scores reported by both genders during equivalent levels of hypoglycemia [2, 5, 6, 16].

6.3 Counterregulation During Exercise

During moderate exercise, similar to hypoglycemia, a decrement in insulin and an increment in glucagon occur, stimulating glucose production to prevent a fall in blood glucose level [17, 18]. When somatostatin, insulin, and glucagon are infused into healthy individuals to prevent changes in hormone levels during exercise, blood glucose falls from 5.5 to 3.4 mmol/l [19]. Likewise, when only insulin is allowed to decrease or only glucagon is allowed to increase, blood glucose still falls. Only when both actions happen is euglycemia maintained. However, because the fall in glucose is still rescued at mild levels of hypoglycemia when insulin and/or glucagon is held constant, it is clear that other hormones are also involved in counterregulation during exercise [19]. In fact, epinephrine and norepinephrine are both important for enhancing glucose production and for limiting the increase in glucose uptake that occurs during exercise [20]. When α-/β- (alpha-/beta-) adrenergic blockade is imposed during exercise in healthy individuals, blood glucose falls as a result of increased glucose utilization but is eventually rescued by decreased insulin secretion and increased glucagon secretion [20]. Preventing catecholamine action and changes in insulin and glucagon through adrenergic blockade and somatostatin infusion causes a precipitous fall in blood glucose during exercise due to diminished glucose production and an early exaggerated increase in noninsulin-mediated glucose utilization [20, 21]. As such, insulin, glucagon, and catecholamines are the primary hormonal regulators of glucose levels during moderate exercise. Sympathetic neural norepinephrine may be the primary glucoregulatory catecholamine during exercise, as opposed to epinephrine during hypoglycemia [20].

When euglycemia is maintained during exercise, a robust counterregulatory response still occurs, as indicated by significant rises in epinephrine and norepinephrine. This suggests that mechanisms that induce hormone secretion during exercise may be at least partially independent of those responsible for counterregulation during resting hypoglycemia [22]. The counterregulatory response to exercise becomes much more intense if blood glucose does fall below fasting levels. Sotsky et al. [22] reported that glucagon, cortisol, norepinephrine, epinephrine, and growth hormone all increased to a significantly greater degree during hypoglycemic exercise compared to euglycemic exercise.

The hormonal response to intense exercise (>80% VO_{2max}) – such as occurs in short bursts in many sports – is much different from the response during moderate exercise. Rather than insulin and glucagon regulating glucose levels, catecholamines are the primary mediators of glucose production and uptake, increasing 14- to 18-fold during intense exercise [23, 24]. Such increases drive a huge increase in glucose rate of appearance (R_a) as glucose is mobilized through hepatic glycogenolysis. Glucose rate of disappearance (R_d) also increases, although to a lesser degree, as catecholamines also stimulate muscle glycogenolysis which moderates glucose uptake. The disproportionate rise in glucose R_a compared to R_d results in hyperglycemia, but insulin concentration during exercise does not change dramatically. Upon cessation of exercise though, catecholamine levels quickly decrease, while insulin increases drastically for up to 60 min to reverse hyperglycemia [24, 25].

6.4   Impaired Cascade of Events in Type 1 Diabetes During Hypoglycemia and Exercise

People with type 1 DM have multiple impairments in the counterregulatory response to hypoglycemia and exercise, placing them at high risk of severe hypoglycemia. Endogenous insulin secretion is absent, and therefore, systemic insulin levels maintained by exogenous delivery cannot be decreased despite changes in energy demand. In some studies, careful replacement of insulin to maintain euglycemia or to allow very slight increases in blood glucose (.5 mmol/l rise in blood glucose during 30 min of exercise) did not cause hypoglycemia during exercise [26, 27]. However, in another study, when basal insulin was infused to generate similar levels of free insulin in healthy controls and type 1 DM, blood glucose fell further in type 1 DM than controls, likely due to other defects in counterregulation [28].

Beyond the first few years of onset of type 1 DM, the glucagon response to hypoglycemia is lost [29, 30]. The mechanism of this defect remains under investigation, but the impairment could be a result of a lack of change in intra-islet insulin concentrations which may be necessary in order to trigger pancreatic α (alpha)-cell glucagon secretion. In support of this theory, infusion of a sulfonylurea into healthy people during a hyperinsulinemic-hypoglycemic glucose clamp to induce a hyperinsulinemic environment within the islet cells resulted in diminished glucagon secretion [31]. In a second study [32], somatostatin was infused to block insulin secretion in healthy people prior to a hyperinsulinemic-hypoglycemic glucose clamp. This prevented a fall in intra-islet insulin concentration upon onset of hypoglycemia. Upon cessation of somatostatin infusion during the clamp glucagon levels increased but were blunted by 30%. The glucagon response to exercise is retained, however, in type 1 DM [26, 33], suggesting a divergence in the signaling mechanisms that control glucagon secretion during hypoglycemia and exercise.

Increments in epinephrine are generally blunted in type 1 DM, both during hypoglycemia and exercise. When controls and type 1 DM exercised at 60–65% VO_{2max} for 60 min at similar blood glucose levels, the epinephrine and norepinephrine response to the ambient hypoglycemia was significantly lower in type 1 DM than in controls [28]. Even when controls exercised at euglycemia, the epinephrine and norepinephrine response tended to be greater compared to type 1 DM subjects exercising under hypoglycemic conditions.

Failure of either the glucagon or the epinephrine response can be mostly compensated for by secretion of the other hormone. Failure of both hormones to increase in response to exercise, however, will result in hypoglycemia in healthy individuals [20]. Moreover, even with an intact glucagon and epinephrine response during exercise, excessive insulin can blunt hepatic glucose production and increase muscle glucose uptake, increasing the risk of hypoglycemia.

Unlike moderate exercise, patients with type 1 DM can mount a normal response to intense exercise as glucoregulation under these conditions is driven primarily by release of catecholamines. The challenge becomes the fact that hyperglycemia arises during intense exercise that requires increments in insulin during the postexercise period. Unless adequate rapid-acting insulin is injected to mimic the normal hyperinsulinemic response in nondiabetic individuals, there will be a prolonged period of hyperglycemia, which carries with it deleterious effects on overall glycemic control and long-term health [34, 35].

6.5 Additional Risk for Hypoglycemia During and After Exercise

In light of an inability to decrease insulin levels and the presence of an altered counterregulatory response, a number of factors further influence the risk of hypoglycemia during exercise in type 1 DM. These factors affect insulin requirements, counterregulatory responses, and symptom identification. Excess insulin and inadequate carbohydrate supplementation and lack of blood glucose monitoring are the primary factors that potentiate the risk of hypoglycemia. Beyond the scope of this chapter, these topics are covered extensively in Chaps. 3, 5, and 7.

6.5.1 Variability in Insulin Uptake and Action

Exogenously administered insulin has intrinsic intra- and interindividual variability in uptake and action [36]. Newer insulin analogs including long-acting (e.g., glargine, detemir) and rapid-acting (e.g., aspart, lispro, glulisine) formulations do however offer less variability and lower risk of hypoglycemia than older treatment options (e.g., NPH, regular) [37–39].

Intramuscular insulin injection exacerbates variability, significantly increasing insulin absorption rate, especially during exercise, resulting in higher free insulin levels and greater insulin action. The difference is likely due to a fivefold increase in skeletal muscle blood flow during exercise, whereas adipose tissue blood flow does not appear to change significantly [40]. There has been a trend toward shorter, smaller-gauge needles since the introduction of subcutaneous insulin injection, thereby reducing the risk of intramuscular injection.

The site at which insulin is injected can also contribute to variability in insulin uptake and action. During leg exercise, absorption of rapid-acting insulin injected into the leg is increased compared to insulin injected into the arm or the abdomen, resulting in higher peak insulin levels and greater decreases in blood glucose [41, 42]. Arm and abdominal injection decreased the risk of hypoglycemia by 57 and 89% [41]. Variable thicknesses of subcutaneous tissue at different sites are likely responsible for variations in insulin absorption, with lower absorption rates occurring in areas where thickness is increased. Some have suggested that this is a function of subcutaneous blood flow, which also decreases with increasing thickness [43], but others have not been able to confirm this [42].

6.5.2 Exercise Duration and Intensity

Both the duration and intensity of exercise will greatly influence insulin and carbohydrate requirements before, during, and after exercise. Perhaps the greatest variability occurs between moderate and intense exercise. As described above, intense exercise generates hyperglycemia, which requires a sustained elevated glucose R_d after exercise to return glucose levels back down to postabsorptive levels. As this requires physiological hyperinsulinemia [34], athletes with type 1 DM may need to cover this postexercise hyperglycemia with extra insulin [35]. This strategy must be carried out carefully, as counterregulation is blunted by exercise and insulin sensitivity is increased, making them vulnerable to hypoglycemia. Repeated bouts of intense exercise can further exacerbate glucose control. The hyperglycemic response to repeated bouts of intense exercise performed after brief rest intervals (5 min) can be additive [23]. If rest periods are longer (i.e., 1 h), the responses to each bout are largely independent of each other in healthy individuals, although hyperglycemia may be lower during repetitions [24]. In type 1 DM however, this pattern may not be so clear, as hyperglycemia from the first bout of exercise could still be present if not sufficiently corrected between bouts.

6.5.3 Temperature

Increased ambient temperature causes increases in skin temperature and enhanced subcutaneous blood flow, which can in turn accelerate insulin absorption [44, 45]. At rest, warmer room temperature (30°C) was associated with a three- to fivefold increase in insulin levels and correspondingly lower blood glucose levels compared to cooler room temperature (10°C). This effect was maintained during exercise, causing larger decrements in blood glucose [46].

Temperature increases can also increase workload (as indicated by increased heart rate and lactate levels), causing a greater reliance on counterregulatory hormones, including cortisol, epinephrine, and norepinephrine [47–49]. Similarly, swimming in cold water can also result in enhanced release of catecholamines, likely as a result of thermoreception [49].

Thermoregulation in cold environments can be compromised by hypoglycemia. Hypoglycemia was induced in healthy men in a cool room (18–19°C) with air blowing to cause sustained shivering [50]. When blood glucose fell to 2.5 mmol/l, shivering subsided and subjects did not feel cold. Despite the cool environment, hypoglycemia-induced peripheral vasodilation and sweating occurred, allowing skin and core temperature to fall to the point that subjects required rewarming. Reciprocally, the colder environment hampered recovery from hypoglycemia.

6.5.4 Age

In healthy older individuals, a greater stimulus may be required for release of glucagon and epinephrine compared to younger people (2.8 versus 3.3 mmol/l) [51]. Hormonal responses to mild hypoglycemia can be less robust as well [51, 52]. These differences disappear at 2.8 mmol/l, indicating that deeper hypoglycemia can still elicit a normal counterregulatory response [52]. However, symptom scores are lower in older versus younger adults during hypoglycemia even when counterregulation is of similar magnitude [53]. Autonomic symptoms appear to be primarily impaired, while neuroglycopenic symptoms remain relatively intact [51]. Thus, diminished symptoms and attenuated counterregulatory responses at milder hypoglycemia mean that older athletes may be more susceptible to larger falls in blood glucose. However, although specific studies of hormonal responses to exercise in older adults with type 1 DM are lacking, healthy older adults are able to mount a similar hormonal response to submaximal exercise as their younger counterparts of similar training level [54]. Deficits did arise in the lactate, growth hormone, and cortisol response to maximal exercise in the older individuals, although the repercussions of such declines are not completely clear.

6.5.5   Increased Insulin Sensitivity

The risk of hypoglycemia is increased immediately and several hours following an exercise session [55]. The more immediate effects of exercise upon glucose uptake and utilization are independent of insulin and are mediated by lasting effects of contraction-stimulated glucose uptake [56, 57]. The increased risk of hypoglycemia beyond the first few hours after exercise is primarily a result of increased insulin sensitivity, which may vary according to duration and intensity of the exercise [56]. Insulin-mediated glucose uptake was increased in healthy, untrained men immediately and 48 h following 60 min of cycle ergometer exercise [58]. Effects are localized, as increases in insulin-stimulated glucose uptake are specific to the exercised muscles [59, 60]. The increased insulin sensitivity is largely a result of a reduced K_m, wherein a lower concentration of insulin is required to induce half-maximal glucose uptake [61]. While some have suggested that glycogen depletion and consequent increased glycogen synthase activity are responsible for driving increases in insulin sensitivity [58, 62], it now seems more likely that enhanced GLUT4 translocation and possibly microvascular perfusion are responsible for these changes. GLUT4 translocation may be regulated by distal portions of the insulin signaling pathway [57]. Clinically, these findings are supported by the fact that extra carbohydrate needs to be taken [63] and/or insulin doses need to be reduced [64, 65] before, during, and following exercise to prevent postexercise hypoglycemia. As a caveat, in a study of marathoners with type 1 DM, whole-body glucose disposal and glucose oxidation rates were decreased despite increased glycogen synthase activity following a competitive marathon [66]. This apparent reduction in insulin sensitivity was attributed to dramatically increased lipid oxidation rates that were observed postexercise. Additionally, muscle damage such as that induced by eccentric contractions can cause insulin resistance [67] due to decreased GLUT4 transcription [68] and/or impaired proximal insulin signaling [69]. Therefore, athletes will need to modify insulin and diet regimens according to variations in workouts and competitions.

Special care may need to be taken to prevent postexercise hypoglycemia in those who participate in afternoon or evening exercise. Glucose requirements following exercise exhibit a biphasic pattern, with increases occurring both immediately and 7–11 h after exercise [70, 71]. Thus, the risk of hypoglycemia is elevated during hours of sleep.

6.5.6 Impaired Symptom Identification

Recognizing a symptom, or perceiving a change in physiological state, is only part of the battle in responding appropriately to hypoglycemia. A person may identify a symptom but still fail to associate that symptom with hypoglycemia. A number of factors can influence a person's ability to rationally establish a link between the symptom and the cause [72]. Specific to athletes, feelings generally associated with hypoglycemia can be masked by normal sympathetic neural and sympathoadrenal responses to exercise. Sweating, for example, is a normal response to both stimuli. Shivering or a cold sweat following exercise in cool environment (i.e., cold water or air) may be interpreted as a normal response, but such physiological responses may also occur during hypoglycemia. Exercise and competition also can cause anxiety, increased heart rate, and fatigue. However, in a study by Nermoen et al. [73], patients exercising at 50% of their maximal heart rate reported symptoms of hypoglycemia during hypoglycemia (2 mmol/l) but not during euglycemia, indicating that the symptoms were actually discernable from those occurring in response to exercise. Symptoms also arose at higher blood glucose levels compared to when hypoglycemia was induced with the subjects lying in bed. As the authors pointed out though, exercise of higher intensity than experienced in the study could obscure the perception of hypoglycemia-associated changes. Moreover, despite altered symptom thresholds in the study, only 6 of 10 subjects answered "yes" when asked if they felt hypoglycemic during hypoglycemic exercise, indicating a disconnect between identification of symptoms and identification of hypoglycemia.

6.5.7 Hypoglycemia-Associated Autonomic Failure and Impaired Hypoglycemia Unawareness

6.5.7.1 Background

While excess insulin levels certainly can cause hypoglycemia, it is often the failure of counterregulatory responses and/or an impaired ability to detect a low blood sugar (hypoglycemia unawareness) that permits the onset of severe hypoglycemia in patients with diabetes. Although overt diabetic autonomic neuropathy (DAN) has been associated with blunted epinephrine and symptom responses to hypoglycemia and exercise [74–76], blunted hormone and symptom responses have been observed in patients without DAN as well [28, 77–81]. Studies have shown that counterregulatory responses during exercise in this population are qualitatively similar but quantitatively reduced compared to healthy individuals [6, 28, 82]. Therefore, it is likely that although DAN contributes to impaired counterregulation and hypoglycemia unawareness [83], a separate condition is responsible for these defects in patients who lack even subclinical DAN [84].

It was observed that patients who suffered from recurring hypoglycemia also exhibited impaired secretion of glucagon, epinephrine, and growth hormone in response to insulin-induced hypoglycemia [85, 86]. This led to the hypothesis that hypoglycemia could be the initial event responsible for impaired counterregulation. It is now widely appreciated that previous autonomic activation (i.e., during hypoglycemia or exercise) is a principal precipitating event for blunted counterregulatory responses to subsequent hypoglycemia and exercise in type 1 DM [79]. This effect has been termed hypoglycemia-associated autonomic failure or HAAF [87]. HAAF is differentiated from DAN, in that the former does not necessarily affect key measures of cardiovascular autonomic function used to assess subclinical or overt DAN, including heart rate variability during deep breathing [88]. Furthermore, a prior hypoglycemic stimulus in healthy nondiabetic people can also blunt glucose counterregulation during hypoglycemia, indicating that blunting effects can occur completely independently of the diabetic disease state [89–91].

To substantiate and elaborate upon the theory of HAAF, researchers have used insulin infusion tests and the hyperinsulinemic glucose clamp technique to experimentally induce and measure the effects of recurrent hypoglycemia in healthy, type 1, and type 2 DM individuals. These studies have uncovered a number of key findings. In healthy individuals, repeated hypoglycemia blunts glucagon, epinephrine, norepinephrine, cortisol, growth hormone, and pancreatic polypeptide responses to hypoglycemia [89, 90]. The blunting of epinephrine and pancreatic polypeptide indicates that both sympathetic and parasympathetic activities, respectively, are attenuated during repeated hypoglycemia. In addition to reduced hormonal responses, metabolic responses (glucose R_a and free fatty acid mobilization) as well as neurogenic and neuroglycopenic symptoms are significantly reduced in healthy individuals during repeated hypoglycemia. Furthermore, the blood glucose levels at which responses are initiated are reset so that blood glucose must fall further in order to induce counterregulation [90, 91].

These findings have been extended to patients with type 1 DM, who also exhibit reduced epinephrine, pancreatic polypeptide, and symptom responses to hypoglycemia along with altered glycemic thresholds after repeated hypoglycemia [79, 92]. Taken together, the above observations promote the unifying concept that multiple factors that contribute to risk of recurring hypoglycemia – blunted counterregulatory responses, hypoglycemia unawareness, and altered counterregulatory thresholds – are largely the result of antecedent hypoglycemia [79, 92]. Importantly, hypoglycemia-induced blunting of counterregulation is not simply an acute phenomenon. When investigators induced hypoglycemia in patients with type 1 DM for 2 h twice a week for 1 month, blunting effects similar to those described above were still significant at the end of the trial [93].

The depth of antecedent hypoglycemia affects the degree to which counterregulation is blunted during subsequent hypoglycemia [94]. In healthy males, two 2-h bouts of hypoglycemia (one morning and one afternoon) at 3.9 mmol/l induced blunting of epinephrine, MSNA, and glucagon during next day hypoglycemia (2.9 mmol/l). When first day hypoglycemia was set at 3.3 or 2.9 mmol/l, norepinephrine, growth hormone, and pancreatic polypeptide responses were also blunted, as well as endogenous glucose production and lipolysis.

The duration of the hypoglycemic stimulus is also of importance. In nondiabetic subjects, two 5-min or 30-min bouts of hypoglycemia blunted hormonal responses to next day hypoglycemia quite similarly to two 2-h bouts of antecedent hypoglycemia [95]. This finding is of clinical significance, as patients who successfully detect and correct a low blood sugar quickly should be aware that their bodies' responses to subsequent bouts of hypoglycemia may still be impaired. Interestingly, the shorter bouts of hypoglycemia did not blunt symptom responses. However, it is unknown whether multiple days of short duration hypoglycemia could become more problematic, eventually blunting symptoms as well.

Even more relevant to athletes with type 1 DM, researchers have found that hypoglycemia and exercise reciprocally blunt counterregulatory responses. Thus, in healthy people and patients with type 1 DM, antecedent hypoglycemia blunts the primary neuroendocrine and metabolic responses to exercise [96, 97]. Similar to above, the depth of antecedent hypoglycemia dose-dependently blunts these responses, with lower blood glucose causing greater blunting effects, which become most apparent after 30 min of exercise [82].

Vice versa, counterregulation during hypoglycemia is blunted by antecedent exercise in a quantitatively similar fashion as antecedent hypoglycemia (see Fig. 6.1). In healthy individuals, day 1 exercise (two 90-min bouts) blunted glucagon, epinephrine, norepinephrine, growth hormone, pancreatic polypeptide, MSNA, and endogenous glucose production responses to day 2 hypoglycemia [98]. When patients with type 1 DM exercised in the morning, epinephrine, MSNA, and endogenous glucose production were blunted during a hypoglycemic clamp in the afternoon of the same day [99].

In the above exercise studies, subjects exercised at ~50% VO_{2max}. It has now been shown that exercise at even 30% VO_{2max} is sufficient to blunt neuroendocrine and metabolic counterregulatory responses during hypoglycemia in type 1 DM [100]. Similar studies of higher exercise intensities are sparse. Because high-intensity exercise causes an increase in blood glucose, some investigators have studied the postexercise glycemic effects of adding bouts of intermittent high-intensity exercise (IHE) during moderate-intensity exercise. In one such study [101], 2 h after 30 min of moderate exercise with IHE, blood glucose was higher in the IHE group compared to a group that exercised continuously at moderate intensity (MOD). However, during sleeping hours, blood glucose levels were significantly lower and hypoglycemia occurred more frequently in the IHE group. Contrarily, other researchers [102] found that nocturnal glucose levels were higher and hypoglycemia was less frequent following IHE compared to MOD. Importantly, in this study, there was a late decrease in blood glucose at ~6 a.m. in the IHE group, suggesting that increased

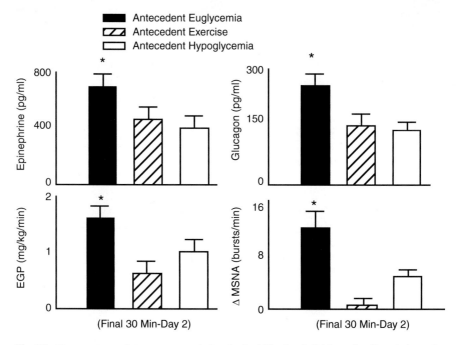

Fig. 6.1 Key counterregulatory responses during the final 30 min of a 2-h hyperinsulinemic-hypogly-cemic (~3.0 mmol/l) glucose clamp on the morning following previous day euglycemia (*solid bars*), exercise (*hatched bars*), and hypoglycemia (*open bars*). Antecedent euglycemia and hypoglycemia studies consisted of two 2-h clamps in the morning and afternoon of day 1. Antecedent exercise con-sisted of two 90-min bouts of moderate intensity (50% VO$_{2max}$) cycling exercise in the morning and afternoon of day 1. *MSNA* muscle sympathetic nerve activity, *EGP* endogenous glucose production; *$p < 0.05$ for antecedent euglycemia versus antecedent hypoglycemia and exercise [98] (Reprinted by permission of the publisher from Galassetti [98], The American Physiological Society)

insulin sensitivity might still occur, albeit in a delayed fashion, after this form of exercise. The discrepancy in findings could be due to several factors. The type of IHE differed between studies, and the former study recruited untrained subjects while trained athletes were studied in the latter. Indeed, trained athletes have altered hormonal and metabolic responses during exercise that could account for differ-ences in the glycemic responses described above and may even have an altered susceptibility to HAAF. Further research is needed to clarify these issues and to determine the underlying metabolic and hormonal factors that contribute to the altered glycemic trends following IHE. Studies of the blunting effects on counter-regulation in type 1 DM athletes are also needed. This information could be critical to both a deeper understanding of the mechanisms of HAAF and the development of better hypoglycemia prevention strategies in athletes with type 1 DM who often exercise at intensities well above 50% VO$_{2max}$.

Nonetheless, the above information illustrates the need for athletes with type 1 DM to pay consistent attention to fluctuations in blood glucose, before, during, and after exercise, both for safety and performance reasons. Sleep is a key period of vulnerability in type 1 DM, with higher rates of prolonged hypoglycemia observed during nighttime than during the day [103–105]. While the mechanism responsible for the increased frequency of severe hypoglycemia during sleep remains to be characterized, it is known that epinephrine, cortisol, and pancreatic polypeptide responses to hypoglycemia during sleep are delayed and reduced in people with type 1 DM [106–108]. Perhaps due to the reduced hormonal response, patients are less likely to awaken during an episode of hypoglycemia [106], preventing them from taking corrective measures. In athletes who have exercised in the previous days, these altered responses will be superimposed upon the blunted responses and increased insulin sensitivity associated with antecedent exercise, exacerbating the risk of hypoglycemia. Despite attenuated counterregulation and lack of awareness during sleep, nocturnal hypoglycemia still blunts counterregulatory hormone and symptom responses to next day hypoglycemia [109, 110]. Therefore, devising strategies to detect low blood glucose levels during the night will not only increase safety during sleep but also will provide information critical to controlling blood glucose in the day ahead.

As noted above, impaired hypoglycemia awareness is often coincident with blunted counterregulation. In fact, the two phenomena are significantly associated [78]. In a study of healthy people and patients with and without a history of hypoglycemia unawareness, a delayed sympathoadrenal response was observed only in those with hypoglycemia unawareness [111]. In diabetes, the glycemic threshold for autonomic symptoms is widely variable and subject to change. Impairment of hypoglycemia awareness occurs along a continuum, with gradually decreasing intensity and/or number of symptoms [81]. Under poor glucose control, symptoms occur at higher blood glucose levels [112]. Conversely, tight glycemic control (often accompanied by increased frequency of hypoglycemia) can cause the threshold for symptoms to be significantly downshifted to lower blood glucose levels [113]. This circumstance is cause for concern, as the thresholds for the onset of symptoms and cognitive dysfunction can become superimposed or even reversed. In subjects with intensively treated diabetes or insulinoma, the onset of autonomic and neuroglycopenic symptoms occurred ~2.0–2.3 mmol/l, compared to ~2.6–3.3 mmol/l in poorly controlled and nondiabetic subjects. Onset of cognitive dysfunction, however, occurred similarly in all groups at ~3.0–3.2 mmol/l [114, 115]. Depending on the severity of neuroglycopenia, impaired cognitive functioning prior to symptom onset may preclude patients from recognizing or responding to their symptoms. Furthermore, a rapid fall in blood glucose leaves little time between the recognition of symptoms and the onset of more severe cognitive dysfunction, thus requiring a rapid, appropriate response to symptoms if they are detected.

6.5.8 Mechanism of Impairment

Why does antecedent hypoglycemia or exercise cause reduced neuroendocrine, metabolic, and symptom responses to subsequent hypoglycemia or exercise? Much effort has been put in to teasing apart the mechanisms by which the body senses and responds to a falling glucose level and the changes that occur within the central nervous system in the face of recurring hypoglycemia. Evidence suggests that changes occur centrally to maintain appropriate substrate levels in the most glucose-sensitive areas of the brain, allowing for continued brain function during lower systemic blood glucose levels. This would shift the initiation of responses to hypoglycemia to lower glycemic levels at which adaptations begin to fail and central glucoprivation ensues. This is an attractive explanation, as the alterations would then reflect an intrinsic protective survival response of the central nervous system to repeated bouts of hypoglycemia. Supporting this theory, mild recurring hypoglycemia (25–40 mg/dl) in awake, unrestrained rats was shown to protect against brain damage (and loss of spatial learning and memory) induced by severe hypoglycemia (10–15 mg/dl) [116].

How does the central nervous system detect a falling blood glucose level? Glucose-sensing neurons appear to be the signaling link between falling glucose levels and the counterregulatory response. The membrane potential of this subset of neurons is altered by changes in ambient glucose level. Glucose-excited neurons increase firing rate as glucose levels increase, while glucose-inhibited neurons decrease firing rate as glucose levels increase. It is believed that fluctuations in the firing rates of these neurons modulate downstream signaling mechanisms that control hormone release. Both types of glucose-sensing neurons are found in regions of the brain that have been implicated in the counterregulatory response, including the lateral hypothalamus [117] and the arcuate and ventromedial nuclei of the ventromedial hypothalamus [118–120]. These neurons are also located in hindbrain [121] in the dorsal motor nucleus of the vagus [122], the nucleus of the solitary tract [123], and the area postrema [124]. Some research also suggests that glucose-sensing neurons are located in the higher processing forebrain. These regions are associated with the blunting effects of repeated hypoglycemia. Localized glucopenia in the ventromedial hypothalamus of rats after chronic hypoglycemia induced lower counterregulatory responses compared to controls not exposed to prior hypoglycemia [125]. Similarly, antecedent injection of 5-thio-glucose into the third ventricle to cause glucoprivation within the hypothalamus resulted in reduced epinephrine and glucagon responses to subsequent hypoglycemia [126].

A number of intracellular elements may be involved in the glucose-sensing mechanism of certain neurons. Glucokinase, a known mediator of glucose sensing in pancreatic β cells, is also located in glucose-sensing neurons in the rat brain [127, 128]. Inhibition of glucokinase slows Ca^{2+} oscillations (an indirect indicator of membrane potential) in glucose-excited neurons and increases Ca^{2+} oscillations in glucose-inhibited neurons [128, 129]. Conversely, pharmacologic activation of glucokinase increases and decreases Ca^{2+} oscillations in glucose-excited and glucose-inhibited neurons, respectively [128]. Glucokinase mRNA expression is increased in the ventromedial nuclei and the arcuate following acute insulin-induced hypoglycemia in rats [130]. This change was associated with reduced epinephrine responses to subsequent hypoglycemia. Accordingly, acute pharmacologic activation of glucokinase in the ventromedial hypothalamus during hypoglycemia was shown to blunt epinephrine, norepinephrine, and glucagon responses [131]. Inhibition of glucokinase or reduction of glucokinase mRNA boosted the epinephrine response to hypoglycemia [131].

Stimulation of AMP-activated protein kinase (AMPK) may also be required for normal glucose sensing. Neuroglucopenia increased AMPK α_1 (alpha$_1$) and α_2 (alpha$_2$) activity in the rat brain [132]. Stimulation of AMPK via injection of 5-aminoimidazole-4-carboxamide ribonucleotide (AICAR) into the ventromedial hypothalamus of rats significantly increased hepatic glucose production during a hyperinsulinemic hypoglycemic clamp [133]. Conversely, downregulation of AMPK via gene silencing blunts counterregulation, with significant reductions in glucagon, epinephrine, and endogenous glucose production responses during hypoglycemia [134]. Gene expression of AMPK α_1 (alpha$_1$) and α_2 (alpha$_2$) was shown to increase after three repeated bouts of hypoglycemia [135], and AMPK activity was blunted after 4 days of repeated neuroglucopenia [132]. Consequent blunted counterregulation (glucagon and epinephrine) can be rescued by injection of AICAR prior to acute or clamped hypoglycemia in both nondiabetic and diabetic rats [132, 135, 136].

ATP-sensitive K+channels, also similar to those found in pancreatic β (beta) cells, are found on glucose-excited neurons [120] and are closed by ATP, which increases with increasing levels of ambient glucose. Closure leads to membrane depolarization, Ca^{2+} influx, and (generally) increased action potential frequency [137]. As would be predicted, pharmacologic closure of ATP-sensitive K+channels using sulfonylureas leads to blunted counterregulatory responses to hypoglycemia [138], while microinjections of K+channel openers significantly enhance counterregulation [139]. Microinjections of diazoxide, another K+channel opener, into recurrently hypoglycemic rats were also found to rescue the epinephrine response to hypoglycemia, resulting in less reliance on exogenously infused glucose [139].

Glucose-sensing neurons must translate a changing glucose signal into a change in synaptic neurotransmitter release to generate a physiological response to the original stimulus. Changes have been observed in a number of neurotransmitters during acute and repeated hypoglycemia, including glutamate, a fast-acting, excitatory neurotransmitter prevalent in the ventromedial hypothalamus. Researchers created a knockout mouse model lacking glutamate synaptic vesicular transporters in SF1 neurons found in the ventromedial hypothalamus. Knockout mice displayed impaired counterregulation during both fasting and insulin-induced hypoglycemia [140]. No information is available however regarding changes in glutamate levels during acute and recurring hypoglycemia.

The inhibitory neurotransmitter γ (gamma)-aminobutyric acid (GABA), on the other hand, has been heavily studied in relation to hypoglycemia. Levels of both GABA and glutamic acid decarboxylase (the enzyme responsible for GABA synthesis) increase in the ventromedial hypothalamus of rats in response to acute and recurring systemic hypoglycemia [141, 142]. The increased levels may partially mediate impaired counterregulation as administration of alprazolam in healthy humans (to induce GABA$_A$ receptor activation) either 90 min or 1 day prior to insulin-induced hypoglycemia results in blunted epinephrine, norepinephrine, glucagon, pancreatic polypeptide, MSNA, growth hormone, ACTH, and metabolic responses [143, 144]. Reciprocally, GABA$_A$ receptor antagonism in the ventromedial hypothalamus of rats enhances the counterregulatory response to hypoglycemia and rescues the blunting effects of repeated hypoglycemia [142, 145]. Norepinephrine synaptically released in the ventromedial hypothalamus may drive increases in GABA, as the first and second peaks of the biphasic rise in GABA during infusion of 2-deoxyglucose were blocked by administration of α_2 (alpha$_2$)- and β (beta)-adrenoceptor antagonists, respectively [146].

The corticotrophin-releasing factor (CRF) family of CRF and urocortins (UCN) I-III may work in opposing fashion to modulate counterregulatory responses. Stimulation of primarily CRF receptor I (CRFRI) via microinjection of CRF amplifies glucagon and epinephrine responses to hypoglycemia in rats [147]. Meanwhile, stimulation of CRFRII via microinjection of UCNI delays and suppresses counterregulation, which can be corrected by infusion of a CRFRII antagonist [147]. The ventromedial hypothalamus contains CRFR I and II, with a greater distribution of CRFRII [148], as well as UCNIII, which is highly selective for CRFRII [147]. Some have hypothesized that it is the balance in the agonism of the two receptors that at least in part dictates the degree of hormonal response during hypoglycemia. Additionally, UCN agonism of CRFRII 24 h prior to hypoglycemia blunts counterregulation, suggesting that activation of this receptor during hypoglycemia could contribute to HAAF [147].

It is likely that the signaling elements described above are affected by many metabolic molecules and thus can integrate several sources of feedback into a unified signaling response. Insulin, lipids, neuropeptides (neuropeptide Y and alpha-melanocyte-stimulating hormone), and leptin, for example, have all been shown to affect a number of signaling pathways and subsequent neurotransmitter release [149–153].

Alterations in brain substrate utilization may also occur during hypoglycemia, thereby subsequently activating signaling cascades to induce a counterregulatory response. The brain increases glycogen utilization during hypoglycemia, as measured by ^{13}C NMR spectroscopy, in both healthy humans [154] and rats [155]. Glycogen is stored primarily within astrocytes and is metabolized to lactate, which can be transferred to axons to support energy demand [156]. In awake rats treated with a glycogen phosphorylase inhibitor that blocked glycogen utilization during euglycemia but not during hypoglycemia, brain glycogen content increased by 88% under euglycemic conditions [157]. Compared to controls, rats treated with the glycogen phosphorylase inhibitor maintained brain functioning longer and had reduced cell death during hypoglycemia (glucose nadir <1 mM), suggesting that glycogen is indeed utilized during hypoglycemia. There is evidence that glycogen supercompensation occurs in both rats [132, 155] and humans [154] after one or multiple bouts of hypoglycemia. These observations have led to the hypothesis that enhanced glycogen utilization during hypoglycemia blunts counterregulatory responses by inhibiting activation of AMPK [132].

In addition to lactate generated from glycogenolysis, lactate appears to be an abundantly available energy source in the brain as a result of astrocyte glucose metabolism stimulated by glutamate released during neuronal activity [158]. Research suggests that lactate is readily metabolized by neural tissue, even in the presence of glucose [159, 160]. Under euglycemic conditions, systemic lactate infusion in humans causes increased brain lactate uptake and metabolism and reduced glucose uptake [161], and lactate metabolism increases under increased neural stimulation [160]. Excess lactate infused into the ventromedial hypothalamus during systemic hypoglycemia dramatically diminishes counterregulatory responses, indicating that normal neuronal signaling responses to hypoglycemia were blocked despite decreasing glucose availability [162]. Consistent with this interpretation, systemic lactate infusion during severe hypoglycemia was shown to maintain neuronal excitability [160]. Adaptations at the blood-brain barrier may occur to increase transport of lactate as well as other monocarboxylic acids (MCA), such as acetate, acetoacetate, and β (beta)-hydroxybutyrate, in response to repeated hypoglycemia. In subjects with well-controlled diabetes and recent recurrent hypoglycemia, alterations in MCA transport were indirectly indicated by twofold increases in brain acetate concentrations, oxidative acetate metabolism, and brain acetate transport [163].

Data are inconsistent regarding changes in brain glucose uptake and metabolism in response to recurrent hypoglycemia. After rats were subjected to 5 days of insulin injection to induce mild hypoglycemia, GLUT1 mRNA and protein were increased in the brain, which could mean that the brain is able to adapt to hypoglycemia by increasing brain glucose transport capacity [164]. Supporting this, in healthy adults, brain glucose uptake fell during a stepped hypoglycemic clamp but was maintained following 56 h of hypoglycemia (3.0 mmol/l) [165]. In diabetes patients with near-normal Hb_{A1c} (and a significantly greater frequency of hypoglycemia), normal levels of glucose uptake were observed, while uptake decreased in patients with higher Hb_{A1c} levels [166]. Additionally, it has been shown that patients with type 1 DM and a history of hypoglycemia unawareness have increased cerebral glucose concentrations compared to healthy controls [167]. However, healthy subjects who underwent three episodes of hypoglycemia (30 min each) over 24 h had no change in brain glucose content [168]. In this study though, the hypoglycemic stimuli may not have been prolonged or severe enough to induce changes in brain glucose uptake, as counterregulatory hormones were not universally blunted among all subjects. In those subjects that did have severe blunting of one or more counterregulatory hormones, brain glucose concentration was increased following antecedent hypoglycemia [168].

Glucose sensors located peripherally in the portal vein [169, 170] and the carotid artery [171] probably also contribute to the signaling response to hypoglycemia. Portal vein afferent denervation or maintenance of portal vein glucose concentrations significantly blunted the epinephrine response to systemic hypoglycemia in rats [172]. Sensing likely occurs in capsaicin-sensitive primary sensory neurons of spinal afferents from the portal vein [173, 174]. The primary site for glucose sensing may shift based on the rate of fall of blood glucose, with the portal vein playing a greater role in counterregulation when the rate of fall of glucose is low [175]. Hypoglycemia increases transmitter secretion from glomus cells in the carotid artery in a concentration-dependent manner, which can in turn stimulate afferent nerve fibers. It has been suggested that transmitter secretion in response to hypoglycemia is mediated by inhibition of K+ channel activity, membrane depolarization, and Ca2+ influx [176]. Resection of carotid bodies in dogs led to reduced counterregulatory responses during clamped hypoglycemia [171], but contradictory evidence exists, showing that low blood glucose does not directly activate carotid body chemoreceptors in the rat [177].

Some have also suggested that reduced β (beta)-adrenergic sensitivity plays a role in the increased risk for hypoglycemia following antecedent hypoglycemia. Patients with type 1 DM who meet the criteria for hypoglycemia unawareness can have reduced sensitivity to isoproterenol, a β (beta)-adrenergic agonist [178, 179] that could be the result of a dysfunction in the proximal $β_2$ (beta$_2$)-adrenergic signaling pathway [180]. Additionally, β (beta)-adrenergic sensitivity is reduced following one bout of hypoglycemia in patients with type 1 DM [181], while avoiding hypoglycemia for a period of 4 months improved both β (beta)-adrenergic and hypoglycemic symptom responses [182].

6.6 Recovering Counterregulatory Responses and Hypoglycemia Awareness

Several studies have focused on reversing deficits in counterregulation and hypoglycemia awareness through strict avoidance of hypoglycemia. In a very short-term study, patients were subjected to an acute bout of hypoglycemia (2.2 mmol/l) once daily for 3 days [183]. Following these repeated episodes of hypoglycemia, patients underwent a hypoglycemic clamp before and after 2 days of avoiding hypoglycemia. During the second clamp, epinephrine, ACTH, cortisol, and symptom scores were all significantly improved compared to the first clamp, indicating that even short-term avoidance of hypoglycemia improves counterregulation. Relaxation of glycemic control over the short term can also reverse counterregulatory deficiencies [182, 184]. In a 3-month study [184], increasing mean daily blood glucose to 8–10 mmol/l decreased episodes of hypoglycemia from 4.7 to 1.9 episodes per person per week. Epinephrine, growth hormone, and symptom responses during a subsequent hypoglycemic clamp were all greater compared to responses preceding the intervention. In a second 4-month study, reducing insulin doses to increase preprandial and bedtime glucose targets from 5.6 to 8.0 and 10.0 mmol/l, respectively, decreased the frequency of hypoglycemia from 8.4 to 1.4 episodes per week. Thereafter, autonomic and neuroglycopenic symptom responses to hypoglycemia were improved [182]. In these studies, Hb_{A1c} increased from 6.9% to 8.0% and from 6.8% to 7.4%, respectively [182, 184]. While preventing severe hypoglycemia is certainly important, the goal is to do so without increasing the risk of microvascular and macrovascular complications that arise with poorer glucose control.

Some argue that recovery of hypoglycemia awareness does not have to compromise glycemic control [185–187]. In a 1-year intervention study [186, 187], subjects with hypoglycemia unawareness who switched from conventional to intensive insulin therapy decreased their frequency of hypoglycemia from 0.5 to 0.045 episodes per patient-day through targeted physiological insulin replacement and intensive education. Improvements in hormone and symptom responses were observed between 2 weeks and 3 months of starting the intervention and were sustained for the duration of the study. Although the study group claimed that glycemic control was not worsened, Hb_{Alc} did increase from 5.83% to 6.94%, indicating that there was some deterioration of mean daily blood glucose levels. In a second study [185], patients under either strict (Hb_{Alc} 6.5%) or poor (Hb_{Alc} 8.2%) glycemic control, all with impaired awareness of hypoglycemia, were provided with education and assistance in modifying diet, exercise, and insulin dosing to avoid hypoglycemia. It took subjects 4 months, on average, to meet the study endpoint of an absence of hypoglycemia for 3 weeks. Epinephrine and symptom scores during hypoglycemia improved and were initiated at higher blood glucose levels. Hb_{Alc} did not significantly increase during the study in either group.

Some research suggests that improvements are only partial. After 3 months of intensively avoiding hypoglycemia, patients exhibited normal symptom responses during hypoglycemia, but neuroendocrine responses, including epinephrine, pancreatic polypeptide, and cortisol, were not recovered [188]. Conversely, another study found an improvement in epinephrine but not symptom responses after a return from intensive to conventional insulin therapy [189]. The reason for these inconsistent observations is still not understood. Some differences may be explained by varying research procedures, including inclusion criteria for hypoglycemia unawareness, hypoglycemic clamp methods, length of interventions, and sample size. However, it is clear that more studies are needed to better identify effective strategies for treating impaired hormone and symptom responses during hypoglycemia. The above studies do indicate that patient education regarding diet, exercise, and fine-tuning insulin replacement as well as regular glucose monitoring can be effective tools for avoiding hypoglycemia and improving counterregulation. Furthermore, relaxing glycemic control, at least temporarily, may be helpful.

6.7 Preventing Severe Hypoglycemia

Hypoglycemia can be severely debilitating, both long- and short term. Avoidance of hypoglycemia is crucial to sustained quality of life in all patients with diabetes. In athletes with diabetes, avoidance of hypoglycemia is vital also to continued athletic success. In those who compete at high speeds, in hazardous environments (i.e., water), and/or in close proximity to others (i.e., basketball, cycling), hypoglycemia can be especially dangerous, increasing the risk for bodily injury to the patient or others. Aspects of visual information processing, including contrast sensitivity, inspection time, visual change detection, and visual movement detection, can be impaired by hypoglycemia [190, 191]. Auditory functioning also changes, with diminished auditory temporal processing and lower ability to discriminate single-tone loudness [192, 193]. Psychomotor function and performance on tasks associated with visual and auditory selective attention are also diminished [194, 195]. These deficits could slow judgment and reaction time and/or result in mistakes.

During a fitness camp developed specifically for active individuals with type 1 DM, continuous glucose monitoring systems were used to follow glycemic fluctuations in 12 subjects over 5 days [196]. On average, subjects were hypoglycemic, hyperglycemic, and euglycemic 7%, 11%, and 82% of the time, respectively. From over ~60 h of data collected in each patient, a total of 75 hypoglycemic episodes were recorded, with at least 1 episode occurring in each person. The wide glycemic variability occurred despite patients demonstrating a substantial degree of knowledge regarding the appropriate use of carbohydrate and insulin during exercise and despite the 24-h availability of expert support staff (i.e., physician, coaches, physician assistants, exercise physiologists). Such is the depth of the ongoing struggle that athletes face in adequately managing their blood glucose levels.

Fear of hypoglycemia is an all too real issue that often arises in type 1 DM. In addition to diminishing quality of life, this fear poses a major barrier to both glycemic control and exercise [197]. The development of a comprehensive plan to prevent hypoglycemia will not only provide individuals with the knowledge to increase safety during exercise and avoid deterioration of glycemic control but also will build confidence in making self-treatment decisions that will hopefully translate into less anxiety.

Does the athlete have impaired hypoglycemia unawareness? This can be assessed by collecting a patient history of frequency of moderate to severe biochemical hypoglycemia with or without associated symptoms [198] or a self-report questionnaire that can be used to generate a more comprehensive understanding of the person's hypoglycemia awareness level. The self-report questionnaire has been shown to correlate well with symptom recognition and thresholds during a stepped hypoglycemic clamp [199]. If impaired hypoglycemia awareness is present, the athlete is very likely to develop hypoglycemia either during or after exercise. Priority should be placed upon correction of this syndrome prior to beginning or continuing training.

Differing disease duration, insulin requirements, diet, training regimens, and choice of sport necessitate an individualized approach to diabetes management. Special attention is required during the initiation of an exercise training regimen and during major shifts in level of activity, diet, or insulin dosage, as these changes tend to increase the frequency of low blood glucose readings [200]. A number of different strategies can be used to minimize the risk of hypoglycemia (see Table 6.2), and the patient and the health-care team should work together to develop the understanding and skills to use each strategy successfully. Regular blood glucose monitoring and adequate adjustment of insulin and carbohydrate intake are crucial to prevention of hypoglycemia, and detailed information regarding these topics is available in Chaps. 3, 5, and 7.

6.7.1   Improving Symptom Identification

Failure to identify symptoms, associate symptoms with hypoglycemia, or respond appropriately to hypoglycemia can lead to more severe hypoglycemia [72]. Thus, a comprehensive understanding of symptoms and how to react to those symptoms is imperative. Patients tend to consistently experience specific sets of symptoms during hypoglycemia [201, 202]. Some studies show that patients tend to rely much more on autonomic than neuroglycopenic symptoms [12]. However, although the onset of

Table 6.2 Strategies for lowering the risk of hypoglycemia during exercise

	Risk factor	Reducing risk
Behavioral		
Insulin injection	Intramuscular injection	Use shorter needles (4–5 mm)
	Injection into working limb	Inject insulin into abdominal subcutaneous tissue, especially if performing leg exercise
	Alternating injection site	Inject into same site but rotate injections within site
Insulin dose	Administering full dose will result in a physiologically hyperinsulinemic state during exercise	Reduce basal and/or bolus doses before, during, and/or after exercise
	Exercising during peak insulin action	Avoid exercise within the first few hours following injection of short- or rapid-acting insulin
		If exercise is unplanned and occurs during peak insulin action, consume extra carbohydrate
Carbohydrate intake	Failure to consume adequate carbohydrate before, during, or after exercise	Consume carbohydrate if blood glucose is <5.6 mmol/l prior to exercise
		Consume additional carbohydrate based on duration and intensity
		Continue monitoring blood glucose during and after exercise to determine if and when more carbohydrate should be taken
Blood glucose monitoring	Failure to detect a low blood glucose	Perform multiple blood glucose measurements before, during (if exercise is of sufficient duration), and after exercise. Alternatively, a continuous blood glucose monitoring system can be used
Biological impairments		
Hypoglycemia-associated autonomic failure	Reduced hormonal, metabolic, and symptom response to exercise and hypoglycemia as a result of a former episode of exercise or hypoglycemia	Reverse hypoglycemia-associated autonomic failure by consistently avoiding hypoglycemic episodes:
		Temporarily relax glycemic control goals in order to avoid hypoglycemia
		Increase preprandial and bedtime glucose targets – reduce insulin doses and/or increase between-meal carbohydrate intake
		Regularly assess trends in blood glucose changes and modify insulin dose accordingly
		Implement or increase frequency of blood glucose monitoring
		Increase understanding of symptoms associated with hypoglycemia and increase ability to identify and react to symptoms

Table 6.2 (continued)

	Risk factor	Reducing risk
Absolute insulin deficiency	Inability to reduce circulating insulin levels	Focus on reducing other risk factors
Environmental		
Extreme temperature	Hot and cold environments can alter hormonal responses to exercise and hypoglycemia as well as obscure symptoms of hypoglycemia	Reduce exposure to temperature extremes Train under environmental conditions similar to those anticipated during competition
Forces of nature	Increased wind, waves, etc., will increase the intensity of the workout	Consume extra carbohydrate Reduce speed to maintain planned intensity
Others		
Travel	Change in activity level, eating pattern, and/or sleep	Plan for travel – pack enough snacks, take regular walking/rest breaks, arrive early enough to rest
Altered competition schedule	Delays, overtime, extra games/matches, etc.	Have extra snacks available, continue monitoring blood glucose, consider reducing insulin and/or consuming more carbohydrate after competition

autonomic and neuroglycopenic symptoms and cognitive dysfunction may occur at different glycemic thresholds regardless of the rate of fall of blood glucose [203], in an everyday life situation, blood glucose may fall at a rate brisk enough that the onset of all symptoms may occur temporally, nearly simultaneously. As such, neuroglycopenic symptoms are frequently reported during hypoglycemia as well [204].

Health-care professionals should help the athlete to identify symptom trends during rest and exercise and to determine which symptoms are most helpful in recognizing hypoglycemia under each condition. The athlete should also learn to monitor for additional symptoms – both autonomic and neuroglycopenic – and factors that can confound identification of symptoms, especially during exercise or competition. When patients have at least one recognizable symptom that typically occurs during hypoglycemia, half of the episodes of blood glucose <3.95 mmol/l can be detected. When the number of recognizable, typical symptoms is increased to four or more, three-quarters of hypoglycemic episodes can be identified [201]. Furthermore, being mindful of the potential for hypoglycemia should help to increase vigilance and sensitivity to physiological changes. In one study of healthy people subjected to a previous episode of insulin-induced hypoglycemia, half of the subjects were told that they would receive insulin during a second session and half were told that they would receive saline. Of those two groups, half were given the opposite intervention of what they expected. Those anticipating insulin infusion had higher symptom scores compared to those expecting saline, regardless of the actual intervention [205].

Teammates, coaches, family members, and friends can also be of major importance in identifying symptoms of hypoglycemia. Education should be provided to members of the athlete's support system regarding signs and symptoms of hypoglycemia and appropriate treatment measures.

6.7.2 Record Keeping

The importance of record keeping should be stressed. With so many variables contributing to fluctuations in blood glucose levels, recording blood glucose levels, insulin dosing (times and doses), meal intake (times and amount of carbohydrate), exercise (duration and intensity), and other relevant details will help the patient to make informed self-treatment decisions, as well as determine reasons for glycemic excursions. A number of record-keeping utilities are now available online, some of which can also be accessed by physicians and health-care professionals to monitor patients' treatment regimens.

6.7.3 Intermittent High-Intensity Exercise

Because intense exercise causes a rise in blood glucose, a group of researchers has studied the antihypoglycemic effects of introducing short bursts of IHE before, during, or after a session of moderate exercise [206–208]. In one group of individuals

[206], performing 4-s sprints every 2 min over the course of 30 min of moderate exercise (40% VO_{2max}) caused blood glucose to fall to a significantly lesser degree compared to a nonsprint group. Furthermore, for 60 min postexercise, glucose continued to fall in the nonsprinters but stabilized in the IHE group. Performing a 10-s maximal sprint before 20 min of exercise (40% VO_{2max}) prevented a fall in blood glucose only during the early recovery period [207], but a 10-s sprint after the same exercise stabilized glucose levels for a full 2 h following exercise [208].

In all three interventions, exercise was performed ~3.5 h after the last meal, beyond peak insulin action and with preexercise blood glucose levels ~11 mmol/l. Therefore, if athletes wish to employ such a preventive strategy, timing and duration of sprints will need to be determined empirically based on prandial state and preexercise blood glucose level. Also, as discussed earlier, evidence is conflicting as to whether or not late-onset exercise-associated hypoglycemia can be avoided using this method [101, 102]. Therefore, glucose monitoring before and throughout sleeping hours is strongly recommended.

6.8 Treatment of Acute Hypoglycemia

When hypoglycemia is detected by symptoms and/or biochemical measurement, treatment will depend on the degree of hypoglycemia and the patient's state of consciousness and his or her willingness and ability to administer or receive treatment (see Table 6.3). Mild to moderate hypoglycemia can generally be initially treated with 15–20 g of simple carbohydrate, such as glucose tablets or gel, soft drinks, or juice [209, 210]. The carbohydrate source should be low in fat so that absorption will not be slowed. If after 15 min symptoms have not abated or blood glucose is still low, the treatment should be repeated [209, 210]. Lower blood glucose (<2.8 mmol/l) should be treated with 30 g of carbohydrate [210]. These recommendations are not specific to athletes who may become hypoglycemic during prolonged, moderately intense exercise. Thus, larger amounts of carbohydrate may be required to treat hypoglycemia under these conditions. Once blood glucose levels return to normal, it is important that the patient consumes a meal including more complex carbohydrate to prevent subsequent bouts of hypoglycemia [209, 210].

During more severe hypoglycemia, glucose gel, jelly, or honey can be used as these substances can be placed in the mouth against the cheek by another person [210] and are readily absorbed through the buccal mucosa. In the unconscious patient, glucagon (1 mg) should be administered subcutaneously or intramuscularly to stimulate hepatic glycogenolysis [209, 210]. Although very effective, glucagon does take approximately 10 min to begin to affect blood glucose levels, which is considerably longer than intravenous glucose. However, unlike intravenous glucose, glucagon, available as a kit, can be safely administered by friends, family members, and coaches with proper education [209–211]. Those who plan to administer glucagon when necessary should receive hands-on training to ensure that glucagon can be

Table 6.3 Recommended interventions for an acute hypoglycemic event

Level of hypoglycemia	Immediate intervention	Comments
Mild to moderate		
Patient is conscious	Consume carbohydrate snack:	
	Blood glucose >2.8 mmol/l	Simple carbohydrate should be used (i.e., glucose tablets or gel, soft drinks, juice)
	15–20 g carbohydrate	Glucose gel, jelly, or honey can be placed against inner cheek
	Blood glucose <2.8 mmol/l	Avoid snacks that contain fat
	30 g carbohydrate	Repeat after 15 min if blood glucose remains low or symptoms have not subsided
Severe		
Patient is unconscious	Glucagon (1 mg) injection	Subcutaneous or intramuscular injection is acceptable
	Call for emergency medical assistance if necessary	Make sure kit is not expired and is readily accessible
		Glucagon has a delayed onset of action (~10 min) compared to glucose
		Do not attempt to administer carbohydrate orally

delivered in an adequate quantity and in a timely manner [211]. Caregivers should be made aware of the location where glucagon kits are stored, and kits should be regularly checked for expiration date [211]. If emergency care is required, medical staff may also administer glucagon 1 mg intramuscularly or intravenously, as well as 50 ml of dextrose (20%) or 25 ml of dextrose (50%) intravenously.

Athletes may need to allow themselves' a recovery period before engaging in exercise following a hypoglycemic episode. In one study, responses to hypoglycemia were not blunted 2 days after induction of a 2-h bout of hypoglycemia [212]. However, the severity and duration of a hypoglycemic event could affect the length of time required to recover full counterregulatory responses.

6.9 Conclusion

Although rapidly improving, the treatment of type 1 DM is not perfect, and the risk of hypoglycemia remains, especially under metabolically challenging conditions such as exercise. Athletes should be sufficiently educated regarding attendant risks and behavioral strategies that can be used to successfully minimize those risks. With practice, athletes can personalize and master such strategies to avoid hypoglycemia as well as enhance performance and the enjoyment of sport and exercise.

References

1. Cryer PE. Hierarchy of physiological responses to hypoglycemia: relevance to clinical hypoglycemia in type I (insulin dependent) diabetes mellitus. Horm Metab Res. 1997;29:92–6.
2. Fanelli C, Pampanelli S, Epifano L, Rambotti AM, Ciofetta M, Modarelli F, et al. Relative roles of insulin and hypoglycaemia on induction of neuroendocrine responses to, symptoms of, and deterioration of cognitive function in hypoglycaemia in male and female humans. Diabetologia. 1994;37:797–807.
3. Mitrakou A, Ryan C, Veneman T, Mokan M, Jenssen T, Kiss I, et al. Hierarchy of glycemic thresholds for counterregulatory hormone secretion, symptoms, and cerebral dysfunction. Am J Physiol. 1991;260:E67–74.
4. Schwartz NS, Clutter WE, Shah SD, Cryer PE. Glycemic thresholds for activation of glucose counterregulatory systems are higher than the threshold for symptoms. J Clin Invest. 1987;79:777–81.
5. Davis SN, Shavers C, Costa F. Differential gender responses to hypoglycemia are due to alterations in CNS drive and not glycemic thresholds. Am J Physiol Endocrinol Metab. 2000;279:E1054–63.
6. Davis SN, Fowler S, Costa F. Hypoglycemic counterregulatory responses differ between men and women with type 1 diabetes. Diabetes. 2000;49:65–72.
7. Sandoval DA, Ertl AC, Richardson MA, Tate DB, Davis SN. Estrogen blunts neuroendocrine and metabolic responses to hypoglycemia. Diabetes. 2003;52:1749–55.
8. DeRosa MA, Cryer PE. Hypoglycemia and the sympathoadrenal system: neurogenic symptoms are largely the result of sympathetic neural, rather than adrenomedullary, activation. Am J Physiol Endocrinol Metab. 2004;287:E32–41.
9. Hoffman RP, Sinkey CA, Anderson EA. Hypoglycemic symptom variation is related to epinephrine and not peripheral muscle sympathetic nerve response. J Diabetes Complications. 1997;11:15–20.
10. Aftab Guy D, Sandoval D, Richardson MA, Tate D, Davis SN. Effects of glycemic control on target organ responses to epinephrine in type 1 diabetes. Am J Physiol Endocrinol Metab. 2005;289:E258–65.
11. Deary IJ. Symptoms of hypoglycemia and effects on mental performance and emotions. In: Frier B, Fisher M, editors. Hypoglycemia in clinical diabetes. 2nd ed. Chichester: Wiley; 2007. p. 25–48.
12. Towler DA, Havlin CE, Craft S, Cryer P. Mechanism of awareness of hypoglycemia. Perception of neurogenic (predominantly cholinergic) rather than neuroglycopenic symptoms. Diabetes. 1993;42:1791–8.
13. Deary IJ, Hepburn DA, MacLeod KM, Frier BM. Partitioning the symptoms of hypoglycaemia using multi-sample confirmatory factor analysis. Diabetologia. 1993;36:771–7.
14. Hermanns N, Kubiak T, Kulzer B, Haak T. Emotional changes during experimentally induced hypoglycaemia in type 1 diabetes. Biol Psychol. 2003;63:15–44.
15. Vea H, Jorde R, Sager G, Vaaler S, Sundsfjord J. Reproducibility of glycaemic thresholds for activation of counterregulatory hormones and hypoglycaemic symptoms in healthy subjects. Diabetologia. 1992;35:958–61.
16. Geddes J, Warren RE, Sommerfield AJ, McAulay V, Strachan MW, Allen KV, et al. Absence of sexual dimorphism in the symptomatic responses to hypoglycemia in adults with and without type 1 diabetes. Diabetes Care. 2006;29:1667–9.
17. Wolfe RR, Nadel ER, Shaw JH, Stephenson LA, Wolfe MH. Role of changes in insulin and glucagon in glucose homeostasis in exercise. J Clin Invest. 1986;77:900–7.
18. Tuttle KR, Marker JC, Dalsky GP, Schwartz NS, Shah SD, Clutter WE, et al. Glucagon, not insulin, may play a secondary role in defense against hypoglycemia during exercise. Am J Physiol. 1988;254:E713–9.
19. Hirsch IB, Marker JC, Smith LJ, Spina RJ, Parvin CA, Holloszy JO, et al. Insulin and glucagon in prevention of hypoglycemia during exercise in humans. Am J Physiol. 1991; 260: E695–704.

20. Hoelzer DR, Dalsky GP, Clutter WE, Shah SD, Holloszy JO, Cryer PE. Glucoregulation during exercise: hypoglycemia is prevented by redundant glucoregulatory systems, sympathochromaffin activation, and changes in islet hormone secretion. J Clin Invest. 1986;77:212–21.
21. Marker JC, Hirsch IB, Smith LJ, Parvin CA, Holloszy JO, Cryer PE. Catecholamines in prevention of hypoglycemia during exercise in humans. Am J Physiol. 1991;260:E705–12.
22. Sotsky MJ, Shilo S, Shamoon H. Regulation of counterregulatory hormone secretion in man during exercise and hypoglycemia. J Clin Endocrinol Metab. 1989;68:9–16.
23. Marliss EB, Vranic M. Intense exercise has unique effects on both insulin release and its roles in glucoregulation: implications for diabetes. Diabetes. 2002;51 Suppl 1:S271–83.
24. Marliss EB, Simantirakis E, Miles PD, Purdon C, Gougeon R, Field CJ, et al. Glucoregulatory and hormonal responses to repeated bouts of intense exercise in normal male subjects. J Appl Physiol. 1991;71:924–33.
25. Marliss EB, Simantirakis E, Miles PD, Hunt R, Gougeon R, Purdon C, et al. Glucose turnover and its regulation during intense exercise and recovery in normal male subjects. Clin Invest Med. 1992;15:406–19.
26. Martin MJ, Robbins DC, Bergenstal R, LaGrange B, Rubenstein AH. Absence of exercise-induced hypoglycaemia in type i (insulin-dependent) diabetic patients during maintenance of normoglycaemia by short-term, open-loop insulin infusion. Diabetologia. 1982;23:336–42.
27. Zinman B, Marliss EB, Hanna AK, Minuk HL, Vranic M. Exercise in diabetic man: glucose turnover and free insulin responses after glycemic normalization with intravenous insulin. Can J Physiol Pharmacol. 1982;60:1236–40.
28. Schneider SH, Vitug A, Ananthakrishnan R, Khachadurian AK. Impaired adrenergic response to prolonged exercise in type I diabetes. Metabolism. 1991;40:1219–25.
29. Gerich JE, Langlois M, Noacco C, Karam JH, Forsham PH. Lack of glucagon response to hypoglycemia in diabetes: evidence for an intrinsic pancreatic alpha cell defect. Science. 1973;182:171–3.
30. Bolli G, de Feo P, Compagnucci P, Cartechini MG, Angeletti G, Santeusanio F, et al. Abnormal glucose counterregulation in insulin-dependent diabetes mellitus. Interaction of anti-insulin antibodies and impaired glucagon and epinephrine secretion. Diabetes. 1983;32:134–41.
31. Banarer S, McGregor VP, Cryer PE. Intraislet hyperinsulinemia prevents the glucagon response to hypoglycemia despite an intact autonomic response. Diabetes. 2002;51:958–65.
32. Gosmanov NR, Szoke E, Israelian Z, Smith T, Cryer PE, Gerich JE, et al. Role of the decrement in intraislet insulin for the glucagon response to hypoglycemia in humans. Diabetes Care. 2005;28:1124–31.
33. Zander E, Schulz B, Chlup R, Woltansky P, Lubs D. Muscular exercise in type I-diabetics. II. Hormonal and metabolic responses to moderate exercise. Exp Clin Endocrinol. 1985; 85:95–104.
34. Purdon C, Brousson M, Nyveen SL, Miles PD, Halter JB, Vranic M, et al. The roles of insulin and catecholamines in the glucoregulatory response during intense exercise and early recovery in insulin-dependent diabetic and control subjects. J Clin Endocrinol Metab. 1993;76:566–73.
35. Sigal RJ, Purdon C, Fisher SJ, Halter JB, Vranic M, Marliss EB. Hyperinsulinemia prevents prolonged hyperglycemia after intense exercise in insulin-dependent diabetic subjects. J Clin Endocrinol Metab. 1994;79:1049–57.
36. Heinemann L. Variability of insulin absorption and insulin action. Diabetes Technol Ther. 2002;4:673–82.
37. Freeman JS. Insulin analog therapy: improving the match with physiologic insulin secretion. J Am Osteopath Assoc. 2009;109:26–36.
38. Miles HL, Acerini CL. Insulin analog preparations and their use in children and adolescents with type 1 diabetes mellitus. Paediatr Drugs. 2008;10:163–76.
39. Hirsch IB. Insulin analogues. N Engl J Med. 2005;352:174–83.
40. Frid A, Ostman J, Linde B. Hypoglycemia risk during exercise after intramuscular injection of insulin in thigh in IDDM. Diabetes Care. 1990;13:473–7.
41. Koivisto VA, Felig P. Effects of leg exercise on insulin absorption in diabetic patients. N Engl J Med. 1978;298:79–83.

42. Ferrannini E, Linde B, Faber O. Effect of bicycle exercise on insulin absorption and subcutaneous blood flow in the normal subject. Clin Physiol. 1982;2:59–70.
43. Hildebrandt P. Skinfold thickness, local subcutaneous blood flow and insulin absorption in diabetic patients. Acta Physiol Scand Suppl. 1991;603:41–5.
44. Hildebrandt P. Subcutaneous absorption of insulin in insulin-dependent diabetic patients. Influence of species, physico-chemical properties of insulin and physiological factors. Dan Med Bull. 1991;38:337–46.
45. Sindelka G, Heinemann L, Berger M, Frenck W, Chantelau E. Effect of insulin concentration, subcutaneous fat thickness and skin temperature on subcutaneous insulin absorption in healthy subjects. Diabetologia. 1994;37:377–80.
46. Ronnemaa T, Koivisto VA. Combined effect of exercise and ambient temperature on insulin absorption and postprandial glycemia in type I patients. Diabetes Care. 1988;11:769–73.
47. Ronnemaa T, Marniemi J, Leino A, Karanko H, Puukka P, Koivisto VA. Hormone response of diabetic patients to exercise at cool and warm temperatures. Eur J Appl Physiol Occup Physiol. 1991;62:109–15.
48. Morris JG, Nevill ME, Boobis LH, Macdonald IA, Williams C. Muscle metabolism, temperature, and function during prolonged, intermittent, high-intensity running in air temperatures of 33 degrees and 17 degrees C. Int J Sports Med. 2005;26:805–14.
49. Galbo H, Houston ME, Christensen NJ, Holst JJ, Nielsen B, Nygaard E, et al. The effect of water temperature on the hormonal response to prolonged swimming. Acta Physiol Scand. 1979;105:326–37.
50. Gale EA, Bennett T, Green JH, MacDonald IA. Hypoglycaemia, hypothermia and shivering in man. Clin Sci (Lond). 1981;61:463–9.
51. Meneilly GS, Cheung E, Tuokko H. Altered responses to hypoglycemia of healthy elderly people. J Clin Endocrinol Metab. 1994;78:1341–8.
52. Ortiz-Alonso FJ, Galecki A, Herman WH, Smith MJ, Jacquez JA, Halter JB. Hypoglycemia counterregulation in elderly humans: relationship to glucose levels. Am J Physiol. 1994; 267:E497–506.
53. Brierley EJ, Broughton DL, James OF, Alberti KG. Reduced awareness of hypoglycaemia in the elderly despite an intact counter-regulatory response. QJM. 1995;88:439–45.
54. Silverman HG, Mazzeo RS. Hormonal responses to maximal and submaximal exercise in trained and untrained men of various ages. J Gerontol A Biol Sci Med Sci. 1996;51:B30–7.
55. MacDonald MJ. Postexercise late-onset hypoglycemia in insulin-dependent diabetic patients. Diabetes Care. 1987;10:584–8.
56. Garetto LP, Richter EA, Goodman MN, Ruderman NB. Enhanced muscle glucose metabolism after exercise in the rat: the two phases. Am J Physiol. 1984;246:E471–5.
57. Maarbjerg SJ, Sylow L, Richter EA. Current understanding of increased insulin sensitivity after exercise - emerging candidates. Acta Physiol (Oxf). 2011;202:323–35.
58. Mikines KJ, Sonne B, Farrell PA, Tronier B, Galbo H. Effect of physical exercise on sensitivity and responsiveness to insulin in humans. Am J Physiol. 1988;254:E248–59.
59. Annuzzi G, Riccardi G, Capaldo B, Kaijser L. Increased insulin-stimulated glucose uptake by exercised human muscles one day after prolonged physical exercise. Eur J Clin Invest. 1991;21:6–12.
60. Frosig C, Sajan MP, Maarbjerg SJ, Brandt N, Roepstorff C, Wojtaszewski JF, et al. Exercise improves phosphatidylinositol-3,4,5-trisphosphate responsiveness of atypical protein kinase C and interacts with insulin signalling to peptide elongation in human skeletal muscle. J Physiol. 2007;582:1289–301.
61. Wojtaszewski JF, Nielsen JN, Richter EA. Invited review: effect of acute exercise on insulin signaling and action in humans. J Appl Physiol. 2002;93:384–92.
62. Bogardus C, Thuillez P, Ravussin E, Vasquez B, Narimiga M, Azhar S. Effect of muscle glycogen depletion on in vivo insulin action in man. J Clin Invest. 1983;72:1605–10.
63. Hernandez JM, Moccia T, Fluckey JD, Ulbrecht JS, Farrell PA. Fluid snacks to help persons with type 1 diabetes avoid late onset postexercise hypoglycemia. Med Sci Sports Exerc. 2000;32:904–10.

64. Sonnenberg GE, Kemmer FW, Berger M. Exercise in type 1 (insulin-dependent) diabetic patients treated with continuous subcutaneous insulin infusion. Prevention of exercise induced hypoglycaemia Diabetologia. 1990;33:696–703.
65. Rabasa-Lhoret R, Bourque J, Ducros F, Chiasson JL. Guidelines for premeal insulin dose reduction for postprandial exercise of different intensities and durations in type 1 diabetic subjects treated intensively with a basal-bolus insulin regimen (ultralente-lispro). Diabetes Care. 2001;24:625–30.
66. Tuominen JA, Ebeling P, Vuorinen-Markkola H, Koivisto VA. Post-marathon paradox in IDDM: unchanged insulin sensitivity in spite of glycogen depletion. Diabet Med. 1997;14:301–8.
67. Asp S, Richter EA. Decreased insulin action on muscle glucose transport after eccentric contractions in rats. J Appl Physiol. 1996;81:1924–8.
68. Kristiansen S, Jones J, Handberg A, Dohm GL, Richter EA. Eccentric contractions decrease glucose transporter transcription rate, mRNA, and protein in skeletal muscle. Am J Physiol. 1997;272:C1734–8.
69. Del Aguila LF, Krishnan RK, Ulbrecht JS, Farrell PA, Correll PH, Lang CH, et al. Muscle damage impairs insulin stimulation of IRS-1, PI 3-kinase, and Akt-kinase in human skeletal muscle. Am J Physiol Endocrinol Metab. 2000;279:E206–12.
70. McMahon SK, Ferreira LD, Ratnam N, Davey RJ, Youngs LM, Davis EA, et al. Glucose requirements to maintain euglycemia after moderate-intensity afternoon exercise in adolescents with type 1 diabetes are increased in a biphasic manner. J Clin Endocrinol Metab. 2007;92:963–8.
71. Tsalikian E, Mauras N, Beck RW, Tamborlane WV, Janz KF, Chase HP, et al. Impact of exercise on overnight glycemic control in children with type 1 diabetes mellitus. J Pediatr. 2005;147:528–34.
72. Gonder-Frederick L, Cox D, Kovatchev B, Schlundt D, Clarke W. A biopsychobehavioral model of risk of severe hypoglycemia. Diabetes Care. 1997;20:661–9.
73. Nermoen I, Jorde R, Sager G, Sundsfjord J, Birkeland K. Effects of exercise on hypoglycaemic responses in insulin-dependent diabetes mellitus. Diabetes Metab. 1998;24:131–6.
74. Bottini P, Boschetti E, Pampanelli S, Ciofetta M, Del Sindaco P, Scionti L, et al. Contribution of autonomic neuropathy to reduced plasma adrenaline responses to hypoglycemia in IDDM: evidence for a nonselective defect. Diabetes. 1997;46:814–23.
75. Hilsted J, Madsbad S, Krarup T, Sestoft L, Christensen NJ, Tronier B, et al. Hormonal, metabolic, and cardiovascular responses to hypoglycemia in diabetic autonomic neuropathy. Diabetes. 1981;30:626–33.
76. Hoeldtke RD, Boden G, Shuman CR, Owen OE. Reduced epinephrine secretion and hypoglycemia unawareness in diabetic autonomic neuropathy. Ann Intern Med. 1982;96:459–62.
77. Boden G, Reichard Jr GA, Hoeldtke RD, Rezvani I, Owen OE. Severe insulin-induced hypoglycemia associated with deficiencies in the release of counterregulatory hormones. N Engl J Med. 1981;305:1200–5.
78. Ryder RE, Owens DR, Hayes TM, Ghatei MA, Bloom SR. Unawareness of hypoglycaemia and inadequate hypoglycaemic counterregulation: no causal relation with diabetic autonomic neuropathy. BMJ. 1990;301:783–7.
79. Dagogo-Jack SE, Craft S, Cryer PE. Hypoglycemia-associated autonomic failure in insulin-dependent diabetes mellitus. Recent antecedent hypoglycemia reduces autonomic responses to, symptoms of, and defense against subsequent hypoglycemia. J Clin Invest. 1993;91:819–28.
80. Berlin I, Grimaldi A, Payan C, Sachon C, Bosquet F, Thervet F, et al. Hypoglycemic symptoms and decreased beta-adrenergic sensitivity in insulin-dependent diabetic patients. Diabetes Care. 1987;10:742–7.
81. Hepburn DA, Patrick AW, Eadington DW, Ewing DJ, Frier BM. Unawareness of hypoglycaemia in insulin-treated diabetic patients: prevalence and relationship to autonomic neuropathy. Diabet Med. 1990;7:711–7.

82. Galassetti P, Tate D, Neill RA, Richardson A, Leu SY, Davis SN. Effect of differing antecedent hypoglycemia on counterregulatory responses to exercise in type 1 diabetes. Am J Physiol Endocrinol Metab. 2006;290:E1109–17.

83. Hoeldtke RD, Boden G. Epinephrine secretion, hypoglycemia unawareness, and diabetic autonomic neuropathy. Ann Intern Med. 1994;120:512–7.

84. Webb SM, Fernandez Castaner M. Glucose counterregulation in diabetic autonomic neuropathy. Clin Physiol. 1985;5 Suppl 5:66–71.

85. Adamson U, Lins PE, Efendic S, Hamberger B, Wajngot A. Impaired counter regulation of hypoglycemia in a group of insulin-dependent diabetics with recurrent episodes of severe hypoglycemia. Acta Med Scand. 1984;216:215–22.

86. Sjobom NC, Adamson U, Lin PE. The prevalence of impaired glucose counter-regulation during an insulin-infusion test in insulin-treated diabetic patients prone to severe hypoglycaemia. Diabetologia. 1989;32:818–25.

87. Cryer PE. Iatrogenic hypoglycemia as a cause of hypoglycemia-associated autonomic failure in IDDM. A vicious cycle. Diabetes. 1992;41:255–60.

88. Kennedy FP, Bolli GB, Go VL, Cryer PE, Gerich JE. The significance of impaired pancreatic polypeptide and epinephrine responses to hypoglycemia in patients with insulin-dependent diabetes mellitus. J Clin Endocrinol Metab. 1987;64:602–8.

89. Davis MR, Shamoon H. Counterregulatory adaptation to recurrent hypoglycemia in normal humans. J Clin Endocrinol Metab. 1991;73:995–1001.

90. Heller SR, Cryer PE. Reduced neuroendocrine and symptomatic responses to subsequent hypoglycemia after 1 episode of hypoglycemia in nondiabetic humans. Diabetes. 1991;40:223–6.

91. Widom B, Simonson DC. Intermittent hypoglycemia impairs glucose counterregulation. Diabetes. 1992;41:1597–602.

92. Lingenfelser T, Renn W, Sommerwerck U, Jung MF, Buettner UW, Zaiser-Kaschel H, et al. Compromised hormonal counterregulation, symptom awareness, and neurophysiological function after recurrent short-term episodes of insulin-induced hypoglycemia in IDDM patients. Diabetes. 1993;42:610–8.

93. Ovalle F, Fanelli CG, Paramore DS, Hershey T, Craft S, Cryer PE. Brief twice-weekly episodes of hypoglycemia reduce detection of clinical hypoglycemia in type 1 diabetes mellitus. Diabetes. 1998;47:1472–9.

94. Davis SN, Shavers C, Mosqueda-Garcia R, Costa F. Effects of differing antecedent hypoglycemia on subsequent counterregulation in normal humans. Diabetes. 1997;46:1328–35.

95. Davis SN, Mann S, Galassetti P, Neill RA, Tate D, Ertl AC, et al. Effects of differing durations of antecedent hypoglycemia on counterregulatory responses to subsequent hypoglycemia in normal humans. Diabetes. 2000;49:1897–903.

96. Davis SN, Galassetti P, Wasserman DH, Tate D. Effects of antecedent hypoglycemia on subsequent counterregulatory responses to exercise. Diabetes. 2000;49:73–81.

97. Galassetti P, Tate D, Neill RA, Morrey S, Wasserman DH, Davis SN. Effect of antecedent hypoglycemia on counterregulatory responses to subsequent euglycemic exercise in type 1 diabetes. Diabetes. 2003;52:1761–9.

98. Galassetti P, Mann S, Tate D, Neill RA, Costa F, Wasserman DH, et al. Effects of antecedent prolonged exercise on subsequent counterregulatory responses to hypoglycemia. Am J Physiol Endocrinol Metab. 2001;280:E908–17.

99. Sandoval DA, Guy DL, Richardson MA, Ertl AC, Davis SN. Acute, same-day effects of antecedent exercise on counterregulatory responses to subsequent hypoglycemia in type 1 diabetes mellitus. Am J Physiol Endocrinol Metab. 2006;290:E1331–8.

100. Sandoval DA, Guy DL, Richardson MA, Ertl AC, Davis SN. Effects of low and moderate antecedent exercise on counterregulatory responses to subsequent hypoglycemia in type 1 diabetes. Diabetes. 2004;53:1798–806.

101. Maran A, Pavan P, Bonsembiante B, Brugin E, Ermolao A, Avogaro A, et al. Continuous glucose monitoring reveals delayed nocturnal hypoglycemia after intermittent high-intensity exercise in nontrained patients with type 1 diabetes. Diabetes Technol Ther. 2010;12:763–8.

102. Iscoe KE, Riddell MC. Continuous moderate-intensity exercise with or without intermittent high-intensity work: effects on acute and late glycaemia in athletes with Type 1 diabetes mellitus. Diabet Med. 2011;28(7):824–32.

103. Iscoe KE, Campbell JE, Jamnik V, Perkins BA, Riddell MC. Efficacy of continuous real-time blood glucose monitoring during and after prolonged high-intensity cycling exercise: spinning with a continuous glucose monitoring system. Diabetes Technol Ther. 2006;8:627–35.

104. The DCCT Research Group. Epidemiology of severe hypoglycemia in the diabetes control and complications trial. Am J Med. 1991;90:450–9.

105. Juvenile Diabetes Research Foundation Continuous Glucose Monitoring Study Group. Prolonged nocturnal hypoglycemia is common during 12 months of continuous glucose monitoring in children and adults with type 1 diabetes. Diabetes Care. 2010;33:1004–8.

106. Banarer S, Cryer PE. Sleep-related hypoglycemia-associated autonomic failure in type 1 diabetes: reduced awakening from sleep during hypoglycemia. Diabetes. 2003;52:1195–203.

107. Jones TW, Porter P, Sherwin RS, Davis EA, O'Leary P, Frazer F, et al. Decreased epinephrine responses to hypoglycemia during sleep. N Engl J Med. 1998;338:1657–62.

108. Matyka KA, Crowne EC, Havel PJ, Macdonald IA, Matthews D, Dunger DB. Counterregulation during spontaneous nocturnal hypoglycemia in prepubertal children with type 1 diabetes. Diabetes Care. 1999;22:1144–50.

109. Veneman T, Mitrakou A, Mokan M, Cryer P, Gerich J. Induction of hypoglycemia unawareness by asymptomatic nocturnal hypoglycemia. Diabetes. 1993;42:1233–7.

110. Fanelli CG, Paramore DS, Hershey T, Terkamp C, Ovalle F, Craft S, et al. Impact of nocturnal hypoglycemia on hypoglycemic cognitive dysfunction in type 1 diabetes. Diabetes. 1998; 47:1920–7.

111. Hepburn DA, Patrick AW, Brash HM, Thomson I, Frier BM. Hypoglycaemia unawareness in type 1 diabetes: a lower plasma glucose is required to stimulate sympatho-adrenal activation. Diabet Med. 1991;8:934–45.

112. Boyle PJ, Schwartz NS, Shah SD, Clutter WE, Cryer PE. Plasma glucose concentrations at the onset of hypoglycemic symptoms in patients with poorly controlled diabetes and in nondiabetics. N Engl J Med. 1988;318:1487–92.

113. Clarke WL, Gonder-Frederick LA, Richards FE, Cryer PE. Multifactorial origin of hypoglycemic symptom unawareness in IDDM. Association with defective glucose counterregulation and better glycemic control. Diabetes. 1991;40:680–5.

114. Amiel SA, Pottinger RC, Archibald HR, Chusney G, Cunnah DT, Prior PF, et al. Effect of antecedent glucose control on cerebral function during hypoglycemia. Diabetes Care. 1991;14:109–18.

115. Maran A, Lomas J, Macdonald IA, Amiel SA. Lack of preservation of higher brain function during hypoglycaemia in patients with intensively-treated IDDM. Diabetologia. 1995;38:1412–8.

116. Puente EC, Silverstein J, Bree AJ, Musikantow DR, Wozniak DF, Maloney S, et al. Recurrent moderate hypoglycemia ameliorates brain damage and cognitive dysfunction induced by severe hypoglycemia. Diabetes. 2010;59:1055–62.

117. Oomura Y, Ooyama H, Sugimori M, Nakamura T, Yamada Y. Glucose inhibition of the glucose-sensitive neurone in the rat lateral hypothalamus. Nature. 1974;247:284–6.

118. Borg MA, Sherwin RS, Borg WP, Tamborlane WV, Shulman GI. Local ventromedial hypothalamus glucose perfusion blocks counterregulation during systemic hypoglycemia in awake rats. J Clin Invest. 1997;99:361–5.

119. Borg WP, Sherwin RS, During MJ, Borg MA, Shulman GI. Local ventromedial hypothalamus glucopenia triggers counterregulatory hormone release. Diabetes. 1995;44:180–4.

120. Song Z, Levin BE, McArdle JJ, Bakhos N, Routh VH. Convergence of pre- and postsynaptic influences on glucosensing neurons in the ventromedial hypothalamic nucleus. Diabetes. 2001;50:2673–81.

121. Andrew SF, Dinh TT, Ritter S. Localized glucoprivation of hindbrain sites elicits corticosterone and glucagon secretion. Am J Physiol Regul Integr Comp Physiol. 2007;292:R1792–8.

122. Balfour RH, Hansen AM, Trapp S. Neuronal responses to transient hypoglycaemia in the dorsal vagal complex of the rat brainstem. J Physiol. 2006;570:469–84.

123. Mizuno Y, Oomura Y. Glucose responding neurons in the nucleus tractus solitarius of the rat: in vitro study. Brain Res. 1984;307:109–16.

124. Funahashi M, Adachi A. Glucose-responsive neurons exist within the area postrema of the rat: in vitro study on the isolated slice preparation. Brain Res Bull. 1993;32:531–5.

125. Borg MA, Borg WP, Tamborlane WV, Brines ML, Shulman GI, Sherwin RS. Chronic hypoglycemia and diabetes impair counterregulation induced by localized 2-deoxy-glucose perfusion of the ventromedial hypothalamus in rats. Diabetes. 1999;48:584–7.

126. Sanders NM, Taborsky Jr GJ, Wilkinson CW, Daumen W, Figlewicz DP. Antecedent hindbrain glucoprivation does not impair the counterregulatory response to hypoglycemia. Diabetes. 2007;56:217–23.

127. Roncero I, Alvarez E, Vazquez P, Blazquez E. Functional glucokinase isoforms are expressed in rat brain. J Neurochem. 2000;74:1848–57.

128. Kang L, Dunn-Meynell AA, Routh VH, Gaspers LD, Nagata Y, Nishimura T, et al. Glucokinase is a critical regulator of ventromedial hypothalamic neuronal glucosensing. Diabetes. 2006;55:412–20.

129. Dunn-Meynell AA, Routh VH, Kang L, Gaspers L, Levin BE. Glucokinase is the likely mediator of glucosensing in both glucose-excited and glucose-inhibited central neurons. Diabetes. 2002;51:2056–65.

130. Kang L, Sanders NM, Dunn-Meynell AA, Gaspers LD, Routh VH, Thomas AP, et al. Prior hypoglycemia enhances glucose responsiveness in some ventromedial hypothalamic glucosensing neurons. Am J Physiol Regul Integr Comp Physiol. 2008;294:R784–92.

131. Levin BE, Becker TC, Eiki J, Zhang BB, Dunn-Meynell AA. Ventromedial hypothalamic glucokinase is an important mediator of the counterregulatory response to insulin-induced hypoglycemia. Diabetes. 2008;57:1371–9.

132. Alquier T, Kawashima J, Tsuji Y, Kahn BB. Role of hypothalamic adenosine 5′-monophosphate-activated protein kinase in the impaired counterregulatory response induced by repetitive neuroglucopenia. Endocrinology. 2007;148:1367–75.

133. McCrimmon RJ, Fan X, Ding Y, Zhu W, Jacob RJ, Sherwin RS. Potential role for AMP-activated protein kinase in hypoglycemia sensing in the ventromedial hypothalamus. Diabetes. 2004;53:1953–8.

134. McCrimmon RJ, Shaw M, Fan X, Cheng H, Ding Y, Vella MC, et al. Key role for AMP-activated protein kinase in the ventromedial hypothalamus in regulating counterregulatory hormone responses to acute hypoglycemia. Diabetes. 2008;57:444–50.

135. McCrimmon RJ, Fan X, Cheng H, McNay E, Chan O, Shaw M, et al. Activation of AMP-activated protein kinase within the ventromedial hypothalamus amplifies counterregulatory hormone responses in rats with defective counterregulation. Diabetes. 2006;55:1755–60.

136. Fan X, Ding Y, Brown S, Zhou L, Shaw M, Vella MC, et al. Hypothalamic AMP-activated protein kinase activation with AICAR amplifies counterregulatory responses to hypoglycemia in a rodent model of type 1 diabetes. Am J Physiol Regul Integr Comp Physiol. 2009;296:R1702–8.

137. Levin BE, Routh VH, Kang L, Sanders NM, Dunn-Meynell AA. Neuronal glucosensing: what do we know after 50 years? Diabetes. 2004;53:2521–8.

138. Evans ML, McCrimmon RJ, Flanagan DE, Keshavarz T, Fan X, McNay EC, et al. Hypothalamic ATP-sensitive K+channels play a key role in sensing hypoglycemia and triggering counterregulatory epinephrine and glucagon responses. Diabetes. 2004;53:2542–51.

139. McCrimmon RJ, Evans ML, Fan X, McNay EC, Chan O, Ding Y, et al. Activation of ATP-sensitive K+channels in the ventromedial hypothalamus amplifies counterregulatory hormone responses to hypoglycemia in normal and recurrently hypoglycemic rats. Diabetes. 2005;54:3169–74.

140. Tong Q, Ye C, McCrimmon RJ, Dhillon H, Choi B, Kramer MD, et al. Synaptic glutamate release by ventromedial hypothalamic neurons is part of the neurocircuitry that prevents hypoglycemia. Cell Metab. 2007;5:383–93.

141. Beverly JL, De Vries MG, Bouman SD, Arseneau LM. Noradrenergic and GABAergic systems in the medial hypothalamus are activated during hypoglycemia. Am J Physiol Regul Integr Comp Physiol. 2001;280:R563–9.

142. Chan O, Cheng H, Herzog R, Czyzyk D, Zhu W, Wang A, et al. Increased GABAergic tone in the ventromedial hypothalamus contributes to suppression of counterregulatory responses after antecedent hypoglycemia. Diabetes. 2008;57:1363–70.
143. Giordano R, Grottoli S, Brossa P, Pellegrino M, Destefanis S, Lanfranco F, et al. Alprazolam (a benzodiazepine activating GABA receptor) reduces the neuroendocrine responses to insulin-induced hypoglycaemia in humans. Clin Endocrinol (Oxf). 2003;59:314–20.
144. Hedrington MS, Farmerie S, Ertl AC, Wang Z, Tate DB, Davis SN. Effects of antecedent GABAA activation with alprazolam on counterregulatory responses to hypoglycemia in healthy humans. Diabetes. 2010;59:1074–81.
145. Chan O, Zhu W, Ding Y, McCrimmon RJ, Sherwin RS. Blockade of GABA(A) receptors in the ventromedial hypothalamus further stimulates glucagon and sympathoadrenal but not the hypothalamo-pituitary-adrenal response to hypoglycemia. Diabetes. 2006;55:1080–7.
146. Beverly JL, de Vries MG, Beverly MF, Arseneau LM. Norepinephrine mediates glucoprivic-induced increase in GABA in the ventromedial hypothalamus of rats. Am J Physiol Regul Integr Comp Physiol. 2000;279:R990–6.
147. McCrimmon RJ. Corticotrophin-releasing factor receptors within the ventromedial hypothalamus regulate hypoglycemia- induced hormonal counterregulation. J Clin Invest. 2006;116:1723–30.
148. Chalmers DT, Lovenberg TW, De Souza EB. Localization of novel corticotropin-releasing factor receptor (CRF2) mRNA expression to specific subcortical nuclei in rat brain: comparison with CRF1 receptor mRNA expression. J Neurosci. 1995;15:6340–50.
149. Cotero VE, Routh VH. Insulin blunts the response of glucose-excited neurons in the ventro-lateral-ventromedial hypothalamic nucleus to decreased glucose. Am J Physiol Endocrinol Metab. 2009;296:E1101–9.
150. Wang R, Cruciani-Guglielmacci C, Migrenne S, Magnan C, Cotero VE, Routh VH. Effects of oleic acid on distinct populations of neurons in the hypothalamic arcuate nucleus are dependent on extracellular glucose levels. J Neurophysiol. 2006;95:1491–8.
151. Paranjape SA, Chan O, Zhu W, Horblitt AM, McNay EC, Cresswell JA, et al. Influence of insulin in the ventromedial hypothalamus on pancreatic glucagon secretion in vivo. Diabetes. 2010;59:1521–7.
152. Wang R, Liu X, Hentges ST, Dunn-Meynell AA, Levin BE, Wang W, et al. The regulation of glucose-excited neurons in the hypothalamic arcuate nucleus by glucose and feeding-relevant peptides. Diabetes. 2004;53:1959–65.
153. Canabal DD, Song Z, Potian JG, Beuve A, McArdle JJ, Routh VH. Glucose, insulin, and leptin signaling pathways modulate nitric oxide synthesis in glucose-inhibited neurons in the ventromedial hypothalamus. Am J Physiol Regul Integr Comp Physiol. 2007;292:R1418–28.
154. Oz G, Kumar A, Rao JP, Kodl CT, Chow L, Eberly LE, et al. Human brain glycogen metabolism during and after hypoglycemia. Diabetes. 2009;58:1978–85.
155. Choi IY, Seaquist ER, Gruetter R. Effect of hypoglycemia on brain glycogen metabolism in vivo. J Neurosci Res. 2003;72:25–32.
156. Brown AM, Ransom BR. Astrocyte glycogen and brain energy metabolism. Glia. 2007;55:1263–71.
157. Suh SW, Bergher JP, Anderson CM, Treadway JL, Fosgerau K, Swanson RA. Astrocyte glycogen sustains neuronal activity during hypoglycemia: studies with the glycogen phosphorylase inhibitor CP-316,819 ([R-R*, S*]-5-chloro-N-[2-hydroxy-3-(methoxymethylamino)-3-oxo-1-(phenylmethyl)pro pyl]-1 H-indole-2-carboxamide). J Pharmacol Exp Ther. 2007;321:45–50.
158. Pellerin L, Magistretti PJ. Glutamate uptake into astrocytes stimulates aerobic glycolysis: a mechanism coupling neuronal activity to glucose utilization. Proc Natl Acad Sci U S A. 1994;91:10625–9.
159. Larrabee MG. Lactate metabolism and its effects on glucose metabolism in an excised neural tissue. J Neurochem. 1995;64:1734–41.
160. Wyss MT, Jolivet R, Buck A, Magistretti PJ, Weber B. In vivo evidence for lactate as a neuronal energy source. J Neurosci. 2011;31:7477–85.

161. van Hall G, Stromstad M, Rasmussen P, Jans O, Zaar M, Gam C, et al. Blood lactate is an important energy source for the human brain. J Cereb Blood Flow Metab. 2009;29:1121–9.

162. Borg MA, Tamborlane WV, Shulman GI, Sherwin RS. Local lactate perfusion of the ventro-medial hypothalamus suppresses hypoglycemic counterregulation. Diabetes. 2003;52: 663–6.

163. Mason GF, Petersen KF, Lebon V, Rothman DL, Shulman GI. Increased brain monocarboxy-lic acid transport and utilization in type 1 diabetes. Diabetes. 2006;55:929–34.

164. Koranyi L, Bourey RE, James D, Mueckler M, Fiedorek Jr FT, Permutt MA. Glucose trans-porter gene expression in rat brain: pretranslational changes associated with chronic insulin-induced hypoglycemia, fasting, and diabetes. Mol Cell Neurosci. 1991;2:244–52.

165. Boyle PJ, Nagy RJ, O'Connor AM, Kempers SF, Yeo RA, Qualls C. Adaptation in brain glucose uptake following recurrent hypoglycemia. Proc Natl Acad Sci U S A. 1994;91: 9352–6.

166. Boyle PJ, Kempers SF, O'Connor AM, Nagy RJ. Brain glucose uptake and unawareness of hypoglycemia in patients with insulin-dependent diabetes mellitus. N Engl J Med. 1995;333:1726–31.

167. Criego AB, Tkac I, Kumar A, Thomas W, Gruetter R, Seaquist ER. Brain glucose concentra-tions in patients with type 1 diabetes and hypoglycemia unawareness. J Neurosci Res. 2005;79:42–7.

168. Criego AB, Tkac I, Kumar A, Thomas W, Gruetter R, Seaquist ER. Brain glucose concentrations in healthy humans subjected to recurrent hypoglycemia. J Neurosci Res. 2005;82:525–30.

169. Hevener AL, Bergman RN, Donovan CM. Novel glucosensor for hypoglycemic detection localized to the portal vein. Diabetes. 1997;46:1521–5.

170. Matveyenko AV, Bohland M, Saberi M, Donovan CM. Portal vein hypoglycemia is essential for full induction of hypoglycemia-associated autonomic failure with slow-onset hypoglyce-mia. Am J Physiol Endocrinol Metab. 2007;293:E857–64.

171. Koyama Y, Coker RH, Stone EE, Lacy DB, Jabbour K, Williams PE, et al. Evidence that carotid bodies play an important role in glucoregulation in vivo. Diabetes. 2000;49: 1434–42.

172. Hevener AL, Bergman RN, Donovan CM. Portal vein afferents are critical for the sympathoa-drenal response to hypoglycemia. Diabetes. 2000;49:8–12.

173. Fujita S, Bohland M, Sanchez-Watts G, Watts AG, Donovan CM. Hypoglycemic detection at the portal vein is mediated by capsaicin-sensitive primary sensory neurons. Am J Physiol Endocrinol Metab. 2007;293:E96–E101.

174. Fujita S, Donovan CM. Celiac-superior mesenteric ganglionectomy, but not vagotomy, sup-presses the sympathoadrenal response to insulin-induced hypoglycemia. Diabetes. 2005;54: 3258–64.

175. Saberi M, Bohland M, Donovan CM. The locus for hypoglycemic detection shifts with the rate of fall in glycemia: the role of portal-superior mesenteric vein glucose sensing. Diabetes. 2008;57:1380–6.

176. Pardal R, Lopez-Barneo J. Low glucose-sensing cells in the carotid body. Nat Neurosci. 2002;5:197–8.

177. Conde SV, Obeso A, Gonzalez C. Low glucose effects on rat carotid body chemoreceptor cells' secretory responses and action potential frequency in the carotid sinus nerve. J Physiol. 2007;585:721–30.

178. Berlin I, Grimaldi A, Landault C, Zoghbi F, Thervet F, Puech AJ, et al. Lack of hypoglycemic symptoms and decreased beta-adrenergic sensitivity in insulin-dependent diabetic patients. J Clin Endocrinol Metab. 1988;66:273–8.

179. Korytkowski MT, Mokan M, Veneman TF, Mitrakou A, Cryer PE, Gerich JE. Reduced beta-adrenergic sensitivity in patients with type 1 diabetes and hypoglycemia unawareness. Diabetes Care. 1998;21:1939–43.

180. Trovik TS, Vaartun A, Jorde R, Sager G. Dysfunction in the beta 2-adrenergic signal pathway in patients with insulin dependent diabetes mellitus (IDDM) and unawareness of hypoglycae-mia. Eur J Clin Pharmacol. 1995;48:327–32.

181. Fritsche A, Stumvoll M, Grub M, Sieslack S, Renn W, Schmulling RM, et al. Effect of hypoglycemia on beta-adrenergic sensitivity in normal and type 1 diabetic subjects. Diabetes Care. 1998;21:1505–10.

182. Fritsche A, Stefan N, Haring H, Gerich J, Stumvoll M. Avoidance of hypoglycemia restores hypoglycemia awareness by increasing beta-adrenergic sensitivity in type 1 diabetes. Ann Intern Med. 2001;134:729–36.

183. Lingenfelser T, Buettner U, Martin J, Tobis M, Renn W, Kaschel R, et al. Improvement of impaired counterregulatory hormone response and symptom perception by short-term avoidance of hypoglycemia in IDDM. Diabetes Care. 1995;18:321–5.

184. Liu D, McManus RM, Ryan EA. Improved counter-regulatory hormonal and symptomatic responses to hypoglycemia in patients with insulin-dependent diabetes mellitus after 3 months of less strict glycemic control. Clin Invest Med. 1996;19:71–82.

185. Cranston I, Lomas J, Maran A, Macdonald I, Amiel SA. Restoration of hypoglycaemia awareness in patients with long-duration insulin-dependent diabetes. Lancet. 1994;344:283–7.

186. Fanelli C, Pampanelli S, Epifano L, Rambotti AM, Di Vincenzo A, Modarelli F, et al. Long-term recovery from unawareness, deficient counterregulation and lack of cognitive dysfunction during hypoglycaemia, following institution of rational, intensive insulin therapy in IDDM. Diabetologia. 1994;37:1265–76.

187. Fanelli CG, Epifano L, Rambotti AM, Pampanelli S, Di Vincenzo A, Modarelli F, et al. Meticulous prevention of hypoglycemia normalizes the glycemic thresholds and magnitude of most of neuroendocrine responses to, symptoms of, and cognitive function during hypoglycemia in intensively treated patients with short-term IDDM. Diabetes. 1993;42:1683–9.

188. Dagogo-Jack S, Rattarasarn C, Cryer PE. Reversal of hypoglycemia unawareness, but not defective glucose counterregulation, in IDDM. Diabetes. 1994;43:1426–34.

189. Davis M, Mellman M, Friedman S, Chang CJ, Shamoon H. Recovery of epinephrine response but not hypoglycemic symptom threshold after intensive therapy in type 1 diabetes. Am J Med. 1994;97:535–42.

190. McCrimmon RJ, Deary IJ, Huntly BJ, MacLeod KJ, Frier BM. Visual information processing during controlled hypoglycaemia in humans. Brain. 1996;119(Pt 4):1277–87.

191. Ewing FM, Deary IJ, McCrimmon RJ, Strachan MW, Frier BM. Effect of acute hypoglycemia on visual information processing in adults with type 1 diabetes mellitus. Physiol Behav. 1998;64:653–60.

192. Strachan MW, Ewing FM, Frier BM, McCrimmon RJ, Deary IJ. Effects of acute hypoglycaemia on auditory information processing in adults with Type I diabetes. Diabetologia. 2003;46:97–105.

193. McCrimmon RJ, Deary IJ, Frier BM. Auditory information processing during acute insulin-induced hypoglycaemia in non-diabetic human subjects. Neuropsychologia. 1997;35:1547–53.

194. Geddes J, Deary IJ, Frier BM. Effects of acute insulin-induced hypoglycaemia on psychomotor function: people with type 1 diabetes are less affected than non-diabetic adults. Diabetologia. 2008;51:1814–21.

195. McAulay V, Deary IJ, Sommerfield AJ, Frier BM. Attentional functioning is impaired during acute hypoglycaemia in people with Type 1 diabetes. Diabet Med. 2006;23:26–31.

196. Iscoe KE, Corcoran M, Riddell MC. High rates of nocturnal hypoglycemia in a unique sports camp for athletes with type 1 diabetes: lessons learned from continuous glucose monitoring systems. Can J Diabetes. 2008;32:182–9.

197. Brazeau AS, Rabasa-Lhoret R, Strychar I, Mircescu H. Barriers to physical activity among patients with type 1 diabetes. Diabetes Care. 2008;31:2108–9.

198. Clarke WL, Cox DJ, Gonder-Frederick LA, Julian D, Schlundt D, Polonsky W. Reduced awareness of hypoglycemia in adults with IDDM. A prospective study of hypoglycemic frequency and associated symptoms. Diabetes Care. 1995;18:517–22.

199. Janssen MM, Snoek FJ, Heine RJ. Assessing impaired hypoglycemia awareness in type 1 diabetes: agreement of self-report but not of field study data with the autonomic symptom threshold during experimental hypoglycemia. Diabetes Care. 2000;23:529–32.

200. Clarke WL, Cox DJ, Gonder-Frederick LA, Julian D, Schlundt D, Polonsky W. The relation-ship between nonroutine use of insulin, food, and exercise and the occurrence of hypoglyce-mia in adults with IDDM and varying degrees of hypoglycemic awareness and metabolic control. Diabetes Educ. 1997;23:55–8.
201. Cox DJ, Gonder-Frederick L, Antoun B, Cryer PE, Clarke WL. Perceived symptoms in the recognition of hypoglycemia. Diabetes Care. 1993;16:519–27.
202. Pennebaker JW, Cox DJ, Gonder-Frederick L, Wunsch MG, Evans WS, Pohl S. Physical symptoms related to blood glucose in insulin-dependent diabetics. Psychosom Med. 1981; 43:489–500.
203. Mitrakou A, Mokan M, Ryan C, Veneman T, Cryer P, Gerich J. Influence of plasma glucose rate of decrease on hierarchy of responses to hypoglycemia. J Clin Endocrinol Metab. 1993;76:462–5.
204. Hepburn DA, Deary IJ, Frier BM, Patrick AW, Quinn JD, Fisher BM. Symptoms of acute insulin-induced hypoglycemia in humans with and without IDDM. Factor-analysis approach. Diabetes Care. 1991;14:949–57.
205. Pohl J, Frohnau G, Kerner W, Fehm-Wolfsdorf G. Symptom awareness is affected by the subjects' expectations during insulin-induced hypoglycemia. Diabetes Care. 1997;20: 796–802.
206. Guelfi KJ, Jones TW, Fournier PA. The decline in blood glucose levels is less with intermit-tent high-intensity compared with moderate exercise in individuals with type 1 diabetes. Diabetes Care. 2005;28:1289–94.
207. Bussau VA, Ferreira LD, Jones TW, Fournier PA. A 10-s sprint performed prior to moderate-intensity exercise prevents early post-exercise fall in glycaemia in individuals with type 1 diabetes. Diabetologia. 2007;50:1815–8.
208. Bussau VA, Ferreira LD, Jones TW, Fournier PA. The 10-s maximal sprint: a novel approach to counter an exercise-mediated fall in glycemia in individuals with type 1 diabetes. Diabetes Care. 2006;29:601–6.
209. Cryer PE, Davis SN, Shamoon H. Hypoglycemia in diabetes. Diabetes Care. 2003;26: 1902–12.
210. Pearson T. Glucagon as a treatment of severe hypoglycemia: safe and efficacious but under-utilized. Diabetes Educ. 2008;34:128–34.
211. Harris G, Diment A, Sulway M, Wilkinson M. Glucagon administration – underevaluated and undertaught. Practical Diabetes Int. 2001;18:22–5.
212. George E, Marques JL, Harris ND, Macdonald IA, Hardisty CA, Heller SR. Preservation of physiological responses to hypoglycemia 2 days after antecedent hypoglycemia in patients with IDDM. Diabetes Care. 1997;20:1293–8.

Chapter 7
Fueling the Athlete with Type 1 Diabetes

Carin Hume

7.1 Introduction

Evidence-based guidelines exist to advise athletes on the appropriate amount, composition, and timing of food intake required to optimize training and performance [1–3]. The nutrition goals and guidelines for training and competition for athletes with and without T1DM are similar, yet there are special considerations for the athlete with T1DM. Maintenance of glycemic control remains an important goal for the athlete with T1DM so as to limit the progression of long-term complications from diabetes [4].

A recent review by the American Dietetic Association shows that medical nutrition therapy can help to reduce the potential for complications of diabetes through improvements in glycemic, lipid, and blood pressure control [5]. Tailored nutritional advice may also be able to have a significant influence both on athletic performance and glycemic control in active individuals with T1DM. In this chapter, we will consider important features of the nutritional guidelines for athletes without diabetes and, then, discuss how these might need to be adjusted for athletes with T1DM.

7.2 Nutrition Guidelines for the Athlete Without T1DM

A summary of nutrition guidelines for athletes without diabetes is presented below. These guidelines serve as a basis for nutritional advice to the athlete with T1DM but will need to be adjusted to accommodate the particular needs of this group.

C. Hume, B.Sc., M.Sc.
Department of Nutrition and Dietetics, Buckinghamshire Hospitals NHS Trust,
Queen Alexandra Rd., High Wycombe, Buckinghamshire
HP11 2TT, UK

I. Gallen (ed.), *Type 1 Diabetes*,
DOI 10.1007/978-0-85729-754-9_7, © Springer-Verlag London Limited 2012

7.2.1 Carbohydrate

- Athletes need to consume a diet containing adequate daily carbohydrate (CHO) to support training and maintain health. CHO in the athlete's diet needs to be considered in terms of whether both the total daily intake and the timing of CHO consumption in relation to exercise maintain an adequate supply of CHO substrate for the muscle and central nervous system [3]. CHO needs will change according to the training load and competition program and are therefore likely to vary from day to day.
- An adequate CHO intake is required to meet the fuel requirements of training and to optimize the restoration of muscle glycogen stores between training sessions. This is essential for high-intensity and long duration training sessions. Daily CHO intake guidelines for athletes are expressed per kilogram body mass and range from 3–12 g/kg BM/day [3]. Athletes partaking in moderate-intensity exercise for approximately 1 h per day should aim for a CHO intake of 5 to 7 g/kg BM/day. CHO recommendations for endurance athletes training at a moderate to high intensity level for 1–3 h per day are 6–10 g/kg BM/day. Athletes partaking in more extreme and moderate- to higher-intensity exercise for more than 4 h per day may require a CHO intake in the range of 8–12 g/kg BM/day. For athletes performing skill-based activities and recreational athletes not performing daily exercise, a CHO intake of 3 g/kg BM/day is probably adequate. It is essential to have an understanding of the type of training undertaken by the athlete and the energy demands of the sport in order that these guidelines may be correctly applied.
- "Carbohydrate loading" is the consumption of extra CHO in the time leading up to an event in order to maximize muscle glycogen stores. Evidence suggests that this may be beneficial for endurance events lasting longer than 90 min [6], in particular when the athlete's daily diet provides <7–8 g CHO/kg BM/day. A CHO-loading regimen may involve 1–3 days of a high-CHO diet, providing between 10–12 g CHO/kg BM/day [7, 8].
- During exercise, the consumption of CHO provides an exogenous fuel source to the muscle and central nervous system. Current guidelines recommend a CHO intake of 30–60 g/h for sports of more than 60 min in which fatigue is likely to occur [1, 2]. This is a general guideline and must be adapted to the needs of the individual and sport.
- In events lasting an hour or less, small amounts of CHO can improve cognitive and physical performance, most likely due to a central nervous system effect [9]. Interestingly, performance improvements have also been shown where athletes simply rinsed their mouth with a CHO drink during a 1-h cycling time trial [10].
- In events lasting longer than 2.5 h, it is suggested that the amount of CHO required to optimize performance ranges from 60–90 g/h and there appears to be a dose-response relationship between CHO intake and performance [11]. When the hourly CHO intake is between 70–90 g/h, it is advisable to use sports products that contain a mixture of CHO sources (i.e., glucose and fructose) in order to maximize CHO oxidation and absorption from the gut [12].

- Where the recovery period is short (i.e., <8 h between intense training sessions), it is advisable to begin consuming CHO as soon as possible after a training session or competition event. In the immediate post-exercise period (0–4 h after exercise), a CHO intake of 1.0–1.2 g/kg BM/h for the first 4 h is required to replace glycogen stores. CHO with a moderate to high glycemic index (see below) may be preferable when rapid restoration of glycogen stores is a priority [13]. The combined ingestion of a small amount of protein (0.2–0.4 g/kg BM/h) with smaller amounts of CHO (0.8 g/kg BM/h) results in similar muscle glycogen synthesis compared to when larger amounts of CHO are ingested alone [14]. The addition of protein to the post-exercise CHO is therefore beneficial when CHO requirements cannot be met. For athletes who rest for a day between intense training sessions, the timing and quantity of CHO consumed immediately post-exercise is of lesser importance, and the focus should be on consuming sufficient CHO during the 24-h period after exercise [15]. Nevertheless, consuming a meal or snack within 60 min post-exercise is important as muscle glycogen synthesis rates are much higher in the immediate post-exercise period.

7.2.1.1   Glycemic Index (GI)

The GI classifies CHO-rich foods based on their postprandial blood glucose response compared with a reference food (usually white bread or glucose), which has a GI value of 100 [16]. GI is calculated by measuring the incremental area under the blood glucose response curve after the ingestion of a reference food containing 50 g of available CHO and a test food also containing 50 g of available CHO. A high GI value indicates rapid absorption and delivery of the CHO into circulation. CHO-rich foods can be classified as high GI (GI>71), moderate GI (GI between 56 and 70), and low GI (GI of 55 or less) [16].

7.2.1.2   The GI and Exercise Performance in the Athlete

Low-GI pre-exercise feedings (1–3 h before exercise) have been shown to result in greater fat oxidation and lower muscle glycogen utilization during exercise compared to high-GI pre-exercise feedings [17]. However, it is debatable whether this apparent metabolic benefit translates into a performance benefit. A small number of studies have shown a performance benefit for a low-GI pre-exercise meal [18], but studies which have supplemented CHO during exercise indicate that the GI of the pre-exercise meal has little impact on athletic performance and show no differences in CHO and fat oxidation when a CHO beverage is ingested during exercise [19]. Given that it is accepted practice for athletes to consume CHO during endurance events and exercise lasting more than 1 h, the practical relevance of including the GI in the pre-exercise nutrition strategy is unclear.

The GI may have a more important impact on post-exercise nutrition. If rapid restoration of glycogen is a priority due to short recovery periods (<8 h between training sessions), a benefit has been demonstrated for higher-GI foods over lower-GI foods [20]. However, as discussed above, the timing, quantity, and rate of CHO ingested after exercise are also all important for rapid glycogen synthesis.

7.2.2 Protein

- The timing of protein intake is important. Foods or snacks containing high-quality protein should be consumed regularly throughout the day and, in particular, soon after exercise to aid in the maintenance or gain of muscle and in the repair of damaged tissues. Consumption of 15–25 g of protein soon after all training sessions will maximize the synthesis of proteins [1].
- A varied diet that meets energy needs will provide adequate protein for most athletes; however, for smaller athletes with lower energy intakes, consideration needs to be given to ensure that adequate protein is consumed.

7.2.3 Hydration

Being adequately hydrated is important for optimizing exercise performance. The American College of Sports Medicine (ACSM) position stand on exercise and fluid replacement [21] forms the basis for the following recommendations.

- It is recommended to ingest 5–7 ml/kg of fluid at least 4 h before exercise.
- During exercise, athletes should drink enough fluid to limit dehydration to <2% of body weight. It is important to avoid excessive fluid ingestion, which can result in hyponatremia and associated problems. Gaining weight during exercise is an important indicator that fluid ingestion is inappropriately high.
- Rates of fluid loss are highly variable. The rate of fluid replacement required will be dependent on a number of factors such as the individual's sweat rate, exercise duration, and opportunities to drink. Extra care needs to be given to avoiding dehydration when exercising in hot and humid environments and at high altitudes.
- Sodium stimulates thirst and fluid retention and should be included in beverages (at a level of 500–700 mg/l) when sweat losses are high and when exercise lasts more than 2 h.
- The CHO concentration of beverages should ideally not exceed 8% in order to maximize gastric emptying and minimize the chance of gastrointestinal upset.
- In the post-exercise period, rapid and complete recovery from excessive dehydration can be achieved by drinking 1.5 l of fluid for every kilogram lost.

7.2.4 Vitamin and Mineral Supplements

- Vitamin and mineral supplements are typically not required if an athlete is consuming adequate energy from a varied diet.

- Adequate calcium and vitamin D play an important role in bone health and in the prevention of stress fractures. Athletes who live at northern latitudes or who train predominantly indoors may be deficient in vitamin D and are therefore likely to benefit from supplementation with vitamin D [22].
- In addition to vitamin D, calcium supplementation may be required in athletes with amenorrhea and weight-conscious athletes with a low energy intake in order to prevent low bone density and the risk of stress fractures [23].

7.3 Specific Challenges in Diabetes

As we have seen in Chap. 2, exercise presents particular metabolic challenges in T1DM, with a significant risk of both hyper- and hypoglycemia depending on the situation. Maintaining blood glucose levels within an acceptable range requires the correct balance between insulin dosing, the consumption of metabolic fuels (particularly carbohydrate), and the energy requirements of the exercise. In practice, the energy requirements are often relatively inflexible, being determined by the training goals or demands of competition. This means that glycemic control is invariably maintained by making adjustments to insulin dosing or carbohydrate replacement. Insulin dosing has been considered elsewhere in this volume (Chap. 3) in conjunction with pre-exercise carbohydrate feeding, and so this chapter will focus on nutritional advice specific to the athlete with T1DM and, in particular, the effects of CHO supplementation.

7.4 Macronutrient Recommendations for the Athlete with T1DM

No specific macronutrient recommendations exist for the athlete with T1DM. Guidance is therefore drawn from both general nutrition practice recommendations for adults with diabetes [5] and recommendations for athletes without diabetes.

7.4.1 Carbohydrate

- As noted above, it is essential to consume adequate CHO to support training in order to optimize sporting performance. Daily CHO recommendations for athletes (as presented earlier) are also applicable to the athlete with T1DM.
- In order to maintain glycemic control in T1DM, this CHO intake needs to be matched with appropriate insulin doses given at the appropriate time. Individuals on MDI and CSII therapy are advised to adjust insulin doses to match CHO intake (insulin-to-CHO ratios) [24].

- Athletes without T1DM are advised to vary energy and CHO intake according to the periodized training load and daily fluctuations in training. For the athlete with T1DM, it is important to consume adequate CHO on a daily basis to ensure that glycogen stores are replenished, which should aid in reducing exercise-associated hypoglycemia. There is evidence to suggest that day-to-day consistency in distribution of CHO intake results in improved glycemic control, although it is debatable whether this applies to individuals who adjust insulin to match CHO [25]. At present, therefore, there is perhaps insufficient evidence to suggest that substantial day-to-day variation in CHO intake is beneficial for the athlete with T1DM, and so a reasonably consistent daily CHO intake may be preferable.
- CHO should be distributed fairly evenly throughout the day, with a particular focus on ensuring that adequate CHO is consumed soon after training sessions to promote glycogen synthesis post-exercise.

7.4.1.1   GI in the Nutritional Management of Diabetes

The use of the GI is recognized as playing an important part in the management of diabetes by various professional organizations, including the Canadian Diabetes Association, Diabetes UK, and Diabetes Australia [26–28]. Using continuous glucose monitoring, a low-GI meal has been shown to reduce postprandial glucose excursions in children and adolescents treated with both MDI and CSII when compared with a high-GI meal [29, 30]. A low-GI diet has also been found to positively affect the daily mean blood glucose concentration [31]. These differences probably explain why low-GI diets can help to lower HbA1c in people with diabetes, and are therefore recommended in this group [32].

A low-GI diet also has the potential to limit insulin requirements, which may be particularly beneficial in the context of exercise. Lower insulin dosing will result in lower levels of circulating insulin which may help to reduce the risk of hypoglycemia both during exercise and in the early postprandial period and also post-exercise when insulin sensitivity is enhanced. Related to this, it is interesting to note that nutrition recommendations for individuals with T1DM frequently focus on "carbohydrate counting" (matching insulin to CHO) but do not take the GI into account. Given that the above evidence suggests that lower-GI CHO requires less insulin than an equal amount of higher-GI CHO, it seems that the GI of CHO should also be taken into account when deciding appropriate insulin dosing.

It is also important to understand that the GI does not tell the whole story about some foods, and so its use should be applied with appropriate consideration. For example, while watermelon has a high GI, the CHO load in a serving is relatively small, and therefore, there does not seem any reason to limit such a food in the diet, even in the context of diabetes. In contrast, adding fat to a high-GI food not only lowers its GI but also alters its overall nutritional value, meaning that there may not be such a strong benefit from the lower-GI food in these circumstances.

7.4.1.2 GI and Exercise in the Athlete with T1DM

As noted elsewhere in this volume (Chap. 3), the findings of two recent studies have looked at the effect of low-GI compared to high-GI CHO in individuals with T1DM and have made recommendations for athletes with T1DM [33, 34]. Isomaltulose, a low-GI CHO, was compared with dextrose, a high-GI CHO. Optimal timing of isomaltulose (and ideal insulin dose reduction) was also considered. The overall outcome was that taking low-GI CHO in the form of isomaltulose 30 min prior to running with a reduced bolus (25% of usual bolus) of rapid-acting analogue insulin was protective against hypoglycemia. A more stable blood glucose response was also observed when compared with dextrose, and a more normal metabolic response was seen with lipid oxidation maintained in spite of CHO ingestion.

Care may be needed in applying these recommendations to individual athletes, as 75 g of CHO, as used in these studies, is a large amount of CHO to ingest 30 min before an exercise such as running (this is unlikely to be a problem for cycling), and so the possibility of gastrointestinal disturbance needs to be considered. Future studies using solid food, mixed macronutrient meals, and smaller pre-exercise CHO feedings are important for seeing how this research will translate into practice. Nonetheless, the results are worthy of attention as they do suggest that the GI of the pre-exercise feeding may be important and is potentially a useful strategy for some individuals with T1DM.

7.4.2 CHO Intake Prior to Training or Competition

Ideally, individuals need to find a pre-event nutrition strategy that safeguards against hyperglycemia in the hours prior to exercise and hypoglycemia before and during exercise. The pre-event meal serves the purpose of maintaining or increasing muscle glycogen stores and liver glycogen content (especially important for early morning events where the liver glycogen stores are depleted from an overnight fast). In order to achieve this, the pre-event meal should be based on high-CHO foods that the individual athlete is comfortable with. In diabetes, there is likely to be a benefit from consuming a low-GI CHO pre-exercise meal for endurance events or longer duration training sessions. The timing of the pre-event meal is individual; a meal 2–4 h before the event is suitable for most athletes. For the individual with T1DM, the benefit of consuming the pre-event meal at least 4 h before the event allows the athlete to start exercise with low circulating insulin levels, which may be advantageous in endurance events and for individuals prone to hypoglycemia. When the pre-exercise meal is <2 h before the event or training session, the meal insulin bolus may need adjusting according to the intensity and duration of the exercise [35] and the individual's glycemic response to competition. Blood glucose may be raised in the hours before competition through stress-associated increases in counterregulatory hormones, and therefore, some individuals may require a slightly larger insulin bolus than usual with the pre-exercise meal.

Consumption of a low-GI CHO drink 30 min before the event or training session, in conjunction with a significant reduction in the meal insulin bolus (a reduction of up to 75% of usual insulin bolus), is another strategy which may be helpful. It remains to be seen whether ingestion of a solid meal containing similarly low-GI CHO at this point might have the same effect. The possibility of GI upset means this strategy may not be practical in all competition situations, but it may be particularly useful in training, especially where the individual chooses not to supplement with CHO during the exercise. The use of common sports drinks as a replacement for a pre-event meal may not be ideal in all circumstances due to the high GI of these products which will promote hyperglycemia in the hours before an event.

Glycemic control must be assessed prior to training and events in order to make a decision whether CHO is required before exercise. The direction of the rate of change in BG is useful in this instance, which has implications for blood glucose testing (see below). If the pre-exercise BG is <5 mmol/l, not rising, and the exercise is primarily aerobic, at least 15 g of CHO should be ingested. In contrast, if the BG is 5–14 mmol/l and stable or increasing, no CHO may be required before exercise. The preferred strategy in these circumstances might be to supplement CHO during exercise (depending on the exercise duration and experience of the glycemic response to exercise).

It is common practice for athletes with T1DM who are prone to hypoglycemia during exercise to preload with high-GI CHO to ensure that blood glucose is sufficiently raised at the start of exercise. This practice is not encouraged as exercising in a hyperglycemic state poses problems with regard to performance, through possible effects on both coordination [36] and metabolism, with hyperglycemia associated with a shift toward CHO oxidation as the main fuel source compared to when exercising in euglycemia [37]. Supplementing with high-GI CHO at regular intervals during exercise (e.g., every 15–20 min) will maintain a more stable and physiological blood glucose level than pre-loading with CHO.

7.4.2.1   CHO Loading

The aim of CHO loading is to maximize muscle glycogen stores prior to endurance events. While CHO loading has been proven to have performance benefits in endurance events in the athlete without T1DM [6], this practice has not been researched in the athlete with T1DM. "Tapering," the reduction in training load immediately prior to an event, may already pose a challenge with maintaining euglycemia in the days leading up to an event. A significant increase in CHO intake prior to an event may therefore exacerbate this challenge. For this reason, CHO loading is currently not encouraged in the athlete with T1DM.

7.4.3   CHO Intake During Training and Competition

CHO intake is known to increase performance during endurance and intermittent high-intensity exercise, allowing for the maintenance of high levels of CHO oxidation throughout the exercise. In the athlete with T1DM, supplementing with

CHO during exercise has been shown to prevent hypoglycemia and is a useful strategy for unplanned activities or when insulin adjustments are not an option (such as in the late postprandial period). Guidelines on CHO supplementation during exercise for the athlete without T1DM are discussed earlier in this chapter. These guidelines can be used for the athlete with T1DM, but consideration needs to be given to various factors (see below).

Consideration must also be given to the type of CHO used. Exogenous CHO oxidation rates have been shown to be higher when ingesting a combination of CHOs that use different intestinal digestion and transport systems compared to when a single CHO source is used [12]. This becomes particularly important in circumstances where more than 70 g CHO/h may be required, such as when performing intense exercise during peak insulin action. The source of CHO consumed should be selected to maximize CHO oxidation and prevent gastrointestinal problems. For example, when a mixture of glucose and fructose is ingested during exercise (in the athlete without T1DM), exogenous CHO oxidation rates have been shown to be as high as 1.7 g/min [38]. In contrast, isomaltulose and fructose are oxidized at low rates (0.6 g/min) and for this reason are not routinely recommended to be ingested during exercise.

There are a number of important factors which need to be taken into account when adapting recommendations regarding CHO intake during exercise to the individual athlete:

1. *The mode of insulin delivery and insulin regimen*

   CSII gives the athlete a greater degree of flexibility for making basal rate adjustments before, during, and after exercise, unlike other regimens, i.e., MDI, and twice daily insulin regimens. CHO needs for individuals on CSII may therefore be at the lower end of suggested recommendations if appropriate insulin adjustments are made.

2. *The timing of exercise in relation to insulin administration*

   CHO needs have been shown to vary according to the levels of circulating insulin. Francescato et al. found that 60 min of moderate-intensity exercise performed 1 h after insulin administration required approximately 1 g CHO/kg BM; the subjects required approximately 0.5 g/kg BM and 0.25 g/kg BM of CHO when the same intensity exercise was performed 2.5 and 4 h after insulin administration, respectively [39]. When the pre-meal rapid insulin dose is adjusted for postprandial exercise (see Table 1 of Rabasa-Lhoret et al. [35]), the CHO needs are likely to be lower than suggested recommendations.

3. *Time of day of exercise*

   CHO needs when exercising in a fasted state are likely to be significantly lower than when exercising at other times in the day, and therefore, CHO supplementation during exercise at this time may not be required.

4. *Blood glucose when commencing exercise*

   The pre-exercise BG will influence the type of CHO and timing of CHO feeding during exercise. When BG is elevated prior to aerobic exercise, for example, above 10 mmol/l, CHO feedings may need to be delayed until BG has lowered or solid foods (e.g., banana, cereal bar), which have a lower GI, can be ingested earlier on in the exercise. In contrast, when the pre-exercise BG is below 6 mmol/l, high-GI CHO such as energy drinks and energy gels may need to be taken on board earlier in the exercise.

Interestingly, since performance improvements have been shown where athletes without T1DM simply rinsed their mouth with a CHO drink [10], this may be a strategy the athlete with T1DM wishes to try when competing with elevated BG. However, it is important to recognize that this has not been investigated in the context of T1DM

5. *The effect of antecedent hypoglycemia and/or prolonged moderate exercise*

Both these factors have been shown to blunt counterregulatory responses during subsequent exercise bouts, thereby making the athlete more susceptible to hypoglycemia. Davis et al. found that nearly threefold greater exogenous glucose infusion rates were required to preserve euglycemia during exercise following a day of antecedent hypoglycemia as compared to a day without hypoglycemia [40]. The athlete therefore needs to be aware that after recent hypoglycemia, CHO needs during subsequent training sessions may be greater than usual.

6. *The type of exercise*

High-intensity (e.g., sprints, weight training) and intermittent high-intensity exercise (e.g., football, hockey) may result in hyperglycemia during and/or after the exercise; therefore, CHO feeding during exercise as per general sports nutrition recommendations will exacerbate the hyperglycemia.

7. *Training status*

The level of fitness of the individual will affect the CHO needs. An untrained individual will require more CHO than someone who is physically fit. If an individual exercises different muscles to the usual muscles used, CHO needs may also be greater.

8. *Environmental conditions*

Training and competing in warm and humid conditions and at altitude may raise BG; consideration must therefore be given to the environmental conditions, especially if they are different to usual conditions.

By considering these factors, in addition to using a trial and error approach, an athlete with T1DM can develop their individual strategy for managing CHO supplementation during exercise. A stable BG before, during, and after exercise suggests that the individual has made the appropriate insulin and CHO adjustments for the activity.

7.4.4   CHO and Protein Intake After Training and Competition

Insulin sensitivity in the athlete with T1DM may last for 12–24 h post-exercise [41, 42], predisposing the athlete to post-exercise late-onset hypoglycemia if muscle glycogen stores are not replenished after exercise. Post-exercise nutrition is also important to facilitate skeletal muscle repair and synthesis. In athletes without T1DM, the co-ingestion of CHO (0.8 g/kg BM/h) with a small amount of protein (0.2–0.4 g/kg BM/h) post-exercise stimulates endogenous insulin release and results in similar muscle glycogen repletion rates to when only CHO (1.2 g CHO/kg BW/h) is ingested [14]. It is speculated that greater postprandial insulin levels after protein co-ingestion may stimulate the storage of CHO in more insulin-sensitive tissues such as the liver and exercised skeletal muscle, therefore promoting more efficient storage of CHO [42]. The athlete with T1DM should consider administering a small insulin bolus with the post-exercise CHO to facilitate rapid glycogen synthesis. The consumption of approximately 20 g of intact protein, which is the equivalent of 9 g of essential amino acids, is sufficient to maximize muscle protein synthesis during the first few hours after exercise. When the athlete has multiple training sessions on the same day, consuming moderate- to higher-GI CHO within the first few hours post-exercise will aid in replenishing muscle glycogen stores. Individuals on a MDI regimen who are prone to post-exercise late-onset hypoglycemia during the night may benefit from consuming a CHO and protein-containing snack at bedtime [43].

7.5 The Role of Blood Glucose Monitoring

There are significant interindividual variations in BG responses to exercise, but there is some stability of intraindividual responses, which means that individuals can use knowledge of their BG responses to make informed decisions about the management of their diabetes for exercise. The gathering of relevant information is key to this process. Frequent BG monitoring before, during, and after exercise is useful as it provides information about how BG values change with exercise. A single reading is rarely helpful in itself. For this reason, continuous glucose monitoring is a useful alternative to finger prick testing and may be particularly beneficial for the recognition of post-exercise hypoglycemia.

Seeing the pattern of how BG changes are affected by a particular type of exercise bout will provide the basis for the insulin and nutrition strategy for future, similar exercise bouts. It may also be useful to record the timing of the exercise, duration and intensity of a training session or event, the dose and timing of any insulin bolus, and CHO intake before, during, and after exercise. Noting the injection site and incidence of hypoglycemia in the preceding 24 h is also likely to be helpful.

7.6 Weight Management for the Athlete with T1DM

Weight control is often an issue for athletes, and there are circumstances where it will be particularly relevant: long distance running where an athlete is required to carry their own weight, cycling where appropriate weight may result in an increase in the power-to-weight ratio, and sports which have weight categories such as lightweight rowing, horse racing, boxing, and martial arts. Unfortunately, controlling weight can be a particular challenge for the athlete with T1DM for a number of reasons. For example, exercising with inappropriately high levels of circulating insulin will increase CHO needs during exercise and also suppress the use of endogenously stored fuel sources.

Losing weight requires setting realistic goals, getting the fine balance between energy intake and expenditure correct, and considering the macronutrient composition and energy density of the diet. A number of strategies are available to the athlete with T1DM to aid with weight control, either by reducing the amount of CHO required at the time of exercise or by affecting substrate utilization:

- Exercise in the morning, in a fasted state (this is not advisable for key, high-intensity training sessions), or in the late postprandial period (i.e., 4–5 h after the meal insulin bolus).
- In the case of CSII, reduce basal insulin infusion rate around exercise in order to minimize CHO requirements during exercise (see Chap. 5).
- If on an MDI regimen, consider the time action profile of the basal insulin; aim to exercise at a time when the basal insulin's action is coming to an end. Using twice daily NPH may help in this instance.
- Reduce the pre-meal insulin bolus when exercising within 90–120 min of the meal.
- Exercise soon after a low-GI meal (e.g., 30 min after meal). Due to the dampened postprandial blood glucose response produced by a low-GI meal, the associated insulin bolus may be significantly reduced or even omitted if the pre-meal blood glucose is in a low to normal range and the exercise is predominantly aerobic.
- Eat a low-GI diet—this may have a small but positive effect on weight control.
- Ingest caffeine before exercise to help prevent hypoglycemia associated with exercise (not advisable when exercising after midday). The dose of caffeine used in the research was 5 mg/kg BM [44]. This large dose may not be practical for most athletes.
- Start exercise in a euglycemic state (BG of 5–9 mmol/l) to maximize fat oxidation.
- Abstain from heavy pre-loading with CHO and instead supplement with CHO during exercise as dictated by BG.

7.7 Hydration

Recommendations regarding fluid intake for athletes with T1DM are similar to those for athletes without T1DM as outlined earlier. However, it is worth noting that exercising with elevated BG will promote fluid loss and therefore fluid requirements will be greater than when exercising in a euglycemic state. When exercising during hyperglycemia, water or CHO-free electrolyte sports drinks should be ingested instead of regular sports drinks.

7.8 Protein

In individuals with T1DM with normal renal function, a protein intake of 15–20% of daily energy intake is recommended [5]. Guidance on the timing of protein intake (as discussed earlier in this chapter) should also be adopted by the athlete with T1DM.

7.9 Fat

In contrast to CHO and protein recommendations, there are at present no reference values for fat intake in exercise.

7.10 Summary

A sound nutritional strategy is an important weapon in the armory of the athlete with T1DM. Many of the general recommendations made for all athletes apply to this population, but there are special considerations which apply to T1DM of which both athletes with T1DM and their health professionals should be aware. The majority of the differences between recommendations for those with and without T1DM come in the consideration of appropriate CHO intake in the diet.

References

1. Burke LM. The IOC consensus on sports nutrition 2003: new guidelines for nutrition for athletes. Int J Sport Nutr Exerc Metab. 2003;13(4):549–52.
2. Rodriguez NR, Di Marco NM, Langley S. American College of Sports Medicine position stand. Nutrition and athletic performance. Med Sci Sports Exerc. 2009;41(3):709–31.
3. Burke LM, Hawley JA, Wong SH, Jeukendrup AE. Carbohydrates for training and competition. J Sports Sci. 2011;29:S17–27.
4. The Diabetes Control and Complications Trial Research Group. The effect of intensive treatment of diabetes on the development and progression of long-term complications in insulin-dependent diabetes mellitus. N Engl J Med. 1993;329(14):977–86.
5. Franz MJ, Powers MA, Leontos C, Holzmeister LA, Kulkarni K, Monk A, et al. The evidence for medical nutrition therapy for type 1 and type 2 diabetes in adults. J Am Diet Assoc. 2010;110(12):1852–89.
6. Hawley JA, Schabort EJ, Noakes TD, Dennis SC. Carbohydrate-loading and exercise performance. An update. Sports Med. 1997;24(2):73–81.
7. Bussau VA, Fairchild TJ, Rao A, Steele P, Fournier PA. Carbohydrate loading in human muscle: an improved 1 day protocol. Eur J Appl Physiol. 2002;87(3):290–5.
8. James AP, Lorraine M, Cullen D, Goodman C, Dawson B, Palmer TN, et al. Muscle glycogen supercompensation: absence of a gender-related difference. Eur J Appl Physiol. 2001;85(6): 533–8.
9. Jeukendrup A, Brouns F, Wagenmakers AJ, Saris WH. Carbohydrate-electrolyte feedings improve 1 h time trial cycling performance. Int J Sports Med. 1997;18(2):125–9.
10. Carter JM, Jeukendrup AE, Jones DA. The effect of carbohydrate mouth rinse on 1-h cycle time trial performance. Med Sci Sports Exerc. 2004;36(12):2107–11.
11. Smith WM, Zachwieja JJ, Peronnet F, Passe DH, Massicotte D, Lavoie C. Fuel selection and cycling endurance performance with ingestion of (13C) glucose: evidence for a carbohydrate dose response. J App Physiol. 2010;108(6):1520–9.
12. Jentjens RL, Jeukendrup AE. High rates of exogenous carbohydrate oxidation from a mixture of glucose and fructose ingested during prolonged cycling exercise. Br J Nutr. 2005;93(4): 485–92.

13. Burke LM, Collier GR, Hargreaves M. Muscle glycogen storage after prolonged exercise: effect of the glycemic index of carbohydrate feedings. J Appl Physiol. 1993;75(2):1019–23.

14. Howarth KR, Moreau NA, Phillips SM, Gibala MJ. Coingestion of protein with carbohydrate during recovery from endurance exercise stimulates skeletal muscle protein synthesis in humans. J Appl Physiol. 2009;106(4):1394–402.

15. Burke LM, Collier GR, Davis PG, Fricker PA, Sanigorski AJ, Hargreaves M. Muscle glycogen storage after prolonged exercise: effect of frequency of carbohydrate feedings. Am J Clin Nutr. 1996;64:115–9.

16. Jenkins DJ, Wolever TM, Taylor RH, Barker H, Fielden H, Baldwin JM, et al. Glycemic index of foods: a physiological basis for carbohydrate exchange. Am J Clin Nutr. 1981;34(3):362–6.

17. Stevenson E, Williams C, Nute M. The influence of the glycaemic index of breakfast and lunch on substrate utilisation during the postprandial periods and subsequent exercise. Br J Nutr. 2005;93(6):885–93.

18. Donaldson CM, Perry TL, Rose MC. Glycemic index and endurance performance. Int J Sport Nutr Exerc Metab. 2010;20(2):154–65.

19. Burke LM, Claassen A, Hawley JA, Noakes TD. Carbohydrate intake during prolonged cycling minimizes effect of glycemic index of preexercise meal. J Appl Physiol. 1998;85(6):2220–6.

20. Blom PC, Hostmark AT, Vaage O, Kardel KR, Maehlum S. Effect of different post-exercise sugar diets on the rate of muscle glycogen synthesis. Med Sci Sports Exerc. 1987;19(5):491–6.

21. Sawka MN, Burke LM, Eichner ER, Maughan RJ, Montain SJ, Stachenfeld NS. American College of Sports Medicine position stand. Exercise and fluid replacement. Med Sci Sports Exerc. 2007;39(2):377–90.

22. Nakagawa K. Effect of vitamin D on the nervous system and the skeletal muscle. Clin Calcium. 2006;16(7):1182–7.

23. Nattiv A, Loucks AB, Manore MM, Sanborn CF, Sundgot-Borgen J, Warren MP. American College of Sports Medicine position stand: the female athlete triad. Med Sci Sports Exerc. 2007;39(10):1867–82.

24. DAFNE Study Group. Training in flexible, intensive insulin management to enable dietary freedom in people with type 1 diabetes: dose adjustment for normal eating (DAFNE) randomised controlled trial. BMJ. 2002;325(7367):746.

25. Wolever TM, Hamad S, Chiasson JL, Josse RG, Leiter LA, Rodger NW, et al. Day-to-day consistency in amount and source of carbohydrate intake associated with improved blood glucose control in type 1 diabetes. J Am Col Nutr. 1999;18(3):242–7.

26. Canadian Diabetes Association. Guidelines for the nutritional management of diabetes mellitus in the new millennium. Can J Diabetes Care. 2000;23:56–69.

27. Connor H, Annan F, Bunn E, Frost G, McGough N, Sarwar T, et al. The implementation of nutritional advice for people with diabetes. Diabet Med. 2003;20(10):786–807.

28. Perlstein RWJ, Hines C, Milsavlevic M. Dietitians Association of Australia review paper: Glycaemic Index in diabetes management. Aust J Nutr Diet. 1997;54:353–5.

29. Ryan RL, King BR, Anderson DG, Attia JR, Collins CE, Smart CE. Influence of and optimal insulin therapy for a low-glycemic index meal in children with type 1 diabetes receiving intensive insulin therapy. Diabetes Care. 2008;31(8):1485–90.

30. O'Connell MA, Gilbertson HR, Donath SM, Cameron FJ. Optimizing postprandial glycemia in pediatric patients with type 1 diabetes using insulin pump therapy: impact of glycemic index and prandial bolus type. Diabetes Care. 2008;31(8):1491–5.

31. Nansel TR, Gellar L, McGill A. Effect of varying glycemic index meals on blood glucose control assessed with continuous glucose monitoring in youth with type 1 diabetes on basal-bolus insulin regimens. Diabetes Care. 2008;31(4):695–7.

32. Thomas D, Elliott EJ. Low glycaemic index, or low glycaemic load, diets for diabetes mellitus. Cochrane Database Syst Rev. 2009;21(1):CD006296.

33. West DJ, Stephens JW, Bain SC, Kilduff LP, Luzio S, Still R, et al. A combined insulin reduction and carbohydrate feeding strategy 30 min before running best preserves blood glucose concentration after exercise through improved fuel oxidation in type 1 diabetes mellitus. J Sports Sci. 2011;29(3):279–89.
34. West DJ, Morton RD, Stephens JW, Bain SC, Kilduff LP, Luzio S, et al. Isomaltulose improves postexercise glycemia by reducing carbohydrate oxidation in type 1 diabetes mellitus. Med Sci Sports Exerc. 2011;43(2):204–10.
35. Rabasa-Lhoret R, Bourque J, Ducros F, Chiasson JL. Guidelines for premeal insulin dose reduction for postprandial exercise of different intensities and durations in type 1 diabetic subjects treated intensively with a basal-bolus insulin regimen (ultralente-lispro). Diabetes Care. 2001;24(4):625–30.
36. Martin DD, Davis EA, Jones TW. Acute effects of hyperglycaemia in children with type 1 diabetes mellitus: the patient's perspective. J Pediatr Endocrinol Metab. 2006;19(7):927–36.
37. Jenni S, Oetliker C, Allemann S, Ith M, Tappy L, Wuerth S, et al. Fuel metabolism during exercise in euglycaemia and hyperglycaemia in patients with type 1 diabetes mellitus–a prospective single-blinded randomised crossover trial. Diabetologia. 2008;51(8):1457–65.
38. Jeukendrup AE. Carbohydrate and exercise performance: the role of multiple transportable carbohydrates. Curr Opin Clin Nutr Metab Care. 2010;13(4):452–7.
39. Francescato MP, Geat M, Fusi S, Stupar G, Noacco C, Cattin L. Carbohydrate requirement and insulin concentration during moderate exercise in type 1 diabetic patients. Metabolism. 2004;53(9):1126–30.
40. Davis SN, Galassetti P, Wasserman DH, Tate D. Effects of antecedent hypoglycemia on subsequent counterregulatory responses to exercise. Diabetes. 2000;49(1):73–81.
41. MacDonald MJ. Postexercise late-onset hypoglycemia in insulin-dependent diabetic patients. Diabetes Care. 1987;10(5):584–8.
42. Beelen M, Burke LM, Gibala MJ, van Loon LJ. Nutritional strategies to promote postexercise recovery. Int J Sport Nutr Exerc Metab. 2010;20(6):515–32.
43. Kalergis M, Schiffrin A, Gougeon R, Jones PJH, Yale JF. Impact of bedtime snack composition on prevention of nocturnal hypoglycemia in adults with type 1 diabetes undergoing intensive insulin management using lispro insulin before bed. Diabetes Care. 2003;26:9–15.
44. Gallen IW, Ballav C, Lumb A, Carr J. Caffeine supplementation reduces exercise induced decline in blood glucose and subsequent hypoglycaemia in adults with type 1 diabetes (T1DM) treated with multiple daily insulin injection (MDI). ADA 70th Scientific Sessions, June 25–29, 2010, 1184–P.

Chapter 8
Diabetes and Doping

Richard I.G. Holt

8.1   Introduction

When humans are placed in a competitive setting, particularly in the sporting arena, they will attempt to gain an advantage over their opponent in order to win. When all legitimate methods have been exhausted and the athlete has reached their peak performance, there is a temptation for some to seek out pharmacological methods to improve performance yet further. Doping not only damages the integrity of sport but may cause significant harm to athletes who use performance-enhancing drugs. The term doping is originally derived from the African Kaffir's word "dop," an alcoholic drink made from grape skins that was used as a stimulant in battle. The use of the word became popular in the early twentieth century when racehorses were illegally drugged when the word was also used as a slang expression for opium.

During exercise, performance is dependent on the combustion of metabolic fuels, such as glucose for short-term high-intensity activity and free fatty acids for more prolonged activity, to release kinetic energy; this process depends on an adequate supply of nutrients and oxygen to the muscle fibers. This process may be enhanced by drugs that increase fuel and oxygen delivery to exercising muscle, increase muscle strength, or any combination of these factors. Given the complexity of the metabolic and cardiovascular changes during exercise, it is unsurprising that there is an extensive range of drugs that have been used by athletes.

The earliest records of doping in sport come from ancient times but with the advent of modern pharmacology and the birth of the field of endocrinology in the nineteenth century, the number and quantity of drugs used to improve strength and overcome fatigue increased dramatically. At the time, this practice was not illegal,

R.I.G. Holt, M.A., M.B., B.Chir., Ph.D., FRCP, FHEA
Human Development and Health Academic Unit,
University of Southampton, Faculty of Medicine,
IDS Building (MP887), Southampton General Hospital, Tremona Road,
Southampton, Hampshire SO16 6YD, UK
e-mail: r.i.g.holt@southampton.ac.uk

I. Gallen (ed.), *Type 1 Diabetes*,
DOI 10.1007/978-0-85729-754-9_8, © Springer-Verlag London Limited 2012

and so there are good records of the regimens that athletes would take. Alongside the benefits, however, came the dangers and several fatalities followed. Gradually, a code to ban performance-enhancing drugs was developed.

This chapter will describe the history of doping and the most commonly abused performance-enhancing drugs, including insulin. The potential beneficial and adverse effects will be discussed, particularly in relationship to type 1 diabetes, where the performance-enhancing drug may adversely affect the action of insulin and glycemic control. The chapter will finally discuss the therapeutic use exemption (TUE), which is required for all elite competitors with diabetes who use insulin.

8.2   History of Doping

8.2.1   Early History of Doping

Despite the perception that doping is a modern phenomenon, there are many examples of substance use dating back to ancient times, when extracts derived from plants, animals, or even humans were taken [1, 2]. One of the first performance-enhancing substances to be tried was testosterone; the effects of castration on animal behavior were well recognized, and this may have provided the incentive for people living in ancient times to eat the testes of animals or humans to improve their own well-being.

The importance of diet on performance was also recognized; one of the earliest reports describes how dried figs were used to improve the performance of Charmis, the Spartan winner of the stade race (~200 yards [183 m]) at the Olympic Games of 668 B.C.

The ancient Greeks also used concoctions of brandy and wine as stimulants as part of their training regimens while Roman gladiators took unspecified stimulants, mostly derived from plants, to overcome fatigue and injury. Examples include bufotenin, a drug derived from the muscarine-containing mushroom, fly agaric (*Amanita muscaria*), *Cola acuminita* and *Cola nitida*, and coca leaves.

8.2.2   Developments in the Use of Stimulants and Anabolic Agents During the Nineteenth Century

There was an escalation in the number and types of performance-enhancing drugs during the latter half of the nineteenth century, in line with development in modern pharmacology and medicine. Stimulants were used to improve muscular work capacity while the anabolic effects of substances that were later classified as hormones began to be recognized.

Caffeine was used to improve brain functioning while alcoholic beverages were considered a relief for stress. As there were no rules prohibiting such substances, athletes did not try to conceal the use of these compounds, and as a result, good records of doping exist for this time. Trainers also developed doping cocktails for their athletes, using various combinations of stimulants, such as strychnine tablets and mixtures of brandy and cocaine.

The continuous "six-day" bicycle races began in the nineteenth century, and a variety of medications were tried to improve the considerable physical strength and stamina needed for the race; French cyclists are reported to have taken mixtures based on caffeine, while the Belgians experimented with sugar cubes dripped in ether, and others used alcohol-containing cordials; the sprinters specialized in the use of nitroglycerine. As the race progressed, the amounts of strychnine and cocaine added to the caffeine mixtures steadily increased sometimes with lethal consequences; Arthur Linton, an English cyclist who is alleged to have overdosed on "tri-methyl" (a compound thought to have contained either caffeine or ether), was the first such fatality in 1886 during a 600-km race between Bordeaux and Paris. There is some dispute over this, as others suggest that Linton actually won the race and died 10 years later from typhoid fever.

Mixtures of champagne, brandy, hot drops of morphine, belladonna, and strychnine were used to maintain high levels of strength and energy during another endurance race, the "ultramarathon" which was a walking and running race over 6 days and 6 nights, with the winner being the person who covered the greatest distance.

Around the same time in 1889, Charles Édouard Brown-Sequard, a renowned physiologist and neurologist, undertook a series of groundbreaking and controversial experiments that led to the birth of the field of endocrinology. Brown-Sequard reported to the Society of Biology in Paris in 1891 that he had experienced significant restoration of strength following a 3-week program of self-injection of "first blood of the testicular veins; secondly semen; and thirdly juice from a testicle… from a dog or a guinea pig." One month after the last injection, however, he "experienced almost a complete return of the state of weakness." Although it is currently accepted that these findings were likely the result of a placebo effect, the idea of hormone replacement was conceived as a result.

It is perhaps unsurprising that the potential of this research was considered for athletic performance, and in 1894, Oskar Zoth and Fritz Pregl investigated the effect of testicular extracts on muscular strength. Although with hindsight it seems improbable that these testicular extracts contributed positively to athletic performance, many athletes, including the German Olympic team at the 1936 Berlin games, allegedly began to take these extracts.

8.2.3 Twentieth-Century Doping

At the beginning of the twentieth century, scientists isolated, characterized, and synthesized testosterone which allowed a greater understanding of its anabolic effects. The first recorded case of the use of testosterone as a means of improving performance was an 18-year-old horse named Holloway who was reported to have "declined to a marked degree in his staying power and during February of 1941 in several attempts at ice racing, failed to show any of his old speed or willingness." Following testosterone administration, the horse won or was placed in a number of races and established a trotting record at the age of 19 years. The widespread use of testosterone and other anabolic steroids that followed resulted in bodybuilders with deformed body shapes and extremely large muscles.

The use of stimulants, such as amphetamines, also began to increase in the mid-1930s, initially among servicemen fighting in the Second World War and college students but latterly by athletes. The use of stimulants was particularly prevalent in cycling during the 1960s and 1970s, and the first televised doping fatality occurred during the 1967 Tour de France, when the English cyclist, Tom Simpson, died with high circulating levels of methamphetamine.

Doping moved to a new level around this time with suspicions abounding that several countries pursued state-sponsored doping. These concerns were subsequently confirmed following the collapse of the Berlin wall when reports emerged from the former German Democratic Republic that PhD programs had been established to develop the ideal regimens to improve performance.

In the 1980s, anabolic steroids and cortisone remained the drugs most commonly abused, but the number of drugs expanded dramatically, and the current World Anti-Doping Agency (WADA) list of prohibited substances is several pages long and includes 12 categories of substances and methods, including anabolic agents, hormones, diuretics and masking agents, stimulants, and narcotics as well as prohibited methods such as blood transfusion (Table 8.1).

8.2.4 The Prevalence of Doping

The true prevalence of doping is unknown, and reports vary widely from 1% to 90% because of the current secrecy surrounding it. The huge financial rewards for professional sportsmen and women, corporate sponsors, the TV broadcast and cable industries and sport-governing bodies, coupled with the ever-increasing pharmacopoeia of performance-enhancing substances, the athlete's drive to win, and the challenges for doping control may all act to encourage athletes to use prohibited substances.

8.3 History of Anti-Doping

Prior to the end of World War I, doping was not considered to be cheating, and so the use of performance-enhancing substances was neither prohibited nor discouraged. In 1928, the International Amateur Athletic Federation (IAAF) became the first international sport body to ban the use of stimulating substances. Others followed the IAAF lead, but the lack of effective tests failed to curb the use of drugs. Around the same time, Otto Rieser, in his work "Doping and Doping Substances"

Table 8.1 Drugs appearing on the 2011 WADA list of prohibited substances

Substances and methods that are prohibited at all times in and out of competition
Anabolic agents
Anabolic androgenic steroids (AAS)
Other anabolic agents, clenbuterol, selective androgen receptor modulators, tibolone, zeranol, zilpaterol
Hormones and related substances
Erythropoiesis-stimulating agents, e.g., erythropoietin (EPO)
Gonadotropins (e.g., LH, hCG), prohibited in males only
Insulins
Corticotrophins
Growth hormone (hGH), insulin-like growth factors (e.g. IGF-I), fibroblast growth factors (FGFs), hepatocyte growth factor (HGF), mechano growth factors (MGFs), platelet-derived growth factor (PDGF), vascular-endothelial growth factor (VEGF)
Beta-2 agonists
Hormone antagonists and modulators
Diuretics and other masking agents
Methods to enhance oxygen transfer
Gene doping
Substances prohibited during competition
Stimulants
Narcotics
Cannabinoids
Glucocorticosteroids
Substances prohibited in particular sports
Alcohol
Beta-blockers

published in 1933, made the first attempts to educate athletes about the dangers of performance-enhancing drugs and discourage their use.

The death of Danish cyclist Knud Enemark Jensen during the Rome Olympic Games in 1960 following the consumption of amphetamine provided a further incentive for sports authorities to introduce drug testing, and in 1966, the International Cycling Union and International Federation of Association Football introduced tests for prohibited substances. The following year, the International Olympic Committee (IOC) established its Medical Commission under the chairmanship of Prince Alexandre de Merode and voted to adopt a drug-testing policy for banned drugs. Tests were first introduced at the Olympic Winter Games in Grenoble and then at the Olympic Games in Mexico in 1968. The IOC began publishing its Prohibited Substances List which became extensive and remains enforceable at all Olympic events.

Despite the example shown by the IOC, many organizations were slow to follow because of the lack of the necessary protocols or equipment to enforce the bans; for example, the US National Football League only introduced anti-doping testing in 1982.

Championed by Professor Manfred Donike, the IOC Medical Commission developed a worldwide network of top class laboratories staffed by chemists and pharmacologists, who were equipped to measure mainly steroids and stimulants in urine. The introduction of a reliable urinary test for anabolic steroids was seen as a major breakthrough in 1974 resulting in a marked increase in the number of drug disqualifications in the late 1970s, notably in strength-related sports such as throwing events and weightlifting. When combined with the introduction of out-of-competition testing, the testing program provided a major disincentive for athletes to use these drugs.

Following a series of high-profile scandals, the IOC convened a World Conference on Doping in Lausanne in February 1999, during which it was recognized that an independent international agency with powers to set unified anti-doping standards and coordinate sporting organizations and public authorities was needed. As a direct result, the World Anti-Doping Agency (WADA) was established on November 10, 1999. The development and implementation of a uniform set of anti-doping rules, the World Anti-Doping Agency Code, together with a list of prohibited substances are credited as the most important achievements in anti-doping.

8.4   The World Anti-Doping Agency List of Prohibited Substances

The WADA List of Prohibited Substances now runs to several pages and is updated annually as more information about the effects of performance-enhancing drugs becomes available. The list is divided into several sections covering drugs that cannot be used at any time, drugs that cannot be used during competition, and drugs, such as alcohol and beta-blockers, which are only banned in certain sports. An exhaustive list of prohibited substances is beyond the scope of this chapter, and readers are recommended to refer to the latest list which is available on the World Anti-Doping Agency website (http://www.wada-ama.org/). The main categories of performance-enhancing drugs are given in Table 8.1.

8.5   Drugs of Abuse and Diabetes

While each of these drugs may cause harm to people with diabetes, some drugs have specific relevance for people with type 1 diabetes because of their effects on insulin action and glycemic control. A more detailed description of these drugs is given below, including information about prevalence of abuse where this is known, how these drugs may enhance performance, the potential for harm, and the relevance for diabetes.

8.6   Anabolic Androgenic Steroids

Anabolic androgenic steroids (AAS) are steroid hormones that have masculinizing and growth-promoting actions and are the most widely abused performance-enhancing drugs. Although the virilizing effects of the testis have been recognized for millennia,

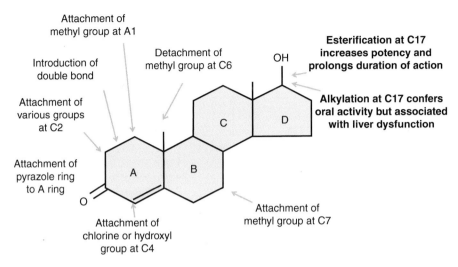

Fig. 8.1 Development of androgenic anabolic steroids. As the half-life of testosterone is short, manipulations at the C17 position of the D ring have led to compounds that are either more potent and longer lasting (esterification) or orally acting (alkylation), marked in *bold*. Further alterations have been tried to alter the relative androgenic and anabolic actions

Table 8.2 Formulations of testosterone available in clinical practice in the UK

Oral
   Testosterone undecanoate (17-β-hydroxyl ester)
Buccal
   Testosterone
Intramuscular (17-β-hydroxyl esters)
   Testosterone enanthate
   Testosterone undecanoate
   Testosterone propionate
   Testosterone phenylpropionate
   Testosterone isocaproate
   Testosterone decanoate
Implant
   Testosterone
Transdermal
   Testosterone

it was not until 1931 that the first androgenic steroid, androsterone, was isolated from urine. An anabolic effect separate from the androgenic effect was then shown in 1935. Following the discovery of testosterone, it became apparent that testosterone only has a short half-life regardless of its route of administration, and so a large number of synthetic molecules were developed subsequently with modified pharmacokinetics. Synthetic androgens predominantly have one of two substitutions on the D ring of native testosterone, either esterification at the 17-β-hydroxy group or alkylation at the 17-α position (Fig. 8.1). Esterification typically results in more potent androgens, with a longer duration of action (Table 8.2), allowing them to be

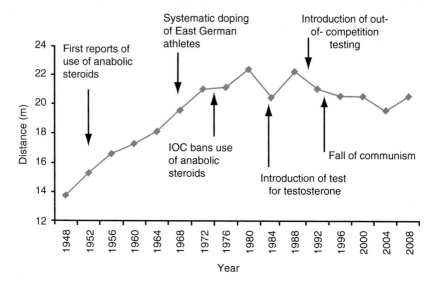

Fig. 8.2 The winning distance in the women's Olympic shot put since 1948

administered by intramuscular injection every 1–4 weeks. The alkylated forms are less potent but can be given orally; however, as they may cause serious liver injury, they are only rarely used clinically. In the late 1990s, topical preparations of testosterone became available. Although more convenient, these may induce skin rashes. Further manipulations of the basic steroid structure have been undertaken to alter the anabolic and androgenic actions (Fig. 8.1).

In addition to the AAS used in clinical practice, there are others available on the "black market." The purity and safety of these compounds is called into question, not least because some of these have been discontinued previously by legitimate pharmaceutical manufacturers because of toxicity.

8.6.1 Prevalence of Anabolic Androgenic Steroid Abuse

Reports of the inappropriate use of AAS first appeared in the 1930s; their use became firmly established in weightlifting during the 1950s before spreading to other sports in the 1960s. For many years, there were debates within the scientific literature about the performance effects of AAS with several articles and reviews commenting on the lack of scientific proof. Despite the skepticism shown by scientists, the benefits were realized by athletes whose performance improved dramatically. For example, between 1956 and 1980, the winning distance in the Olympic women's shot put increased from 15.28 to 22.41 m (Fig. 8.2). Since the introduction of effective testing in the early 1980s, the winning distance in the women's shot put has fallen progressively to the point where the winner in Beijing in 2008 would not have made the final in Moscow in 1980.

During the Cold War, supported by sophisticated scientific research, there was systematic state doping of East German athletes with AAS. Doping was not confined to East Germany, and there have been plenty of examples of abuse of AAS in Western countries. Perhaps the most famous case was Ben Johnson who was disqualified from the 100-meter race at the 1988 Olympic Games in Seoul when stanozolol was detected in his urine. Another example comes from US National Football League where, in 2009, nearly 1 in 10 retired players admitted using AAS in a confidential survey.

Following an undercover investigation by Lance Williams and Mark Fainaru-Wada, two reporters working in San Francisco, the Bay Area Laboratory Co-operative (BALCO) company headquarters was raided on September 3, 2003. Officially, BALCO was a service company for blood and urine analysis and food supplements, but evidence was found that it had supplied performance-enhancing drugs, including AAS, to many high-profile American and international athletes. Its owner Victor Conte was imprisoned for 4 months for his role in the scandal. Designer AAS, such as tetrahydrogestrinone (THG), norbolethone, and desoxymethyltestosterone, had been manufactured by Patrick Arnold, an organic chemist, and supplied to BALCO. THG is remarkable as a highly potent agonist for the testosterone and progesterone receptor, which was undetectable at the time. After Don Catlin, the former director of the Olympic Analytical Laboratory in Los Angeles, succeeded in identifying the molecule and developing a test, the complexity of the underlying chemistry shocked anti-doping agencies but testified to the lengths that some athletes and their supporters would pursue to achieve a performance benefit.

In addition to athletes, AAS appear to be widely used in the general population, most commonly for cosmetic purposes with only ~20% of all users participating in competitive sports or bodybuilding. 0.5% of the adult US population admitted to using AAS regularly while ~2.5% of boys and 0.6% of girls attending US high school reported having taken AAS at some point during their lives. Misuse is commonest among young middle-class heterosexual men. The widespread and increasing use led President George Bush in the mid-1990s to pass the first Anabolic Steroid Control Act, which made it illegal to possess or distribute AAS for non-medical purposes. In the UK, AAS are regulated under the Misuse of Drugs Act which sets out three separate categories, Class A, Class B, and Class C dependent on the drug's capacity to cause harm, with Class A being the most dangerous; AAS are classified as Class C drugs alongside benzodiazepines among others.

8.6.2 Why Do Athletes Abuse Anabolic Androgenic Steroids?

Androgenic anabolic steroids increase muscle mass and strength through a number of mechanisms including the stimulation of protein synthesis, inhibition of protein breakdown, recruitment of satellite cells, production of cytokines, and increase in androgen receptor number. Clinical trials have shown that AAS improve both muscle mass and strength in a dose-dependent manner, and these effects are additive to resistance training alone. It appears that the arms and upper torso are more responsive to the effects of AAS than the lower limbs. The full potential of AAS, however, has almost certainly not been realized in these trials because of the limited doses used because of medical and ethical concerns about potential side effects. By contrast, athletes are reported to take combinations of AAS in doses that are up to 30 times higher than the physiological replacement dose.

There are many websites and printed manuals giving details about the use and supply of AAS. Steroid use usually involves techniques such as "cycling" and "stacking." AAS appear to lose effectiveness with time through adaptation of the androgen receptor, and athletes have learned to obtain a greater benefit through using the steroids intermittently in a cycle over 5–10 weeks. Stacking involves the use of two or more steroids concomitantly in order to obtain a synergistic effect.

8.6.3   Adverse Effects of Androgenic Anabolic Steroids

8.6.3.1   Endocrine Function

The most marked side effect of AAS is virilization [3, 4]. In both men and women, this manifests as acne, an increase in body hair and male pattern baldness. The acne results from excess stimulation of sebaceous glands on both the face and the body. In men, prostatic enlargement may occur leading to urinary hesitancy and poor flow, and there are concerns about the long-term risk of prostate cancer. Gynecomastia may develop as excessive testosterone is converted to estradiol under the action of the aromatase enzyme. In women, the virilizing effects may be even more marked, including a decrease in breast size, cliteromegaly, and enlargement of the larynx causing a deepening of the voice. These changes can be permanent.

The administration of AAS may reduce fertility through suppression of LH and FSH secretion from the anterior pituitary gland. In the absence of gonadotropin drive, gonadal function declines. In men, sperm count falls and testicular atrophy may occur. In women, there is reduced endogenous estrogen production, ovulation is impaired, and irregular or absent menstrual cycles may ensue. These effects on reproductive function are prolonged taking many months to return to normal after AAS discontinuation.

8.6.3.2   Hepatotoxicity

Orally administered AAS impair the filtration and excretion of metabolic waste products by the liver leading to cholestasis, jaundice, and hepatocellular necrosis. Nonalcoholic fatty liver may develop as a result of altered lipid metabolism. Peliosis hepaticus, a rare condition characterized by hemorrhagic blood-filled cysts that are prone to rupture, may also occur. With long-term use, there is an increased risk of hepatocellular carcinoma. Abnormal liver function usually returns to normal a few months after treatment discontinuation.

8.6.3.3 Cardiovascular Disease

The incidence of myocardial infarction is increased in young men taking AAS. The mechanisms are not fully understood, but echocardiography has shown abnormal cardiac enlargement and impaired function following AAS use. There is also evidence that AAS abuse may increase the risk of hypertrophic cardiomyopathy in genetically predisposed individuals.

In addition to these structural changes, AAS misuse is associated with the development of dyslipidemia. The concentration of high-density lipoprotein (HDL) cholesterol is reduced by 40–70% while low-density lipoprotein (LDL) cholesterol increases. These effects vary with dose and type of AAS but seem most marked with oral administration. The changes in lipid profile are particularly relevant for people with diabetes who are already at increased risk of atherosclerotic cardiovascular disease.

8.6.3.4 Psychiatric Effects

The use of AAS is associated with an increase in irritability, aggressiveness, and symptoms of mania. By contrast, depression is also common affecting 10–40% of users. Depression may also occur after AAS withdrawal, particularly when high doses have been used, and may lead to suicide attempts.

8.6.3.5 Anabolic Androgenic Steroids and Diabetes

The effect of AAS on diabetes appears to be dependent on the type and dose of AAS. Oral 17-α alkylated AAS seem to have the most marked effect by inducing insulin resistance, inhibiting its actions on glucose and lipid metabolism. There are case reports of individuals developing diabetes during treatment with AAS although a causative link is uncertain [5], not least because athletes often take a cocktail of drugs, including growth hormone, which may have a much greater effect on glucose metabolism than AAS (see below). Testosterone deficiency is often seen in men with the metabolic syndrome and type 2 diabetes, and under these circumstances, testosterone replacement is associated with improved lipid and glycemic control and reduced insulin resistance. These findings may not, however, be applicable to athletes taking supraphysiological doses.

8.7 Erythropoietin and Blood Transfusion

Erythropoietin (EPO) is a hormone produced in the peritubular cells of the proximal tubules of the kidney and stimulates erythrocyte production by the bone marrow.

8.7.1 Prevalence of Erythropoietin Administration

Blood doping is thought to have started during the 1970s and was first prohibited in the 1970s. Before the ban was introduced, it was openly and commonly used by middle- and long-distance runners as well as cyclists. It is alleged that the US cycling team employed this method during the 1984 Olympics.

Since its prohibition, there have been a number of high-profile cases involving athletes who have used either EPO or blood transfusion. These include Niklas Axelsson who tested positive for EPO in 2000 and Tyler Hamilton who used a homologous blood transfusion in 2004. The Spanish Operación Puerto in 2006 investigated allegations of blood doping in hundreds of athletes while several members of the Astana Team in the 2007 Tour de France tested positive for homologous blood transfusion leading to the withdrawal of the team. The German speed skater and fivefold Olympic gold medalist Claudia Pechstein was banned for 2 years in 2009 for alleged blood doping.

8.7.2 Why Do Athletes Abuse Erythropoietin?

Exogenous EPO, which is available as a recombinant protein or as an analogue, is abused by endurance athletes as the increase in red blood cells improves oxygen transport to muscles. Its administration results in a slow and sustained increase in erythrocyte volume, which is associated with improved performance. Endogenous EPO production can be induced by training at high altitude, and this leads to a similar increase in erythrocyte volume and performance. Only about 50% of competitive athletes respond to altitude training, and it is notable that nonresponders do not improve their aerobic capacity [6].

An alternative method used by athletes to expand erythrocyte volume is autologous or homologous blood transfusion. Blood is removed and erythrocytes are harvested, stored, and then reinfused at a later date. Handling of the blood is important as this can influence erythrocyte function and survival. In contrast to EPO administration, following a blood transfusion, the erythrocyte volume is only increased for a few weeks. In the future, blood dopers may use oxygen-carrying molecules in place of hemoglobin.

8.7.3 Adverse Effects of Erythropoietin and Blood Transfusion

The main adverse effect of an increased erythrocyte volume is an increased risk of thrombotic events. However, there are also additional risks of infection associated with blood transfusion, particularly when this occurs in an unregulated fashion.

8.7.4   *Erythropoietin and Blood Transfusion and Diabetes*

The risks of EPO and blood transfusion appear to be similar for people with diabetes. However, the response to EPO may differ in people with diabetes as both IGF-I and insulin augment the effect of EPO on erythroid progenitors. In some situations, this has resulted in marked polycythemia in people with type 1 diabetes and end-stage renal disease receiving EPO [7]. Whether this is relevant for athletes is unclear.

8.8   Growth Hormone (hGH)

Growth hormone (GH) is a naturally occurring peptide hormone produced by the anterior pituitary gland. Studies of people with GH deficiency have shown that GH plays a pivotal role in maintaining body composition, well-being, physical performance, and cardiovascular health in adults as well as children. These features make the hormone an attractive option for elite athletes wishing to improve their performance.

8.8.1   *Prevalence of GH Abuse*

Exactly when and where GH was first used to enhance performance is unknown but "The Underground Steroid Handbook" written by Dan Duchaine in 1982 was the earliest publication to advocate its use, at least a decade before clinical endocrinologists began treating adults with GH deficiency. Since then, a number of high-profile athletes have been caught or have admitted taking GH. Following the Seoul Olympic Games doping scandal, Justice Charles Dubin led an inquiry into drug abuse in sport which concluded that, despite the tight regulations surrounding its use, GH was widely available and was being used by athletes. In a more recent investigation, US Senator George Mitchell found that GH was used extensively by Major League Baseball players to improve their performance and to assist their recovery from injury and fatigue; the use of GH was believed to have risen because, unlike AAS, it was largely undetectable and was readily available, for example, through "antiaging" centers using prescriptions from physicians whom the athletes had never met.

8.8.2   *Why Do Athletes Abuse Growth Hormone?*

Despite its apparent widespread use, there is little scientific evidence to support its use as an ergogenic aid [7]. Nevertheless, the actions of GH to increase muscle mass and reduce fat mass are attractive to athletes, and two recent studies have suggested that GH may improve performance.

8.8.2.1 Delivery of Fuels

Growth hormone is an insulin antagonist; it increases fasting hepatic glucose output, by increasing hepatic gluconeogenesis and glycogenolysis, and decreases peripheral glucose utilization. Although the effect on peripheral glucose uptake may not appear advantageous for performance, GH also increases the production of insulin-like growth factor-I (IGF-I), which in turn stimulates peripheral glucose uptake and utilization (see below).

Growth hormone stimulates lipolysis, both directly and indirectly by increasing adipocyte sensitivity to other lipolytic factors such as catecholamines. Endogenous nocturnal or exercise-induced GH secretion leads to a rise in fasting free fatty acid (FFA) concentration which peaks around 2 h after the GH spike. Likewise following exogenous GH administration, FFA rises and peaks with a similar pattern. Studies of fatty acid turnover in people with GH deficiency suggest that GH plays a crucial role in FFA delivery to exercising muscle.

Overall, the net effect of GH appears to increase the availability of glucose and fatty acids for exercising muscle and probably explains why endurance athletes, as well as strength athletes, have used GH.

8.8.2.2 Muscle and Bone Anabolism

GH stimulates muscle and whole body protein synthesis, partly through a direct local action and partly by the generation of IGF-I, which in turn inhibits whole body protein breakdown and stimulates protein synthesis. The mechanism of action is different from AAS, and so there are additive effects when these agents are used in combination. Insulin (see below) is also used with GH as it inhibits protein breakdown and promotes anabolism. As well as muscle, GH has profound anabolic effects on bone and soft tissue which may speed healing following an injury.

8.8.2.3 Cardiovascular Effects

Growth hormone therapy in adults with GH deficiency increases left ventricular posterior wall thickness, stroke volume, and left ventricular ejection fraction during exercise thereby ensuring an adequate blood supply to muscle. It is unclear, however, whether these cardiovascular effects are relevant for healthy young adults.

8.8.2.4 Thermoregulation

Growth hormone is involved in the maintenance of body temperature during exercise as impaired thermoregulation occurs during heat exposure and exercise in untreated adults with GH deficiency. By contrast, a change in body temperature may be one of the mechanisms that induces GH secretion during exercise.

8.8.2.5 Effects on Whole Body Physiology

The effects of GH on whole body physiology have been demonstrated through a series of randomized controlled trials of GH replacement in people with GH deficiency. In the absence of GH, body composition changes with a loss of lean tissue and accumulation of fat, in particular visceral fat. Skeletal muscle mass and strength is reduced with a consequent impairment of physical performance, exercise capacity, and VO_2 max (aerobic capacity or the maximum ability to take in and use oxygen).

Following treatment with recombinant human GH (rhGH), there is an impressive normalization of body composition; on average, lean body mass, mainly skeletal muscle, increases by 6 kg while there is a concomitant loss of fat mass. These body composition changes are accompanied by improvements in quality of life, particularly in the area of "increased energy" and performance enhancements. Although a meta-analysis found that short-term rhGH treatment had no effect on muscle strength, a further meta-analysis demonstrated that maximal power output, VO_2 max, and maximum work rate all improved following GH replacement.

8.8.2.6 Effect of Growth Hormone in Healthy Adults

Until recently, most studies in normal young healthy subjects have not found a performance benefit following GH treatment. Although GH administration is frequently associated with increased lean body mass and decreased fat mass, important exercise variables such as respiratory quotient, maximal oxygen uptake, bicycling speed, power output, energy expenditure, or strength are not improved [8].

These studies may not be suited to assess the effects of GH in individual athletes who often use higher doses than those used in the randomized controlled trials and who often combine GH with other performance-enhancing drugs.

The first trial to show a performance benefit for GH in young healthy adults was undertaken in abstinent anabolic steroid users. As well as the previously observed changes in body composition, 6 days of GH treatment lead to significant improvements in strength, peak power output, and maximal oxygen uptake. It is possible that, unlike previous studies, this study found a benefit because the prior use of steroids may have rendered the athletes particularly sensitive to the anabolic actions of GH.

A more recent placebo-controlled RCT of 6-week treatment found that GH improved sprint capacity in both men and women. There was a further synergistic effect with testosterone in men, but the effect on performance was short-lived and had disappeared by 6 weeks after GH discontinuation. Other performance measures, however, including VO_2 max and strength, were unchanged.

Overall, it appears that in recreational athletes, GH has a modest performance-enhancing effect, particularly when combined with testosterone, but whether these effects can be extrapolated to elite athletes is unknown.

8.8.3   Adverse Effects of Growth Hormone

The side effects associated with GH administration in adults with GH deficiency are well documented and may also affect any athlete abusing GH; however, as anecdotal evidence suggests that many athletes are taking doses that are much than those used therapeutically, it is reasonable to predict that athletes may develop features of acromegaly with prolonged use. The long-term effects may therefore include fluid retention (causing ankle swelling, hypertension, and headache), diabetes, and a cardiomyopathy, which is characterized by abnormalities in cardiac muscle structure and function. Although controversial, there is a potential for increased risk of certain cancers, including colorectal, thyroid, breast, and prostate cancer.

All pharmaceutically available GH is now made by recombinant DNA technology, but supplies of pituitary-derived GH are still available to athletes on the black market, increasing the risk of the prion-induced Creutzfelt-Jacob Disease.

8.8.4   Growth Hormone and Diabetes

Under normal physiological conditions, insulin is the prime regulator of glucose metabolism, but there is increasing evidence that GH and IGF-I play an important contributory role. A role for GH in glucose metabolism was first postulated in the 1930s, when Houssay and Biasotti found that hypophysectomy reduced the hyperglycemia seen in canine models of diabetes. The diabetogenic factor isolated from pituitaries was also found to have growth-promoting activity and named "growth hormone." The experimental administration of GH to animals and humans confirmed its diabetogenic properties, but it was only after the development of reliable GH assays that the importance of GH in glucose metabolism was fully appreciated in both healthy subjects and people with type 1 diabetes.

Pituitary GH secretion is increased in individuals with diabetes leading to concentrations that are up to 2–3 times higher than healthy subjects. Portal insulin concentrations play a key role in the regulation of hepatic IGF-I generation; in the absence of portal insulin, a state of acquired hepatic GH resistance develops with reduced IGF-I production and negative feedback at the pituitary gland. GH administration to people with type 1 diabetes has little effect on serum IGF-I concentration while residual insulin secretion, as reflected by plasma C-peptide concentration, determines the degree of GH hypersecretion.

Nocturnal GH hypersecretion may play a role in the early morning worsening of insulin sensitivity and plasma glucose as people with type 1 diabetes and GH deficiency do not exhibit the "dawn phenomenon" while even a single bolus of GH to these individuals decreases morning insulin sensitivity.

8.8.4.1 Growth Hormone and the Microvascular Complications of Diabetes

In 1953, Poulsen presented the case of a woman with type 1 diabetes and background diabetic retinopathy, which regressed after she developed panhypopituitarism after postpartum pituitary necrosis. This observation led to the use of pituitary ablation in the 1960s to treat diabetic retinopathy until the development of the safer photocoagulation. A role for GH in development of microvascular complications is also suggested by the decreased incidence of retinopathy in people with type 1 diabetes and GH deficiency. This area is controversial as there is no evidence that GH replacement therapy causes an increased incidence of retinopathy in GH-deficient adults with or without diabetes. Furthermore, the role of GH is complicated by the many other growth factors, which have been implicated in the development of microvascular complications.

In conclusion, it would appear that GH is likely to be less effective as a performance-enhancing drug in people with type 1 diabetes because of the GH-resistant state; it is also likely to be associated with additional harm through impaired glycemic control and possible worsening of diabetic complications.

8.9 Insulin-Like Growth Factor-I

Insulin-like growth factor-I is a single chain peptide, which has structural homology with proinsulin. Although IGF-I is synthesized widely, the majority of circulating IGF-I is produced in the liver under the regulation of GH, insulin, and nutritional intake. It has profound effects on cell proliferation and differentiation in many tissues as well as metabolic effects, which are broadly similar to those of insulin including actions on glucose metabolism.

8.9.1 Prevalence of Abuse with IGF-I

The prevalence of IGF-I abuse is probably much lower than for GH because, unlike GH, there is no readily available natural source, and, therefore, all IGF-I is manufactured through recombinant DNA technology. As the tests for detecting GH abuse develop, however, there are anecdotal reports that athletes, for example, weightlifters, are increasingly turning to IGF-I as an alternative performance-enhancing agent [9].

Two therapeutic preparations of IGF-I have been approved since 2005 for the treatment of growth failure in children with severe primary IGF-I deficiency or with GH gene deletion who have developed neutralizing GH antibodies. The first product is recombinant human IGF-I (Mecasermin), and the second is a combination of rhIGF-I and its major binding protein, IGFBP-3 (Mecasermin Rinfabate). Although these drugs are still in relatively short supply, IGF-I is manufactured for cell culture and other uses, and this laboratory grade material is available to athletes. The widening availability of IGF-I together with an appreciation of the efforts to detect GH abuse is likely to increase illicit use of IGF-I, despite its inclusion on the WADA List of Prohibited Substances.

8.9.2   Why Do Athletes Abuse IGF-I?

IGF-I has a number of effects on carbohydrate, lipid, and protein metabolism in a wide range of target tissues, some of which may prove beneficial to the competing athlete. Although a positive correlation between serum IGF-I concentration and physical fitness has been observed, there is no published evidence that rhIGF-I administration improves physical performance or indeed alters body composition. Recent studies undertaken in Southampton, however, suggest that IGF-I increases the maximal uptake of oxygen in healthy recreational athletes.

The actions of IGF-I have been demonstrated in people with rare inherited defects of the GH receptor. The condition is characterized by severe postnatal growth failure and rhIGF-I therapy leads to substantial improvements in linear growth. There are significant increases in protein synthesis rates with increased lean body mass and decreased adiposity. Rates of lipolysis and lipid oxidation increase with rhIGF-I therapy. More recently important effects of rhIGF-I on intermediate metabolism have been shown in healthy individuals.

8.9.2.1   Protein Metabolism

IGF-I infusion in healthy individuals results in the insulin-like property of inhibiting proteolysis inhibition and the GH-like property of stimulating protein synthesis. The intracellular pathways of IGF-I action are not fully understood, but it appears that IGF-I acts, at least in part, by stimulating amino acid uptake into cells. The combined actions of IGF-I, GH, and insulin could result in synergistic effects on protein metabolism and may explain why athletes take cocktails of these potent hormones [10].

8.9.2.2   Carbohydrate Metabolism

IGF-I has direct actions on glucose metabolism that are similar to insulin and causes hypoglycemia by increasing peripheral glucose uptake and decreasing hepatic glucose production when administered to healthy volunteers. A single intravenous dose of 100 $\mu g \cdot kg^{-1}$ results in the rapid onset of symptomatic hypoglycemia and is equipotent to 0.15 IU·kg⁻¹ of insulin. A continuous intravenous infusion of IGF-I causes a 50% fall in C-peptide concentration despite the maintenance of euglycemia. The onset of hypoglycemia is slower with subcutaneous IGF-I administration than with insulin, because of the presence of circulating IGF binding proteins which buffer the IGF-I action. IGF-I infusion also inhibits GH secretion through negative feedback, which may contribute to the improvements in insulin sensitivity.

The potential benefit to the athlete is the stimulation of muscle glycogen synthesis replenishing nutrient supplies; physical endurance at high work intensities relies on skeletal muscle glycogen stores, and so IGF-I may improve performance and accelerate recovery in endurance sports such as long-distance running or cycling.

8.9.3 Adverse Effects of IGF-I

The side effect profiles of the commercial preparation of rhIGF-I include hypoglycemia, jaw pain, headache, myalgia, and fluid retention. The combined rhIGF-I-rhIGFBP-3 (Mecasermin Rinfabate) is associated with less hypoglycemia because the IGFBP-3 appears to buffer the acute effects of IGF-I and increase its half-life. Side effects of Mecasermin Rinfabate include local injection-site erythema and lipohypertrophy though headaches and altered liver function tests have also been reported.

There are limited long-term data about the safety of IGF-I. Tonsillar and adenoidal tissue hypertrophy was reported in nearly a quarter of children with GH insensitivity syndrome treated with rhIGF-I for up to 12 years. In addition, there were changes in the facial appearance in some children, although these regressed partially after therapy was withdrawn. By contrast, rhIGF-I treatment in adult patients with severe insulin resistance for 16 months did not result in changes in physical appearance. The clinical features of acromegaly are, however, possible with prolonged use. Epidemiological studies have linked certain cancers with increased serum IGF-I concentration, and, like GH, it is possible that the administration of uncontrolled doses of IGF-I may increase the risk of cancer.

There are also concerns about the use of laboratory grade IGF-I because of the reduced purity.

8.9.4 IGF-I and Diabetes

Serum IGF-I is reduced in people with type 1 diabetes because of the acquired hepatic GH resistance. Intensive insulin treatment by subcutaneous injection does not completely normalize IGF-I, but when insulin is given to people with type 1 diabetes by continuous intraperitoneal infusion directly into the portal circulation (as occurs normally in vivo), using an implantable pump, portal insulin concentration increases, and there is near-normalization of IGF-I.

There has been interest in treating type 1 diabetes with IGF-I at a replacement dose to correct the derangements of the GH-IGF axis and exploit its hypoglycemic actions. When a single dose of IGF-I (40 mcg/kg) was administered to adolescents with type 1 diabetes, hepatic insulin sensitivity increased and the glucose production rate fell. Over 7 days, IGF-I increased peripheral glucose uptake and reduced proteolysis, despite a reduced insulin requirement to maintain euglycemia. After 3 months treatment with rhIGF-I at night, insulin sensitivity and glycated hemoglobin improved in adolescents with type 1 diabetes in association with a fall in insulin requirement [11]. Although these improvements were not sustained over the 6 months of the study, it was thought that the deterioration in control was related to poor concordance with the multi-injection regimen rather than a reduction in the biological effect of IGF-I. The improvement in metabolic control is achieved through both reduced GH secretion and through a direct hypoglycemic action of IGF-I.

Despite these early promising findings, the development of IGF-I as a treatment for diabetes was halted because of concerns that increased serum IGF-I concentrations are associated with progression of retinopathy in people with diabetes.

Overall, there is no published evidence that IGF-I improves performance although metabolic studies suggest it has features that may be beneficial to athletes. The administration of IGF-I to people with type 1 diabetes may affect insulin requirement and increase the risk of hypoglycemia. There are also concerns that it may increase the incidence and progression of retinopathy.

8.10   Insulin

Insulin is a 51-amino-acid peptide hormone comprising two polypeptide chains, the A and B chains, which are linked by disulfide bridges. Insulin is synthesized in the β-cells of the islets of Langerhans in the pancreas. It has major effects on intermediate metabolism and may be considered as the hormone that signals the "post-meal" fed state. During this period, it is pivotal in the regulation of cellular energy supply and macronutrient balance and directing anabolic processes.

Autoimmune destruction of the β-cells leads to the development of type 1 diabetes. Insulin is used therapeutically to treat all people with type 1 diabetes and some people with type 2 diabetes. It was first isolated from the pancreas in 1921 by Banting and Best, and the first person with diabetes was treated in 1922. Initially, the only source of insulin was from animals, and both bovine and porcine insulin are still used, albeit in diminishing amounts. The advent of recombinant DNA technology led to a major advance in the production of insulin; the *insulin* coding sequence is inserted into bacteria such as *Escherichia coli* allowing large quantities of insulin (including animal insulin) to be produced in a highly purified manner.

The half-life of intravenous soluble insulin is only 4 min, but apart from the treatment of diabetic emergencies, insulin administered in clinical practice is by subcutaneous injection. When soluble insulin is injected subcutaneously, it forms a hexamer which delays its absorption from the injection site. It therefore acts more slowly than endogenously secreted insulin, and so the pharmacokinetic profile does not match endogenous requirements; periods of both hypoglycemia and hyperglycemia can therefore ensue. In order to address this problem, attempts have been made to shorten the onset and duration to provide a suitable mealtime insulin and also to lengthen the profile to provide a more appropriate background insulin. The first modifications were the addition of protamine and zinc in the 1930s and the 1950s, respectively, to form isophane insulin which has a prolonged duration of action. Recombinant DNA technology first permitted the production of human soluble insulin and then the development of both short- and long-acting insulin analogues. The shortest-acting insulin analogues appear in the circulation within 5–10 min of injection and are cleared within 4–6 h while the latest long-acting insulin analogues in development are present for over 24 h.

8.10.1 Prevalence of Insulin Abuse

There are only sketchy details about the use of insulin by professional athletes [10]. It is alleged that short-acting insulin is used to increase muscle bulk in body builders, weightlifters, and powerlifters. After concerns raised by the Russian medical officer at the Nagano Olympic Games, the International Olympic Committee (IOC) immediately banned its use in those without diabetes. Athletes with insulin-requiring diabetes may use insulin with a medical exemption.

8.10.2 Why Do Athletes Abuse Insulin?

Insulin has major anabolic actions on intermediate metabolism, affecting glucose, lipid, and protein metabolism with the most important insulin-sensitive tissues being the liver, skeletal muscle, and adipose tissue.

8.10.2.1 Glucose Metabolism

Under normal physiological conditions, insulin, together with its principal counter-regulatory hormone glucagon, is the prime controller of glucose metabolism and plasma glucose concentration. It is involved in the regulation of carbohydrate metabolism at many steps, increasing glucose uptake into cells, promoting glycolysis and glycogen synthesis while inhibiting glycogen breakdown and gluconeogenesis. These actions would allow an athlete to replenish muscle glycogen stores after a bout of exercise in a similar manner to that described for IGF-I.

8.10.2.2 Lipid Metabolism

Insulin increases the rate of lipogenesis in several ways in adipose tissue and liver, and controls the formation and storage of triglyceride. The critical step in lipogenesis is the activation of the insulin-sensitive lipoprotein lipase in the capillaries, which releases fatty acids from circulating chylomicrons or very low-density lipoproteins to be taken up by adipose tissue. Fatty acid synthesis is increased, while fat oxidation is suppressed. Lipogenesis is also facilitated by the glucose uptake, because its metabolism by the pentose phosphate pathway provides NADPH which is needed for fatty acid synthesis. Triglyceride synthesis is stimulated by esterification of glycerol phosphate, while triglyceride breakdown is suppressed by dephosphorylation of hormone-sensitive lipase.

8.10.2.3   Protein Metabolism

Insulin stimulates the uptake of amino acid into cells, thereby promoting protein synthesis in a range of tissues; however, the major action of insulin is to inhibit protein breakdown. The similarities between IGF-I and insulin suggest that these proteins act in a coordinated manner to regulate protein turnover. Furthermore, many of the intracellular signaling mechanisms of insulin and IGF-I, such as IRS-I, are shared. There are differences, however, in their respective dose-response curves. Low physiological insulin concentrations inhibit protein breakdown and increase glucose disposal into skeletal muscle while higher, nonphysiological concentrations are required to stimulate protein synthesis. In contrast, increases in IGF-I that have no effect on glucose uptake stimulate protein synthesis while higher concentrations are required to inhibit protein breakdown. The precise mechanism by which these similar but divergent pathways interact is not fully understood.

8.10.3   Adverse Effects of Insulin

The side effects of insulin are well documented from the extensive experience in treating people with diabetes. The commonest side effect is hypoglycemia, but weight gain is also a problem in people with diabetes. This may be less problematic for athletes whose diet and training regimen is closely monitored. There is evidence that hyperinsulinemia per se may induce insulin resistance, which has been implicated in the development of cardiovascular disease; this remains contentious but argues that people with diabetes should not receive more insulin than is needed to control their hyperglycemia.

8.10.4   Insulin and Diabetes

Unlike the other hormones described in the preceding sections, insulin forms an essential part of the treatment of an athlete with diabetes. The main issue for an athlete with type 1 diabetes is the need to obtain a therapeutic use exemption, which is described below.

8.11 Antihypertensives

Beta-blockers, which may be used in people with diabetes as antihypertensive agents, are prohibited in competition in certain sports during competition (Table 8.1). The main concern about these drugs in diabetes is that they may mask the symptoms of hypoglycemia; they may also worsen glycemic control, particularly if combined with thiazide diuretics.

8.12 Therapeutic Use Exemption

Like all individuals, athletes may develop illnesses or conditions that require them to take prescribed medications. When these appear on the WADA Prohibited List, as is the case for insulin, an athlete must apply for a Therapeutic Use Exemption (TUE) to allow them to take the medicine before and during competition. The International Standard for Therapeutic Use Exemptions (ISTUE) is regulated by WADA to ensure that the process of granting TUEs is coordinated across sports and countries. There are a number of criteria that must be fulfilled before a TUE is granted:

• The athlete would experience significant health problems without taking the prohibited substance or method.
• The therapeutic use of the substance would not produce significant enhancement of performance.
• There is no reasonable therapeutic alternative to the use of the otherwise prohibited substance or method.

In the case of type 1 diabetes, the first and third criteria are clearly fulfilled as insulin is an essential part of the treatment of diabetes without which the athlete would die rapidly from diabetic ketoacidosis. However, it is important to obtain accurate medical records to demonstrate the diagnosis, and this may be difficult if the diagnosis was made several decades previously. The second criterion is more difficult to prove as insulin may be performance enhancing; however, the decision to award a TUE must balance this possibility with the severity of the condition and the appropriateness of the medication. The athlete may be required to provide evidence of recent blood glucose monitoring and other measures of glycemic control.

TUEs may be granted by either International Sporting Federations, which administers applications from all international level athletes, or National Anti-Doping Organizations for national level athletes. Both types of body are required by WADA to have an established process to administer TUE applications. It is important that an athlete should submit an application to only one organization and not to WADA.

The TUE application is usually fairly simple and involves the athlete submitting an electronic or paper application to the relevant International Federation or National Anti-Doping Organization. WADA has developed the Anti-Doping Administration and Management System (ADAMS), a web-based database management system to simplify the process. It is easy to use and is freely available in English, French, Spanish, German, Japanese, Russian, Italian, Dutch, and Arabic. ADAMS stores data on laboratory results, TUEs, and information on Anti-Doping Rule Violations (ADRVs) and facilitates the sharing of information between relevant organizations.

All TUE applications should be supported by a physician's statement and other supporting documentation confirming that the criteria for a TUE are met. The application should be submitted at least 30 days before participating in an event. Following the submission of an application, it is assessed by an independent panel of physicians, known as the Therapeutic Use Exemption Committee. If a TUE is denied by the committee, an athlete has the right to appeal to WADA or ultimately to the Court of Arbitration for Sport.

A TUE is granted for a specific medication with a defined dose and for a specific period of time and may contain conditions that should be adhered to. During a doping control procedure, the athlete should declare the medication being used, and although not mandatory, it is helpful to show the doping control officer the TUE approval form.

As the WADA-accredited laboratories are blinded to the athlete's identity during testing and medical information disclosed in a TUE application is kept strictly confidential, they may report an adverse analytical finding to the doping control authority; however, as long as the TUE is still in effect and that the results of the analysis are consistent with the TUE granted (i.e., the nature of medication, route of administration, dose, time frame of administration are deemed appropriate), the result of the test will be recorded as negative.

Acknowledgments I would like to thank Michael Stow of UK Anti-Doping for his helpful comments on the chapter.

References

1. Holt RI, Erotokritou-Mulligan I, Sonksen PH. The history of doping and growth hormone abuse in sport. Growth Horm IGF Res. 2009;19(4):320–6.
2. Yesalis CE, Bahrke MS. History of doping in sport. In: Bahrke MS, Yessalis CE, editors. Performance-enhancing substances in sport and exercise. 1st ed. Champaign: Human kinetics; 2002. p. 1–20.
3. Wilson JD. Androgen abuse by athletes. Endocr Rev. 1988;9(2):181–99.
4. Bagatell CJ, Bremner WJ. Androgens in men–uses and abuses. N Engl J Med. 1996; 334(11):707–14.
5. Geraci MJ, Cole M, Davis P. New onset diabetes associated with bovine growth hormone and testosterone abuse in a young body builder. Hum Exp Toxicol. 2011;30(12):2007–12.
6. Sawka MN, Muza SR, Young AJ. Erythrocyte volume expansion and human performance. In: Fourcroy JL, editor. Pharmacology, doping and sports. a scientific guide for athletes, physicians, scientists and administrators. Abingdon: Routledge; 2009. p. 125–34.
7. Fernandez-Reyes MJ, Selgas R, Bajo MA, Jimenez C, Del PG, Sanchez MC, et al. Increased response to subcutaneous erythropoietin on type I diabetic patients on CAPD: is there a synergistic effect with insulin? Perit Dial Int. 1995;15(6):231–5.

8. Liu H, Bravata DM, Olkin I, Friedlander A, Liu V, Roberts B, et al. Systematic review: the effects of growth hormone on athletic performance. Ann Intern Med. 2008;148(10):747–58.
9. Guha N, Sonksen PH, Holt RI. IGF-I abuse in sport: current knowledge and future prospects for detection. Growth Horm IGF Res. 2009;19(4):408–11.
10. Holt RI, Sonksen PH. Growth hormone, IGF-I and insulin and their abuse in sport. Br J Pharmacol. 2008;154(3):542–56.
11. Acerini CL, Patton CM, Savage MO, Kernell A, Westphal O, Dunger DB. Randomised placebo-controlled trial of human recombinant insulin-like growth factor I plus intensive insulin therapy in adolescents with insulin-dependent diabetes mellitus. Lancet. 1997; 350(9086): 1199–204.

Further Reading Books

Fainaru-Wada M, Gotham LW. Game of shadows: Barry Bonds, BALCO, and the steroids scandal that rocked professional sports. 1st ed. 2006; pp. 352. ISBN-10: 9781592401994.
Fourcroy JL. Pharmacology, doping and sports: a scientific guide for athletes, coaches, physicians, scientists and administrators. 1st ed. Routledge; 2008, pp. 240. ISBN-10: 0415578221.

Themed Journal Issues

McGrath I, Cowan D, Guest Editors. Drugs in sport. Br J Pharmacol. 2008; 154(3).
Sonksen PH, Holt RIG, Guest Editors. The abuse of growth hormone in sport and its detection: a medical, legal and social framework. Growth Hormone IGF Res. 2009;(4).

Useful Websites

UK Anti-Doping: http://www.ukad.org.uk/
US Anti-Doping Agency: http://www.usantidoping.org/
World Anti-Doping Agency: http://www.wada-ama.org/

Chapter 9
Synthesis of Best Practice

Ian Gallen

In the preceding chapters, we have seen elegant discussions of the hormonal and metabolic responses to exercise and how these responses are altered by type 1 diabetes and insulin therapy. In Chap. 1, we have seen how exercise exerts a great demand on the capacity of the human body to maintain blood glucose homeostasis. The normal physiological counterregulatory hormone response generated by exercise produces a coordinated endocrine response which switches the physiological state from the postabsorptive to the exercise state, enabling release of the nutrients required to support increased work. Increased glucose utilization by skeletal muscle proportionate to the duration and intensity of exercise is counteracted by a complex and well-coordinated endocrine response. Hepatic glucose production (through increased glycogenolysis and gluconeogenesis) mediated through increased glucagon and a fall in insulin concentrations in the portal vein are important stimulators of hepatic glucose production during low- and moderate-intensity exercise. Further counterregulatory catecholamine responses during high-intensity exercise are important in intense exercise and with modest hypoglycemia in nondiabetic intervals. It is perhaps surprising that even in nondiabetic individuals, preexercise hypoglycemia is associated with blunted counterregulation during subsequent exercise, and prior exercise blunts the counterregulatory response to subsequent hypoglycemia. There are further age-, gender-, and obesity-related difference in these responses. It is therefore entirely predictable that diabetes and insulin treatment is likely to have very significant effects on the ability to perform exercise though changes in glycemic and counterregulatory responses.

In Chap. 2, we read how a number of endocrine disturbances can influence glucose regulation during exercise, making the management of glycemia challenging for patient and caregiver. While aerobic exercise frequently results in a reduction in blood glucose concentration, intense and anaerobic exercise can promote transient hyperglycemia.

I. Gallen, B.Sc., M.D., FRCP
Diabetes Centre, Wycombe Hospital,
High Wycombe, UK
e-mail: ian.gallen@buckshealthcare.nhs.uk

I. Gallen (ed.), *Type 1 Diabetes*,
DOI 10.1007/978-0-85729-754-9_9, © Springer-Verlag London Limited 2012

In diabetes, we have seen the effect of relative overinsulinization during exercise, which when combined with the impaired physiological response of the counterregulatory hormones results in impaired endogenous glucose production coupled with increased glucose utilization. The net effect of these variations in normal physiology leads to the classical glycemic response during endurance exercise of progressive falling blood glucose values and risk of hypoglycemia [1, 2]. In contrast, short bursts of intense exercise may produce a relative excess counterregulatory hormone response relative to available insulin which may lead to hyperglycemia during exercise [3, 4].

We have seen how this exercise-induced state may protect against hypoglycemia following shorter periods of endurance exercise [5, 6]. However, for both forms of exercise particularly if the exercise is intermittent, increased glucose disposal into skeletal muscle as a result of increased expression of GLUT4 transporters [7, 8] and resultant improvement in insulin sensitivity can lead to increased insulin sensitivity in the late postexercise period [2, 9]. This is particularly important when combined with the reduction in counterregulatory hormone response to hypoglycemia seen following exercise (particularly in men), as it may predispose to severe nocturnal hypoglycemia [10–16].

Given the well-recognized and strong tendency to dysglycemia with exercise, how can the practicing clinician best advise their patient? The routine clinical review appropriately focuses on glycemic control, on the adverse consequences of insulin treatment (hypoglycemia and weight gain), on the surrogate markers for complications of diabetes (HbAlc, blood pressure, microalbuminuria, eGFR, and lipids), and on examination to detect signs of the complications of diabetes. This leaves little time for dealing with questions about how to manage exercise, and these may not routinely be given the attention that they might deserve. Having said this, patients with diabetes are encouraged to perform regular exercise, and it is therefore incumbent on the clinician to equip himself or herself with the skills that are necessary to advise their patient [17].

Over the last decade, we have developed a specialist diabetes and sports clinic for young people who are outstanding athletes from throughout the UK. The skills and practice gained from this clinic, when combined with the excellent clinical research described in the previous chapters, offer us the opportunity of suggesting a clinic model to health-care professionals to help people manage diabetes and exercise more effectively. We have found that patients attending the service complain of three main groups of symptoms:

1. Seemingly inexplicable dysglycemia during and immediately following exercise
2. Unexpected and severe hypoglycemia particularly at night
3. Excessive fatigue, impaired physical performance, and increased muscle weakness and cramps when compared to their prediabetic state or with peers (this is probably the most subtle of the three groups of symptoms)

To deal with these issues, we conduct a standardized clinical interview. The aim of the interview is to reduce day-to-day variation in insulin therapy and to improve insulin dosage relative to carbohydrate intake. A focus on detail is extremely important, as we frequently find that much of the apparently inexplicable variation in glycemic control is not due to exercise but due to these factors:

1. General history of the person's diabetes in which the duration, treatment, and complications of diabetes, along with control, are assessed.
2. A detailed review of injection technique particularly focusing on needle length, site of injection, and inspection of injection sites for lipohypertrophy and sclerosis is made. Care is taken in identifying suitable sites for injection of basal and bolus insulin doses, particularly in the context of the proposed exercise. When NPH insulin is used, a review of the technique of resuspension is frequently required.
3. A careful review of calorie intake and techniques for dose adjustment (carbohydrate counting) is made, along with a review by our specialist dietician as to the appropriate calorie intake for the individual's estimated energy expenditure. Patients coming to our service frequently report insufficient calorie intake to support their exercise which will increase the risk of late hypoglycemia and cause fatigue and impaired performance. In contrast, where patients are overweight and desirous of weight loss, reducing energy intake can be helpful, and estimating energy expenditure allows appropriate dietary advice to be given. Carbohydrate intake should be spaced throughout the week, avoiding carbohydrate preloading prior to exercise for which there is no evidence of benefit in diabetes. Advice to ensure the accuracy of the carbohydrate intake and appropriate insulin is also given.
4. A detailed history of the sporting/exercise program is made. Particular attention is paid to the timing, duration, intensity, and type of exercise on each day of the week. This allows the exercise to be characterized so that the anticipated effect on blood glucose levels can be identified. In general, the exercise is classified as endurance (in which case blood glucose can be predicted to fall), high intensity (where blood glucose is likely to rise), or mixed exercise such as team sports where the effect may be variable from day to day, depending on the intensity of each event (although the general effect tends to be a fall in blood glucose levels which is attenuated when compared with pure endurance exercise). Importantly, the timing of each event in relation to the bolus dose of insulin is identified as well as any adjustments which are made to this dose.
5. Particular care and attention is paid to symptoms suggestive of hypoglycemic unawareness. Severe hypoglycemia particularly in young adults who are sleeping on their own is of special concern and where found requires specific attention [18]. The risk of exercise-induced nocturnal hypoglycemia is carefully explained, and avoidance of alcohol on days following exercise emphasized. We recommend that people with diabetes set alarms to wake in the early hours of the morning to check blood glucose. When possible, we seek other members of the household to advise on signs of severe hypoglycemia and the appropriate use of glucagon. If exercise is planned to occur after an episode of hypoglycemia, we advise that it is delayed or reduced in intensity and takes place in a safe environment.
6. In our interviews, we also focus on measures of physical performance and fatigue. Identification of variability in performance, such as slowing during timed endurance events or variability in ability to deal with opponents during team

games. This is an area which may not be familiar to diabetes teams but is readily assessable on questioning. Open questions about perceived excess fatigue or poor performance suggest problems with antecedent hyperglycemia prior to or during exercise [19–22] or insufficient food intake. There is also good evidence that fuel oxidation is markedly variable in type 1 diabetes during exercise [23–27], and it is likely that this will contribute to impaired physical performance particularly during endurance sport, but this is amenable to management.

9.1 Potential Strategies

There are limited strategies currently available to improve glycemic control and performance. These are centered on variation in the timing and dosage of insulin therapy and adjustment in carbohydrate intake. Our experience is that it is not possible to manage most patients who are performing regular physical activity on premixed twice-daily insulin without frequent exercise-induced hypoglycemia or conversely hyperglycemia on nonexercise days. For those using such a regimen, we transfer the majority of our patients on to a multiple daily injection regime using rapidly acting analogue injection (insulin aspart (Novo Nordisk), lispro (Eli Lilly), or glulisine (Sanofi-Aventis)) [28]. The basal component of the multiple daily injection regimens uses human NPH insulin (Insulatard (Novo Nordisk) or Humulin I (Eli-Lilly)) or analogue insulin glargine (Sanofi-Aventis) or insulin detemir (Novo Nordisk).

Short-acting insulin analogues enable more predictable postprandial glucose control with reduced risk of late postprandial hypoglycemia in the context of increased calorie intake seen in subjects performing regular exercise. Longer-acting basal analogue insulin therapy has become a mainstay of insulin therapy for many people with type 1 diabetes. The longer duration of action of these therapies, while advantageous during routine treatment, may result in relative excess insulin during exercise. As a result, both insulin glargine and detemir may increase the tendency to hypoglycemia during endurance exercise. There is some evidence to suggest that insulin detemir and NPH insulin may be less likely to cause hypoglycemia with exercise than insulin glargine [28, 29]. Ongoing studies are needed to demonstrate if these differences in this tendency between the two types of insulin are to be confirmed.

Reducing basal insulin on the day preceding endurance exercise leads to prolonged preexercise hyperglycemia and late postexercise hyperglycemia, both of which add substantially to impaired glycemic control. We therefore do not advise preexercise reductions of basal insulin on the night preceding exercise [30]. However, we have found that for some patients who are performing prolonged endurance exercise (e.g., marathon running) on one or two days in the week, particularly in the morning, it may be advantageous to have those patients managed on twice-daily NPH insulin. Normal morning NPH insulin dose can be significantly reduced or omitted on the day of the endurance exercise. This reduces the risk of hypoglycemia and the requirement for additional carbohydrate ingestion, without causing the antecedent nocturnal hyperglycemia which would occur if the nocturnal basal insulin dose was reduced. It may be necessary to give a reduced dose of basal insulin following exercise to avoid later postprandial hyperglycemia.

For patients treated using multiple daily insulin injections, if exercise occurs within 90 min of the insulin injection, it is possible to markedly reduce the preprandial insulin dose [31–33]. This will reduce the tendency to exercise-induced hypoglycemia albeit at the cost of preexercise hyperglycemia [33]. However, if the exercise is more than 2 h after the bolus dose of insulin, this strategy is not beneficial. If patients are of normal body weight and weight control is not an issue, late postprandial exercise can be successfully managed by ingestion of carbohydrate before and during exercise [9, 22, 34–37]. Evidence from the preceding chapters does suggest that complex carbohydrates with low glycemic index may be successful at reducing hypoglycemia during exercise without causing late postexercise hyperglycemia, but these carbohydrates are not currently widely available. More simple forms of carbohydrate such as glucose can be ingested in regularly accessible form during exercise, and we recommend ingestion during endurance up to the dose of approximately 1 g/kg/h of exercise so that typically a 70-kg adult may be ingesting 20 g of glucose every 20 min during exercise. There is considerable evidence that the ability to absorb glucose during exercise is limited to as little as 60 g/h [38]. This implies that excess carbohydrate above this value will not assist in the avoidance of hypoglycemia but merely add to postexercise hyperglycemia. We advise that where exercise is under 1 h duration, simple carbohydrates are taken. When exercise is more prolonged, there is the opportunity to ingest more palatable complex foods. The strategy of ingesting frequent small quantities of glucose during the exercise, where possible, is effective at maintaining euglycemia [39]. This may not be practical for some exercises, and where this is the case, ingestion of the low-glycemic-index carbohydrate isomaltulose is also effective in maintaining euglycemia without antecedent hyperglycemia [40].

If exercise is intermittent (i.e., less than every other day), we advise reduction in basal insulin dose on the night following exercise of between 10% and 20%. Clearly, this may lead to the potential of hyperglycemia in the morning, and where this is present, additional blood sugar monitoring at 2–3 a.m. is useful to ensure that there is no nocturnal hypoglycemia. For patients performing exercise frequently, such dose reductions, once they have occurred, do not need to be repeated.

For patients who are trying to use exercise to lose weight, calculated dietary intake needs to be significantly lower than the energy expenditure and alternates to carbohydrate ingestion during exercise need to be pursued. We find that a brief burst of high-intensity exercise prior to endurance effort and adding intermittent high-intensity exercise during endurance exercise both protect against hypoglycemia following exercise without ingesting extra carbohydrate [4–6]. However, when compared to endurance exercise alone, adding intermittent high-intensity exercise during endurance exercise increases the risk of nocturnal hypoglycemia [18]. Ingestion of sympathomimetic agents including caffeine or β2-adrenoreceptor agonist may potentially offer an additional treatment option for people who wish to do exercise in the late postprandial period and would like to reduce or avoid taking additional carbohydrate. Acute caffeine ingestion 30 min before prolonged endurance exercise reduced hypoglycemia duration and following exercise in type 1 diabetes [41]. Terbutaline may also protect nocturnal hypoglycemia in children following exercise.

Continuous subcutaneous insulin infusion (CSII) enables reduction or suspension of normal basal insulin infusion rates before and during exercise. This reduction may restore some of the physiological response to exercise and reduce the need for carbohydrate ingestion. CSII infusion rates can be restored or increased prior to or following the end of exercise to deal with postexercise glycogenic peak. Nocturnal basal CSII infusion rates can also be reduced if exercise is infrequent. CSII treatment seems an attractive option for people with diabetes who are exercising regularly or who have complex or variable exercise programs which are less amenable to adjustment of MDI regimes. At present, guidance on how CSII infusion rates are to be adjusted is dependent on clinical experience, with little significant evidential base.

The advent of commercially available continuous glucose monitoring (CGMS) equipment may seem at first sign a significant advance in the management of exercise and type 1 diabetes. These devices measure subcutaneous interstitial glucose values following calibration with synchronous capillary glucose measurement [42, 43]. Blood glucose values change very rapidly during exercise, and unfortunately, there is little reliable correlation between the CGMS and capillary glucose, which means that CGMS is not a useful tool for identifying significant glucose changes, particularly hypoglycemia, in real time. However, CGMS may have a role in alerting the user as to the trajectory and speed of glucose responses [44–46], and the high frequency of nocturnal hypoglycemia [47], and is often useful to an individual for identifying the pattern of glucose change which occurs when they are exercising.

9.2 Safety

Clearly prior to assessment, the status of diabetic complications needs to be assessed. Regular physical exercise does not appear to cause deterioration in either early diabetic retinopathy or diabetic nephropathy [48–51], although it seems sensible to caution again intense physical exercise in patients with preproliferative retinopathy and in particular in those with intraretinal and other neovascular abnormalities.

A detailed inspection of the feet is required. While early peripheral neuropathy does not preclude regular physical exercise, detailed advice on foot care needs to be given with regular foot inspections. However, for patients with foot shape abnormality and marked reduction in peripheral sensation or peripheral vascular disease, upright physical exercise with increased workload on the feet and legs is unlikely to be appropriate.

For patients who are seeking advice on how they might increase physical exercise who have had a long duration of diabetes and who have risk factors for vascular disease such as hypertension, smoking history, or hypercholesterolemia, it is sensible to seek detailed cardiological investigations. An exercise ECG or a stress echocardiogram is likely to be necessary before advising people to embark on a new program of exercise.

Where exercise is to be outside, it is sensible to advise on personal safety during exercise. People with diabetes need to carry with them readily accessible simple carbohydrates, ensure adequate hydration, and ideally avoid exercising alone. Where this is not practical, ideally a mobile phone should be carried at all times. Furthermore, others should be informed where they will be and, in particular, when they should be expected to return.

The skills to assist the health-care professionals to manage type 1 diabetes and exercise are transferable to any diabetes service and if applied will reduce dysglycemia and improve physical performance and quality of life for those people.

References

1. Gallen I. Exercise in type 1 diabetes. Diabet Med. 2003;20:2–5.
2. Lumb AN, Gallen IW. Diabetes management for intense exercise [Review, 44 refs]. Curr Opin Endocrinol Diabetes Obes. 2009;16(2):150–5.
3. Mitchell TH, Abraham G, Schiffrin A, Leiter LA, Marliss EB. Hyperglycemia after intense exercise in IDDM subjects during continuous subcutaneous insulin infusion. Diabetes Care. 1988;11:311–7.
4. Guelfi KJ, Ratnam N, Smythe GA, Jones TW, Fournier PA. Effect of intermittent high-intensity compared with continuous moderate exercise on glucose production and utilization in individuals with type 1 diabetes. Am J Physiol Endocrinol Metab. 2007;292(3):E865–70.
5. Bussau VA, Ferreira LD, Jones TW, Fournier PA. The 10-s maximal sprint: a novel approach to counter an exercise-mediated fall in glycemia in individuals with type 1 diabetes. Diabetes Care. 2006;29(3):601–6.
6. Bussau VA, Ferreira LD, Jones TW, Fournier PA. A 10-s sprint performed prior to moderate-intensity exercise prevents early post-exercise fall in glycaemia in individuals with type 1 diabetes. Diabetologia. 2007;50(9):1815–8.
7. Kennedy JW, Hirshman MF, Gervino EV, Ocel JV, Forse RA, Hoenig SJ, Aronson D, Goodyear LJ, Horton ES. Acute exercise induces GLUT4 translocation in skeletal muscle of normal human subjects and subjects With type 2 diabetes [Miscellaneous article]. Diabetes. 1999;48:1192–7.
8. Kraniou GN, Cameron-Smith D, Hargreaves M. Effect of short-term training on GLUT-4 mRNA and protein expression in human skeletal muscle. Exp Physiol. 2004;89:559–63.
9. McMahon SK, Ferreira LD, Ratnam N, Davey RJ, Youngs LM, Davis EA, Fournier PA, Jones TW. Glucose requirements to maintain euglycemia after moderate-intensity afternoon exercise in adolescents with type 1 diabetes are increased in a biphasic manner. J Clin Endocrinol Metab. 2007;92(3):963–8.
10. Galassetti P. Reciprocity of hypoglycaemia and exercise in blunting respective counterregulatory responses: possible role of cortisol as a mediator [Review, 70 refs]. Diabetes, Nutr Metab Clin Exp. 2002;15(5):341–7; discussion 347–8, 362.
11. Galassetti P, Tate D, Neill RA, Morrey S, Davis SN. Effect of gender on counterregulatory responses to euglycemic exercise in type 1 diabetes. J Clin Endocrinol Metab. 2002;87(11):5144–50.
12. Galassetti P, Tate D, Neill RA, Morrey S, Wasserman DH, Davis SN. Effect of antecedent hypoglycemia on counterregulatory responses to subsequent euglycemic exercise in type 1 diabetes. Diabetes. 2003;52(7):1761–9.
13. Galassetti P, Tate D, Neill RA, Morrey S, Wasserman DH, Davis SN. Effect of sex on counterregulatory responses to exercise after antecedent hypoglycemia in type 1 diabetes. Am J Physiol Endocrinol Metab. 2004;287(1):E16–24.

14. Galassetti P, Tate D, Neill RA, Richardson A, Leu SY, Davis SN. Effect of differing antecedent hypoglycemia on counterregulatory responses to exercise in type 1 diabetes. Am J Physiol Endocrinol Metab. 2006;290(6):E1109–17.

15. Sandoval DA, Guy DL, Richardson MA, Ertl AC, Davis SN. Effects of low and moderate antecedent exercise on counterregulatory responses to subsequent hypoglycemia in type 1 diabetes. Diabetes. 2004;53(7):1798–806.

16. Sandoval DA, Guy DL, Richardson MA, Ertl AC, Davis SN. Acute, same-day effects of antecedent exercise on counterregulatory responses to subsequent hypoglycemia in type 1 diabetes mellitus. Am J Physiol Endocrinol Metab. 2006;290(6):E1331–8.

17. American College of Sports Medicine and American Diabetes Association joint position statement. Diabetes mellitus and exercise. Med Sci Sports Exerc. 1997;29(12):i–vi.

18. Maran A, Pavan P, Bonsembiante B, Brugin E, Ermolao A, Avogaro A, Zaccaria M. Continuous glucose monitoring reveals delayed nocturnal hypoglycemia after intermittent high-intensity exercise in nontrained patients with type 1 diabetes. Diabetes Technol Ther. 2010;12(10): 763–8.

19. Almeida S, Riddell MC, Cafarelli E. Slower conduction velocity and motor unit discharge frequency are associated with muscle fatigue during isometric exercise in type 1 diabetes mellitus. Muscle Nerve. 2008;37(2):231–40.

20. Baldi JC, Cassuto NA, Foxx-Lupo WT, Wheatley CM, Snyder EM. Glycemic status affects cardiopulmonary exercise response in athletes with type I diabetes. Med Sci Sports Exerc. 2010;42(8):1454–9.

21. McKewen MW, Rehrer NJ, Cox C, Mann J. Glycaemic control, muscle glycogen and exercise performance in IDDM athletes on diets of varying carbohydrate content. Int J Sports Med. 1920;20:349–53.

22. Tamis-Jortberg B, Downs Jr DA, Colten ME, 5. Effects of a glucose polymer sports drink on blood glucose, insulin, and performance in subjects with diabetes. Diabetes Educ. 1996;22:471–87.

23. Chokkalingam K, Tsintzas K, Snaar JE, Norton L, Solanky B, Leverton E, Morris P, Mansell P, Macdonald IA. Hyperinsulinaemia during exercise does not suppress hepatic glycogen concentrations in patients with type 1 diabetes: a magnetic resonance spectroscopy study. Diabetologia. 2007;50(9):1921–9.

24. Chokkalingam K, Tsintzas K, Norton L, Jewell K, Macdonald IA, Mansell PI. Exercise under hyperinsulinaemic conditions increases whole-body glucose disposal without affecting muscle glycogen utilisation in type 1 diabetes. Diabetologia. 2007;50(2):414–21.

25. Harmer AR, Chisholm DJ, McKenna MJ, Hunter SK, Ruell PA, Naylor JM, Maxwell LJ, Flack JR, 11. Sprint training increases muscle oxidative metabolism during high-intensity exercise in patients with type 1 diabetes. Diabetes Care. 2008;31:2097–102; Erratum appears in Diabetes Care. 2009;32(3):523.

26. Jenni S, Oetliker C, Allemann S, Ith M, Tappy L, Wuerth S, Egger A, Boesch C, Schneiter P, Diem P, Christ E, Stettler C. Fuel metabolism during exercise in euglycaemia and hyperglycaemia in patients with type 1 diabetes mellitus – a prospective single-blinded randomised crossover trial. Diabetologia. 2008;51(8):1457–65.

27. Robitaille M, Dube MC, Weisnagel SJ, Prud'homme D, Massicotte D, Peronnet F, Lavoie C, 1. Substrate source utilization during moderate intensity exercise with glucose ingestion in type 1 diabetic patients. J Appl Physiol. 2007;103:119–24.

28. Yamakita T, Ishii T, Yamagami K, Yamamoto T, Miyamoto M, Hosoi M, Yoshioka K, Sato T, Onishi S, Tanaka S, Fujii S. Glycemic response during exercise after administration of insulin lispro compared with that after administration of regular human insulin. Diabetes Res Clin Pract. 2002;57(1):17–22.

29. Arutchelvam V, Heise T, Dellweg S, Elbroend B, Minns I, Home PD. Plasma glucose and hypoglycaemia following exercise in people with Type 1 diabetes: a comparison of three basal insulins. Diabet Med. 2009;26(10):1027–32.

30. Tsalikian E, Mauras N, Beck RW, Tamborlane WV, Janz KF, Chase HP, Wysocki T, Weinzimer SA, Buckingham BA, Kollman C, Xing D, Ruedy KJ. Diabetes research in children network

DirecNet Study Group: Impact of exercise on overnight glycemic control in children with type 1 diabetes mellitus. J Pediatr. 2005;147(4):528–34.

31. Bracken RM, West DJ, Stephens JW, Kilduff LP, Luzio S, Bain SC. Impact of pre-exercise rapid-acting insulin reductions on ketogenesis following running in Type 1 diabetes. Diabet Med. 2011;28:218–22.

32. Mauvais-Jarvis F, Sobngwi E, Porcher R, Garnier JP, Vexiau P, Duvallet A, Gautier JF. Glucose response to intense aerobic exercise in type 1 diabetes: maintenance of near euglycemia despite a drastic decrease in insulin dose. Diabetes Care. 2003;26(4):1316–7.

33. Rabasa-Lhoret R, Bourque J, Ducros F, Chiasson JL. Guidelines for premeal insulin dose reduction for postprandial exercise of different intensities and durations in type 1 diabetic subjects treated intensively with a basal-bolus insulin regimen (ultralente-lispro). Diabetes Care. 2001;24(4):625–30.

34. Francescato MP, Geat M, Fusi S, Stupar G, Noacco C, Cattin L. Carbohydrate requirement and insulin concentration during moderate exercise in type 1 diabetic patients. Metabolism. 2004;53(9):1126–30.

35. Francescato MP, Zanier M, Gaggioli F. Prediction of glucose oxidation rate during exercise. Int J Sports Med. 2008;29(9):706–12.

36. Ramires PR, Forjaz CL, Strunz CM, Silva ME, Diament J, Nicolau W, Liberman B, Negrao CE. Oral glucose ingestion increases endurance capacity in normal and diabetic (type I) humans. J Appl Physiol. 1997;83(2):608–14.

37. Riddell MC, Bar-Or O, Hollidge-Horvat M, Schwarcz HP, Heigenhauser GJ. Glucose ingestion and substrate utilization during exercise in boys with IDDM. J Appl Physiol. 2000;88(4):1239–46.

38. Jeukendrup AE, Jentjens R. Oxidation of carbohydrate feedings during prolonged exercise: Current thoughts, guidelines and directions for future research. Sports Med. 2000;29(6): 407–24.

39. Perrone CA, Rodrigues CA, Petkowicz RO, Meyer F. The effect of 8 and 10% carbohydrate drinks on blood glucose level of type 1 diabetic adolescents during and after exercise. Med Sci Sports Exerc [Abstract]. 2004;36:S272.

40. West DJ, Morton RD, Stephens JW, Bain SC, Kilduff LP, Luzio S, Still R, Bracken RM. Isomaltulose improves postexercise glycemia by reducing CHO oxidation in T1DM. Med Sci Sports Exerc. 2011;43(2):204–10.

41. Gallen IW, Ballav C, Lumb A, Carr J. Caffeine supplementation reduces exercise induced decline in blood glucose and subsequent hypoglycaemia in adults with type 1 diabetes (T1DM) treated with multiple daily insulin injection (MDI). Diabetes Care. 2010;59:184-P.

42. Davison R, Aitken G, Charlton J, McKnight J, Kilbride L. Comparison of patient blood glucose monitoring with continuous blood glucose monitoring during exercise. Diabetic Medicine Conference: Diabetes UK Annual Professional Conference; 2010 Mar 3–5; Liverpool, UK

43. Aitken G, Charlton J, Davison R, Hill G, Kilbride L, McKnight J. Reproducibility of the glucose response to moderate intensity exercise in people with type 1 diabetes exercise. Diabetologia Conference: 45th EASD Annual Meeting of the European Association for the Study of Diabetes Vienna Austria Conference; 2009 Sep 29–Oct 2; Vienna, Austria

44. Cauza E, Hanusch-Enserer U, Strasser B, Kostner K, Dunky A, Haber P, 12. Strength and endurance training lead to different post exercise glucose profiles in diabetic participants using a continuous subcutaneous glucose monitoring system. Eur J Clin Invest. 2005;35:745–51.

45. Cauza E, Hanusch-Enserer U, Strasser B, Ludvik B, Kostner K, Dunky A, Haber P, 9. Continuous glucose monitoring in diabetic long distance runners. Int J Sports Med. 2005;26:774–80.

46. Kapitza C, Hovelmann U, Nosek L, Kurth HJ, Essenpreis M, Heinemann L. Continuous glucose monitoring during exercise in patients with type 1 diabetes on continuous subcutaneous insulin infusion. J Diabetes Sci Technol. 2010;4(1):123–31.

47. Iscoe KE, Corcoran M, Riddell MC, 3. High rates of nocturnal hypoglycemia in a unique sports camp for athletes with type 1 diabetes: Lessons learned from continuous glucose monitoring systems. Can J Diabetes. 2008;32:182–9.

48. Svarstad E, Gerdts E, Omvik P, Ofstad J, Iversen BM. Renal hemodynamic effects of captopril and doxazosin during slight physical activity in hypertensive patients with type-1 diabetes mellitus. Kidney Blood Press Res. 2001;24(1):64–70.
49. Tuominen JA, Ebeling P, Koivisto VA. Long-term lisinopril therapy reduces exercise-induced albuminuria in normoalbuminuric normotensive IDDM patients. Diabetes Care. 1998;21(8):1345–8.
50. Viberti G, Pickup JC, Bilous RW, Keen H, Mackintosh D. Correction of exercise-induced microalbuminuria in insulin-dependent diabetics after 3 weeks of subcutaneous insulin infusion. Diabetes. 1981;30:818–23.
51. Kruger M, Gordjani N, Burghard R. Postexercise albuminuria in children with different duration of type-1 diabetes mellitus. Pediatr Nephrol. 1996;10(5):594–7.

Chapter 10
The Athlete's Perspective

10.1 Chris Pennell, Professional Rugby Player

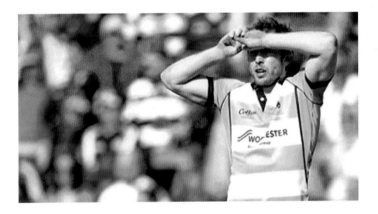

How and when were you diagnosed with type 1 diabetes?

CP: "From the age of nine I became very passionate about Rugby Union. I feel extremely privileged to be in a position where Rugby is my profession and livelihood. I was diagnosed with Type 1 Diabetes aged 19 following a routine blood test at the rugby club. Now aged 24, I currently captain The Worcester Warriors in the Aviva Premiership after earning promotion in the 2010/2011 season."

I. Gallen (ed.), *Type 1 Diabetes*,
DOI 10.1007/978-0-85729-754-9_10, © Springer-Verlag London Limited 2012

How do you train?

CP: "I am on multiple daily insulin injections. I can effectively breakdown my insulin treatment into three categories, which I can slide between when required:

1. Fully fit; this is when my insulin dependency is quite low. My metabolism is fast as I am active most days and competing in my sport on weekends. My basal dosage drops to 8–10 units. My bolus dosage will change depending on the format of my training day. I will only need 1–2 units with a large bowl of porridge along with sipping sports drinks during my morning training. My Blood glucose levels will stay consistently between 5 and 8 mmol/L during this training period. Depending on the intensity of the afternoon session, I may not take any bolus insulin with my meal despite eating a small portion of carbohydrate. These sessions tend to commence 1-½ hours after eating. In this afternoon session I can regulate my blood glucose by sipping sports drinks over the training period in accordance with the type of training session and its intensity. If I have no training, I will take 1 unit per 30 grams of carbohydrate and continue this dosage for any further food until dinner. At 8pm I will take my basal insulin. I like to go to bed at a level between 6 and 7 mmol/L and tend to wake up between 4.5 and 6 mmol/L. Regular blood testing allows me to spot if I need any extra carbohydrate during training sessions. Glucose tablets work very well in pushing my levels up during more demanding sessions.

2. Injured. Being injured presents a huge challenge as a diabetic especially when there is a sudden change from being fully fit to bed ridden. During this time, unsurprisingly my insulin requirements shoot up. I very quickly increase my basal dosage to 16–20 units. My bolus dosage goes up to 1 unit per 15 grams of carbohydrate. Again, regular testing allows small amendments to be made and prevents any serious hypoglycemic or hyperglycemic episodes.

3. Transition. This is the period of time between beginning to exercise after injury and returning to full fitness. During this period I have found a steady change in my insulin dependency in direct correlation to my activeness during training. In the early stages of recovery where training intensity remains fairly low, my insulin requirement stays high. Through the natural progression of returning to fitness, my insulin requirements drop accordingly. During this time I test very regularly and make small adjustments over the weeks until I return to full fitness.

I have become acute to the different requirements of different training sessions and I have learned to adjust the amount of glucose I intake through sports drinks depending on the type of training and its intensity. This method has allowed me to control my blood glucose levels whilst coping with a different variety of training intensities and periods."

CP: "Over the last 5 years my HbA1c results have come down from 7.0 to the most recent being 5.4, a normal reading for a non-diabetic. I largely put this down to keeping active but also sticking to a strict diet. I have always enjoyed eating healthily and staying in shape. However, the main changes in my diet have been around the choices of carbohydrates I eat and the balance of food on my plate. I have an even measure of protein, fibrous carbohydrate and starchy carbohydrate. This balance of food provides me with all the nutrients and fuel I need to maintain a regular body fat percentage and weight. Instead of eating white pasta, white rice, white potato and white bread, I have swapped for whole meal pasta, rice and bread. I believe this small change in choice has been the reason my HbA1c has come down to that of a non-diabetic. The steady drip of glucose into my blood stream forms a smooth blood glucose curve throughout the day."

What kind of problems have you encountered during training and how were they solved?
CP: "The nature of my sport and position means I must have the ability to perform in both an aerobic and anaerobic capacity to a very high level. In a fully fit state I am able to adjust my glucose intake without changing my insulin requirements. During aerobic training, my glucose requirement goes up and additional supplementation is sometimes needed on top of the sports drinks to avoid hypoglycaemia. This is often in the form of glucose tablets. During anaerobic training I have found little or no need to top up my glucose levels due to the hormone response from the body. I have however found need to monitor my blood glucose levels after very intense anaerobic training, something I only really experience during preseason."

CP: "Match day is another time when things change slightly for me. My body's response to playing in big matches in front of big crowds of course makes my glucose levels shoot up. In the early stages I would go into matches having done everything the same as a training day. I would go into a game with my blood glucose level between 6 and 8 mmol/L and sip glucose drinks during stoppages. I stopped drinking the sports drinks and stuck to water. This had very little effect. I then injected 1 unit 5 minutes before kick-off and 1 unit again at half time but because of my sensitivity to insulin I was worried that I would simply induce hypoglycaemia. However, this had the desired result and I would finish games between 6 and 9 mmol/L."

10.2   Jen Alexander, Marathon Swimmer

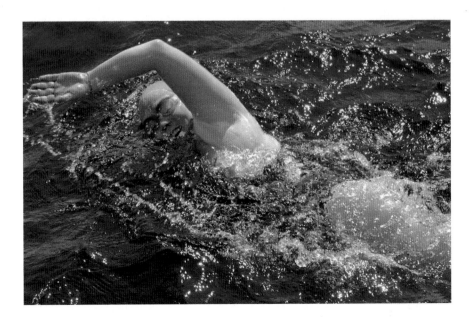

How and when were you diagnosed with type 1 diabetes?

JA: "I've had type one diabetes since 1988 and have swum for most of my life. I live and train in Halifax, Nova Scotia, Canada, swimming outdoors April-November. I've swum 18+ hours on a couple of occasions. In 2008, I was awarded the Diabetes Exercise and Sports Association's 'Athlete of the Year' award. I use an insulin pump."

How do you train?

JA: "Swim-specific diabetes management starts 5 hours before the scheduled start. I don't eat *anything*. I recognize that this isn't the greatest strategy for preserving muscle glycogen, but it works for me in terms of managing my diabetes. I swim with a waterproof insulin pump. My general strategy is to run my basal rate high enough that I don't need to bolus for carbs. I turn my basal rate up to 150% and test my blood glucose just before I am about to jump into the water. From this blood test and until the swim ends, we react to each blood test in the same way:

- If my blood glucose is <6 mmol/L, I get 40 grams of carbs.
- If my blood glucose is 6–8 mmol/L, I get 30 grams of carbs.
- If my blood glucose is 8–10 mmol/L, I get 15 grams of carbs.
- If my blood glucose is >10 mmol/L, I get water.

I test and feed every 30 minutes, with 50 grams of flavored sugar crystals/Gatorade in 750 ml of water to give a solution that's 6.7% carbohydrate. I receive three feeds of flavored crystals and then one feed of Gatorade. I don't have the same need to replace electrolytes because I'm not sweating much, if at all. We'll mix in liquid acetaminophen every 4–6 hours for pain, and we deduct this from my carb allowance.

If my blood glucose level has trended downward or upward for two consecutive tests, my crew prompts me to adjust my basal rate. Even though I start my swims at 150%, I'll titrate down to about 50%. Severe nausea can be part of open water swimming, and I've dealt with this by turning my pump off for 30 minutes and consuming ginger chews. Other than this, I don't consume solids during my swim. This plan works extremely well for me until hypothermia begins to affect my blood sugar as acute hypothermia elevates glucose levels due to catecholamine-induced glyconeogenesis.[1]"

What kind of problems have you encountered during training and how were they solved?

JA: "The 'standard' challenges of blood glucose levels affecting performance still apply. Hypoglycemia causes me to pull through the water less strongly. Both hypoglycaemia and hyperglycemia reduce my stroke rate. Furthermore swimmers with diabetes face additional risks: hypothermia complicates hypoglycaemia. Core

---

[1] Granberg. Human endocrine responses to the cold. Arct Med Res. 1995;54:91–103.

body temperature falls during hypoglycaemia,[2] and recovery from hypoglycaemia is impaired at low body temperatures.[3] Conversely, hypoglycaemia complicates hypothermia: a small study of people without diabetes suggests that blood glucose levels under 2.5 mmol/L suppress both shivering and the sensation of being cold.[4] A swimmer unable to shiver to generate body heat risks advancing through the stages of hypothermia. Therefore swimming safely demands careful diabetes management."

JA: "Tight control over blood glucose levels is critical, and finding a way to test blood while swimming was an exceptional challenge! Open water swimmers around the world adhere tightly to the code of England's Channel Swimming Association: the swim is disqualified if the swimmer touches the boat, or a crew member touches the swimmer. Neither continuous glucose monitors nor heart rate monitors transmit properly in the salt water, so blood glucose levels must be measured by finger stick. Additional challenges included waves, sea spray, wind blowing so loudly that I couldn't hear my meter beep, test results being skewed by water on my finger, and the daunting challenge of being able to squeeze enough blood from a finger vasoconstricted by hypothermia.

To get my test kit to me, we've constructed a 'fishing pole' of sorts. On the boat, my crew has an aluminum painter's extension pole. Instead of twisting a paint roller onto its end, however, we've twisted the marine version of a carabineer onto the pole, then twisted a cap on top of that to ensure the hook doesn't move. We roll 25 meters of rock-climbing rope around a kite-string winder, then thread the rope through the carabineer. My crew attaches items to the rope, extends the pole, and then unwinds the rope to lower the item(s) to me. This is 'legal' in the open water world as long as the rope remains slack.

We use a waterproof container made of transparent plastic to house two meters, a facecloth, and a lancing device stuck to the side of the container with Velcro. During the early hours of a swim, we use a standard lancing device, but switch to larger, disposable lancets (and then blades) as needed. When it's time to test, my crew prepares my test kit by putting a strip in each meter, and then activating the finger flashlight. The boat pulls close and my crew dangles my test kit over my head using the pole and rope. I grab the kit, open the lid, and dry off my finger with the facecloth. I lance my finger, and apply blood to each strip until the finger flashlight turns off (which confirms enough blood has been applied). Sometimes there is too much seaspray to see clearly into the container, and sometimes the wind blows too loudly to hear the meters beep to signal they have enough blood, so watching the finger flashlight turn off is the only way I know the tests are working. I reseal the plastic container, drop it into the water, and resume swimming. My crew then pull the test kit back on the boat and read the results."

---

[2] Gale, Bennett, Green and MacDonald. Hypoglycaemia, hypothermia and shivering in man. Clin Sci. 1981;61:463–9.

[3] Ibid.

[4] Ibid.

10.3   Mark Blewitt, Long-Distance Swimmer

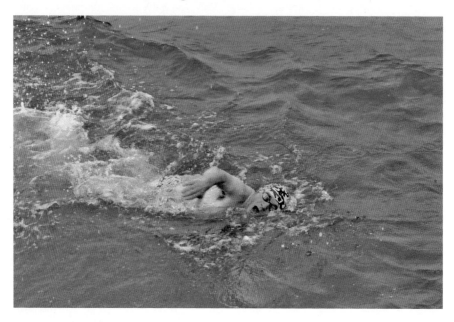

How and when were you diagnosed with type 1 diabetes?

MB: "I was diagnosed with Type 1 Diabetes in 1980 at the age of thirteen. In the mid 1990s after reading an article on the profile of athletes competing in the London Marathon, I decided to get fit. My fitness regime started with a casual visit once a week to my local swimming pool. The following summer I would partake in my first open water swimming race, and I was hooked and would return to this venue several years' later and win the four mile men's race outright."

How did you train?

MB: "I started to think about taking part in the longest annually held race in the British swimming calendar, one length, or 10.5 miles of Windermere in the annual British Long Distance Swimming Association championship. When undertaking longer swims I had realised that I needed less and less insulin and more food. All my insulin was given by multiple daily injections (MDI) which consisted of three fast-acting injections and one slow-acting injection. In 1998 at the time of my Windermere swim I was most probably taking Actrapid and Ultratard."

MB: "I had only been able to get to the start line of such a swim though hours of training and competition. I am also sure that the highs and insulin-driven lows that are found with MDI drove me to eat through the lows, resulting in my carrying the little extra weight. The key is to feed appropriately for the sport you are undertaking and whether on MDI or pump therapy you are in a position to change your insulin amounts to match the food intake you need and exercise that you are undertaking and target weight you need to be at."

MB: "In 1988 I completed my inaugural Windermere swim, fourth in the men's race. Later I realised that my finishing time would make me eligible for selection in the world's longest annually held swimming race, the race around Manhattan Island, New York. I would complete the length of Windermere a further ten times over the next few years, including the Two-Way 21 mile swims on three separate occasions (in 2003 I smashed the breaststroke record for the course)."

What kind of problems did you encounter during training and how were they solved?

MB: "An attempt on the English Channel was made in the July of 2002 but despite reduced insulin, injecting during the swim in the water, my attempted ended in the southern shipping lane. I found my blood glucose level low but in defeat I had learned a lot and decided in the few hours that it took to get back to Dover that I would be having another go. With support from my consultant, Dr Ian O'Connell at Wigan Infirmary and nurse, Judith Campbell, who would be in my escort boat, we worked out a new insulin and feeding regime. Judith is a diabetes nurse and had asked around for advice on what we were trying to achieve and was usually told in no uncertain terms that it would not be possible. However, this time my swim was successful. I stumbled up the beach before clearing the water line 16 hours and 20 minutes after leaving Shakespeare Beach, Dover."

MB: "Later I would learn that the a few hours from the end of the swim the escort pilot was concerned about the way I was swimming. Judith asked, 'Do others (non-diabetics) show such fatigue at this point in a swim?' And when the reply came in the affirmative, Judith persuaded them that all I needed was tiny amount of insulin to pick me up. A compromise was reached. Collectively they would let me carry on swimming and no insulin would be administered. On completing the swim, my Blood Glucose levels were monitored every hour for the next twelve hours through the night. The following day I resembled a Cabbage Patch Kid[R] as my face was swollen with jelly fish stings and my eyes sunken."

10.4   Russell Cobb, Long-Distance Runner

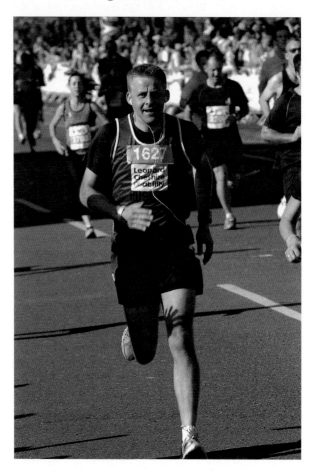

How and when were you diagnosed with type 1 diabetes?
RC: "I was originally diagnosed with Type 1 diabetes whilst training to be a Royal Air Force pilot in 1984. My main performance sport is running, although I play golf and sail dinghies as well."

How do you train?
RC: "I run to keep in good shape and health. I enter at least two half marathons a year and also compete in 2 or 3 10ks whilst training for these. Typically I run 3 to 4 times a week of which 2 or 3 are short runs before work and one longer run of 8–10 miles on a weekend.

My 'fear' during sport is that I will have hypoglycemia so, for much of the time, this is the focus but it is vital to keep blood sugars within an effective range in order to perform. Anything above 10 or 11 mmol/L and the 'leaden' effect takes over and affects performance. Anything under 5 mmol/L and I can sense that the 'tank' is nearly empty. Both affect performance.

In a race, getting blood sugar right is vital if I want to run a good time. On my PB, at the Silverstone Half Marathon in 2008, I started and finished the race with 6 mmol/L blood glucose. This clearly links good control with good performance. Timing of the race matters to strategy. A late morning race and you can eat breakfast normally, with normal dosage and then just before the race 'fuel up' with a bottle of Powerade and a Mars bar. I also reduce basal to about 25% for the first hour. This means I start with a good blood sugar, can establish a good pace early and then in the second half of the race start to step it out. Leave too long between fuelling and the start and blood sugar rises and affects performance until you have 'run it off.'

For an early race I will not eat breakfast at home but take a banana sandwich, or something similar to the race with me, and then eat this about 30 to 45 minutes before the start without any bolus and then rely on the lack of bolus insulin in my body to enable me to get round on this fuel with blood sugar at a good level. I will typically test once whilst running and adjust either basal rate up or down depending on the result and I carry 'Go-gel's' with me if I need to top up."

What kind of problems have you encountered during training and how were they solved?

RC: "Training requires less thought in advance but if you don't think ahead it can also catch you out. I have had low blood sugars by heading off for a quick run without taking any carbohydrate on board or adjusting basal down and then gone slightly further than intended and suddenly I know I am down to less than 4 mmol/L and with a mile or so to home this is no fun! Running in the morning with no remaining bolus insulin present generally means, if you do get it wrong and end up low, then it will generally be 'gentle' and a single Go-gel and slowing the pace down will sort it out. Spontaneous runs around two hours after a normal meal with normal bolus are typically the ones that will catch me out even if I do have additional carbohydrate and stop basal, so I try to avoid these and plan my runs."

RC: "In golf I have linked high blood sugars with poor play. For a three-and-a-half-hour round, carrying clubs on a hilly course I will eat normally, whether breakfast or lunch, approx 50/60 carbohydrates, but reduce bolus by 50% (provided blood sugar is in normal range beforehand) and also reduce basal to about 65% for approx 90 minutes. Get this right and keep blood sugar stable within 7–9 range this removes high blood sugar as a detriment to a poor round."

10.5 Sebastien Sasseville, Ironman Competitor and Mountain Climber

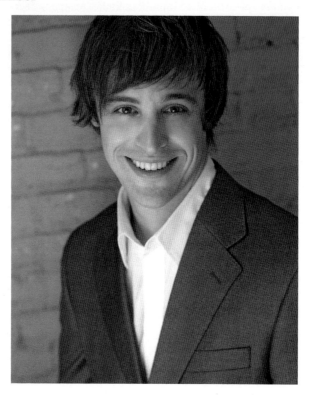

How and when were you diagnosed with type 1 diabetes?

SS: "When I first trekked to Mount Everest base camp in 2001, I promised myself that one day I would come back and climb Everest all the way to the top. What was initially a dream quickly became a project and I went back to Nepal four times in the following seven years. Along the way, I was given the gift of diabetes and I say that with no irony whatsoever. Both the obstacle that I chose, Everest, and the one I didn't choose, diabetes, made me stronger."

How did you train?

SS: "Climbing in high altitude is a demanding and risky endeavor. Add managing type one diabetes to the mix and it becomes a monumental challenge. I believe three key words can make everything a lot simpler and safer: education, preparation and experimentation. In that order and in a continuous circle."

SS: "Education. To complete my journey it has been crucial to take ownership of my diabetes and proactively educate myself about it. Two minutes in my doctor's office three times a year wasn't going to cut it. I decided to learn as much as I could about type one diabetes from as many sources as possible. When exercising, understanding how everything works is fundamental. When insulin peaks, how long it is active for, understand the concept of insulin on board, how blood glucose monitors works, their limitations, know how to count carbohydrates, know how different types of carbohydrates absorb, understand how my pump works, etc. The list goes on indefinitely.

Preparation. Climbing Mount Everest is a 60-day expedition. Needless to say a lot went into planning my diabetes strategy. I packed about 15 blood glucose monitors, 2 pumps, 12 months worth of insulin, insulin pens, 1500 test strips and a LOT of treatment for hypoglycemia. Having a back up plan is one thing, but the strategy doesn't stop there. Transportation, storage and repartition of the supplies are all very important. For example, no matter how much insulin I have, if it's all in the same place and freezes I'm in trouble. During the expedition, I broke down my insulin stock in three thermos. I kept one on me at all times, one at base camp and one in a clinic in Katmandu. No matter how short you exercise for, always have something to treat hypoglycaemia. When prepared properly, hypoglycemia is simply a discomfort. On the other hand, if unprepared, hypoglycemia can be catastrophic if not life threatening.

Experimentation. Every time I do something new I learn a lot. It took me 5 years of preparation to feel my diabetes strategy was ready to scale Mount Everest. I started with weekend camping trips, then went for short expeditions, then started climbing more seriously, then added altitude in the mix, went on several 30-day expeditions and eventually felt ready. By building slowly but surely, the next step is always just a little bit higher and seems achievable."

What kind of problems did you encounter during training and how were they solved?
SS: "The Ironman race is grueling, a 2.4 mile swim, 112 mile bike ride and a 26 mile marathon. Needless to say that training for such an event with type one diabetes is a challenge. Starting slow is key. You need to figure out what to do on a 30 minute run before going on a 2 hour run. The more you measure something the more you understand it. I could not imagine testing my blood glucose fewer than ten times a day. I test pre and post meals, before, during and after exercise and whenever I'm not sure of what my blood glucose is. From this you can figure out why you are high, low or within range. Identify what you have done right and what needs to be changed. In a race that can be as long as 17 hours, preventing a low blood sugar often starts hours before the race. On the flip side, my current blood sugar impacts how I will perform in several hours."

SS: "One thing is crucial to understand and to accept: diabetes is different for everyone and different every day. What works one day isn't likely to work the next day. Instead, think of diabetes and exercise as an equation with variables that constantly change. Some variables are obvious, duration and intensity for example. I have listed several different variables that impact on my diabetes during exercise. Some variables don't have an actual impact on my blood glucose but they impact my strategy and the way I prepare for the outing. Time of the day, type of activity, overall goal (recreation, weight loss or performance), stress, insulin on board, recovery, risk of disappointment, risk to safety, and temperature are just a few. Every day the equation adds up to a different strategy."

10.6   Fred Gill, Rower

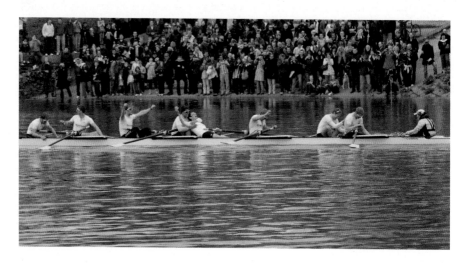

How and when were you diagnosed with type 1 diabetes?

FG: "I was diagnosed with Type 1 Diabetes aged 21 at the start of my 3rd year at Newcastle University. While I had been a very keen sportsman in almost every sport at school it took me until my first year at Newcastle to find a sport that I was naturally good at in rowing. I was very tall and fit and progress was rapid until the start of my third year where it tailed off drastically. After losing 5 kilos and with an insatiable thirst I went for a blood test and that was the start of my diabetic challenge."

"I had of course heard of Steve Redgrave winning his 5th Olympic Gold aged 38 as a diabetic so there was never any question as to whether I would continue my rowing or not. However, having been diagnosed on the Monday and taking a few days to get to terms with the life change my coach then, Angelo Savarino, rung me up on the Wednesday demanding why I was not at training and telling me that he had known 'hundreds' of diabetic athletes in Italy and I should stop feeling sorry for myself and start training properly again straight away. This proved to me the perfect mindset for me as I attacked my training just as I had before and within a month was producing scores similar to those prior to my diagnosis."

"That year I had also managed to make an application to Cambridge University and was lucky enough to be accepted. The training program at Cambridge, however, was completely different to the one I had come from and was far more based on training at low intensity and for long periods of time. For instance, our two main ergometer sessions in the week were 70–80 mins at a low rate and intensity with one short break at half way. This is the method of training employed at most nation levels where athletes can train full time and thus spend longer periods training and recovering."

How did you train?
FG: "The training implemented at Newcastle was an Italian-style program where all training was to maximum intensity. Through the winter we would do long low-rate work such as 3–4 x 6k, 3–5 x 4k, 8–10 x 3k and our least favourite 14–16 x 1500 metres. All these pieces were started with one minute flat out before coming down onto a low rate that was carried on through the rest of the distance. I did not know it at the time but it was these one minute high intensity starts that staved off any hypos. I have only recently heard of the maximal sprint technique as a defense against hypos and have brought it into my current training. Therefore, because of these one minute flat out starts to all the pieces in my time at Newcastle I did not have a single session ruined by hypoglycemia. At the end of that first season I won four gold medals at the British Universities' regatta and for the first time in the club's history, won the Student fours at Henley Royal Regatta. My pairs partner and I also managed to achieve a 6th place finish at the national trials which meant we were in the Great Britain under 23 eight that came 5th at the under 23 World Championships later that summer."

What kind of problems did you encounter during training and how were they solved?
"At Cambridge, the training program was completely different being far more based on training at low intensity and for long periods of time. For instance our two main ergometer sessions in the week were 70–80 mins at a low rate and intensity with one short break at half way. This is the method of training employed at most nation levels where athletes can train full time and thus spend longer periods training and recovering. However with no one minute flat out start and the low intensity of the training I was hypoing almost every time we would do these sessions. I would be exhausted with 10 mintues of the workout and subsequently used to dread them and not understand why I was so exhausted and everyone else was far less fatigued at the end of the ergo sessions. I found out that it is the low intensity use of large muscle areas such as quads, glutes and back that lead to lowering blood sugar and hypogly-cemia after sustained periods such training with no glucose."

"I struggled through my first year a Cambridge constantly exhausted, falling asleep in lectures and producing very inconsistent performances throughout. Some of my high-intensity work was at the top end of the squad and I was therefore given a good chance of being in the 'Blue Boat' for the boat race but after some bad per-formances and a spectacularly bad 5 k ergo score I was named in the reserve boat. It was after losing the reserve boat race in 2009 that lead me to plan a new insulin regime where I would take half my normal amount of insulin if I was training within one hour of eating and take glucose, in the form of drinks and gels, every 20 or so minutes throughout low intensity training to keep my blood sugar levels stable."

"My new regimen worked almost immediately so that through the summer I was able to train hard and effectively and attack the new year with renewed gusto. I was far more consistently producing scores near the top end of the squad and started being regarded as a genuine boat blue candidate and even potential stroke man, which carries with it added glory and responsibility. I hypoed far less in training and the coaches faith in me was shown as they named me in the stroke seat of the provisional blue boat 3 months before the boat race."

"In the week leading up to the Race our training decreased as we tapered towards the big day and with it my insulin sensitivity. My blood sugar cycled throughout the day and night as I found it hard to live and eat with non-diabetics and carry out a different routine to the one I had got used to in training. However, with help from the club doctor I kept to a personalised diet of low glycemic indexed (GI) foods and was able to regain some control in the days before the race. I was obviously extremely worried about what might happen if I hypoed or hypered during the race but tried to ignore it and put my energy into organising exactly what I would do hour by hour on the day so I would arrive on the start line with stable blood sugars."

"As it turned out even the best plans do not play out how they should. My blood sugar was quite high in the hours before the race and were about 13–14 mmol/L at the start. As it turned out my control was just about good enough as I stroked Cambridge around the outside of the Surrey bend a length down to then come through to take the inside of the last bend and win by a length. Since the boat race in 2010 I have continued my rowing with the aim of making the senior team. Having come 9th in both national trial regattas in 2011 I have not made the team for the forthcoming Olympics in London but will continue with rowing and hopefully make the team for the next Olympiad and Rio 2016."

10.7   Monique Hanley, Professional Cyclist

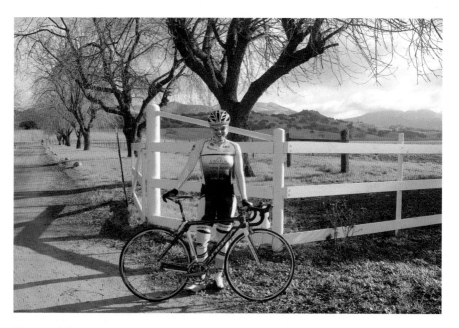

Photo credit to Mark Suprenant

How and when were you diagnosed with type 1 diabetes?

MH: Monique Hanley was diagnosed with type 1 diabetes in 1998. Based in Melbourne, Australia, she became 2007 State track champion in the individual pursuit and points score. She raced with the US-based cycling team, Team Type 1, as a professional cyclist from 2007 to 2009. She was the only female member of Team Type 1's eight-person team, which won the 2007 Race Across AMerica (RAAM) and set a new world record.

MH: "My life on the bike began shortly after a stern lecture from my endocrinologist. I was 22 at the time and had just 'retired' from playing basketball. I played at Australian Women's National Basketball League (WNBL) level but struggled with form and passion following my diagnosis with type 1 diabetes two years earlier. I lacked a lot of understanding on how type 1 diabetes could affect my on-court performance, and received little sympathy from teammates and coaching staff. At the end of a disappointing second season and with all passion for the sport gone, I walked away and never returned."

MH: "The impacts on my life were immediate. With more time to work and party, life moved from being centered around exercise and performance. My conditioning fell away rapidly and my weight blossomed, with an A1c shooting up past 8. Cycling met my needs, replaced my mode of transport and offered me a door into another life. And it still remains the best fun I have ever had while exercising!"

How did you train?

MH: "I first completed a number of recreational cycling challenges including riding across Canada (7,800 km) and around France (2,700 km). I followed le Tour on my own, with a one man tent and a month's supply of test strips and insulin. I was fascinated to discover that after four days of heavy exercise and constant reduction of insulin needs, the fifth day onwards I would require slightly more. It seemed to take the four days to get the body adjusted to the new regime, and from there it would say, 'okay, got the hang of this. I actually need a little bit more to keep going'. Racing became my next goal. Starting with local road races, I progressed to open women's racing and eventually moved onto the track which resulted in finding my true passion in the sport and achieving success at an elite level in Australia. During this time I was invited to race for Team Type 1 in their 2007 and 2008 Race Across AMerica teams. We competed in the eight person team category, and I was the only female member. We won the event in 2007 and in the process set a new world record for the crossing. I spent three years in the USA racing on the professional women's circuit, specializing in criterium racing."

What kind of problems did you encounter during training and how were they solved?

MH: "These are my key management strategies. I use a pump and CGM. I switched to the pump in 2004 and found it far more useful for training and racing. When you need to be flexible, as life often is, the pump is there to move with you! I have to admit that I still find long races difficult to master, and I struggle with being able to guess my blood sugar after two hours on the bike. A continuous glucose monitor is the best thing for bike racing and recovery.

I reduced basal rate for criterium racing. It was easier to develop my diabetes 'formula' in criteriums thanks to trialing it every weekend in local races. I am resistant to complete removal of my pump during races or to reduce insulin rate in the lead up to the start of a race. Races can be delayed due to crashes in a previous race, sudden change in weather (we were once delayed by a hail storm), or simply at the discretion of officials. A 50% basal reduction to cover the length of the race on the start line with some top up fuel ready to go (usually 20–25 g high GI food in my back pocket) is ideal for me. Usually the adrenaline of a criterium start will spike my blood glucose early on, and as long as I eat around the 40 minute mark of a race, my levels will be okay until the sprint finish (this is assuming a one hour race, no racing or heavy strain in the previous days, and general cycling good fortune).

I reduced basal rate for Racing Across AMerica. Every shift during this crazy race required a different basal rate. Combining the intense physical output (short bursts at almost maximum effort) with next to no sleep meant the body had no real chance to recover. A 'good' sleep was three hours. During one shift when I was hurting at my very worst, my basal needs increased, but typically my basal reduction was between 50–80%. Constant glucose monitoring was essential. After five and a half days, it was an experience like no other.

(Try to) Manage your mind. Mental preparation is essential in track racing, and I quickly learnt the price you pay from adrenaline-induced high blood sugars. My performances are impacted the further north my meter reading is from 10 mmol/L. My challenge became how to focus on the racing goal while at the same time open to 'variations' in the event, such as a puncture or reschedule. This helped me minimize the surge in blood glucose levels from adrenaline. Engaging a sports psychologist was extremely beneficial. I learnt how to visualize performance goals and adopted breathing techniques which made a huge difference.

Start at a low base. Once I realized just how much my blood sugars soared from adrenaline, I adopted a new strategy: if I start at a low base, the adrenal jump wouldn't land me into the evil realms of life above 13 mmol/L. The trick was to ensure that the blood sugar wasn't *too* low. It was a fine line to walk, and it required plenty of monitoring during warmup. If it did drop too low, there was always sports drink or lollies on hand to get it up enough for race time.

Manage your hypos. It is extremely important to manage post-exercise hypos. During preparation for the Australian track season, I encounter a fair share of extreme hypos. They usually happen following a heavy training period, but never immediately following the conclusion of training and so tend to 'sneak up' on me. Anywhere up to 48 hours afterwards I am subject to severe lows, and with my focus on keeping my blood sugar relatively low for track performance I am especially vulnerable. You can never test enough."

Index

A

AAS. *See* Anabolic androgenic
    steroids (AAS)
Aerobic exercise
  definition, 31
  hyperglycemia, 33–34
  hypoglycemia, 32, 33
Alpha-/beta-adrenergic blockade, 118
Anabolic androgenic steroids (AAS)
  adverse effects of
    AAS and diabetes, 177
    cardiovascular disease, 177
    endocrine function, 176
    hepatotoxicity, 176–177
    psychiatric effects, 177
  athletes abuse, 175–176
  development of, 173
  prevalence of, 174–175
  testosterone, formulations of, 173–174
Anaerobic exercise, 34–35
Anti-doping
  history of, 170–172
  World Anti-Doping Agency, prohibited
    substances, 171, 172
Anti-doping administration and management
    system (ADAMS), 189–190
Antihypertensives, 189
Athletes
  abuse
    AAS, 175–176
    EPO, 178
    growth hormone, 179–182
    insulin, 187–188
    insulin-like growth factor-I, 184–185
  carbohydrate

intake after training and competition,
    160–161
intake during training and competition,
    158–160
intake prior to training, 157–158
loading, 158
with type 1 diabetes, 155–157
without type 1 diabetes, 152–154
nutrition guidelines, without type 1 dia-
    betes
  carbohydrate, 152–154
  hydration, 154
  protein, 154
  vitamin and mineral supplements,
    154–155
with type 1 diabetes
  blood glucose monitoring, 161
  carbohydrate, 155–161
  fat, 163
  hydration, 162
  protein, 162–163
  weight management, 161–162
Autonomic symptoms, hypoglycemia,
    116–117

B

Basal insulins, 52
Beneficial effects, physical activity
  cardiovascular benefits, 79–80
  psychological well-being, 77–79
Blood transfusion
  adverse effects of, 178
  and diabetes, 179
  prevalence of, 178

I. Gallen (ed.), *Type 1 Diabetes*,
DOI 10.1007/978-0-85729-754-9, © Springer-Verlag London Limited 2012

C

Caffeine
  dosage, 110
  in hypoglycemi, 108
  uses, 168
Carbohydrate
  athletes
    intake after training and competition,
      160–161
    intake during training and competition,
      158–160
    intake prior to training, 157–158
    loading, 158
    with type 1 diabetes, 155–157
    without type 1 diabetes, 152–154
  childhood diabetes
    amount of, 89
    exercise types, 88
    ingestion, 88
    management, 90
    pre-exercise meal/snack
      suggestions, 89
    type of, 89–90
  ingestion of, 64–65
  post-exercise hypoglycemia, 60–61
  pre-exercise timing, 61–63
Cardiovascular benefits, physical activity,
    79–80
CGM. *See* Continuous glucose
    monitoring (CGM)
Childhood diabetes
  assessment, 75–76
  carbohydrate, 88–90
  cardiovascular benefits, 79–80
  competition and travel, 94–95
  diabetes management, 82–83
  endurance sports, 94
  energy requirements, 86–88
  fat, 91
  fluid, hydration and thermoregulation,
    91–92
  fluid management, 92
  glucose and glycemic control, 80–82
  management of, 84–86
  nutrition and exercise, 83
  patterns, 76–77
  physical activity and developmental
    changes, 74–75
  power/strength sports, 94
  protein, 90–91
  psychological well-being, 77–79
  supplements and ergogenic aids, 93
  team sports, 94

  training/competitive sports, 86
  unplanned and spontaneous, 83–84
  vitamins and minerals, 93
Clamp procedure, 51
Continuous glucose monitoring (CGM)
  challenges, 105
  limitations, 105–106
  and nocturnal hypoglycemia, 106–107
  uses, 105
Continuous subcutaneous insulin infusion
    (CSII) therapy
  basal insulin infusion, 104
  in children, 103
  and nocturnal hypoglycemia, 106–107
Counterregulatory responses
  and glucose ingestion, 15–18
  hypoglycemia, 12–14
  recovery, 132–133
CSII therapy, Continuous subcutaneous insulin
    infusion (CSII) therapy

D

Dietary reference values (DRVs), 84
Doping
  early history, 168
  origin of, 167
  prevalence of, 170
  stimulants and anabolic agents,
    use of, 168–169
  twentieth-century doping, 169–170

E

Early post-exercise hyperglycemia, 35
Endurance sports, 94
Endurance training, 39
Erythropoietin (EPO)
  athletes abuse and adverse
    effects of, 178
  and diabetes, 179
  prevalence of, 178
Exercise
  CGM, 104–106
  characteristics of, 47–48
  counterregulation, 117–118
  CSII therapy
    basal insulin infusion, 104
    in children, 103
    and nocturnal hypoglycemia, 106–107
  endocrine and metabolic responses
    aerobic exercise, 31–34
    anaerobic exercise, 34–35

blood glucose responses, 30
early post-exercise hyperglycemia, 35
energy metabolism and fuel
    utilization, 2–5
exercise and hyperinsulinemia, 5–7
gender differences, 14–15
glucose ingestion, 15–18
glucose metabolism, hormonal
    regulation of, 8–11
hypoglycemia, 12–14
insulin action, 7–8
late post-exercise
    hypoglycemia, 35–36
endurance training, 39
fuel utilization, abnormalities in, 36–37
hypoglycemia (*see* Hypoglycemia)
type 1 diabetes individual
    effects, 37–38
    endurance exercise-induced
        hypoglycemia, 48
    intermittent exercise, 49–50
    post-exercise hypoglycemia
        (*see* Post-exercise hypoglycemia)
    resistance exercise, 50–51
    safety factors, 64–66
    sprint exercise, 49

F
Fatigue, 15

G
Glucokinase, 128–129
Glucose ingestion, 15–18
Glycemic control
    in childhood diabetes, 80–82
    potential strategies, 196–198
    resistance exercise, 50
    variational factors, 195–196
Glycemic index (GI)
    and exercise performance, 153–154, 157
    in nutritional management, 156
    post-exercise hypoglycemia, 60–61
Growth hormone (GH)
    adverse effects, 182
    athletes abuse
        cardiovascular effects, 180
        fuel delivery, 180
        in healthy adults, 181–182
        muscle and bone anabolism, 180
        thermoregulation, 180–181
        whole body physiology, 181

and diabetes, 182–183
features, 179
prevalence of, 179

H
HAAF. *See* Hypoglycemia-associated
    autonomic failure (HAAF)
Hepatic glycogenolysis, 9
Hexokinase II (HKII), 7
Hyperglycemia
    aerobic exercise, 33–34
    early post-exercise hyperglycemia, 35
Hyperinsulinemia, 5–7
Hyperinsulinization, 115–116
Hypoglycemia
    acute hypoglycemia treatment, 138–139
    aerobic exercise, 32, 33
    autonomic symptoms, 116–117
    counterregulation and hypoglycemia
        awareness, 132–133
    counterregulatory responses to, 12–14
    impaired cascade of events, 118–119
    late post-exercise hypoglycemia, 35–36
    normal cascade of events, 116–117
    post-exercise hypoglycemia
        (*see* Post-exercise hypoglycemia)
    prevention, strategies for, 107–108
    risk factors
        age, 121–122
        AMP-activated protein kinase, 129
        corticotrophin-releasing factor, 130
        exercise duration and intensity,
            120–121
        gamma-aminobutyric acid, 129–130
        glucokinase, 128–129
        glucose-sensing neurons, 128
        HAAF and hypoglycemia unawareness,
            123–127
        impaired symptom identification, 123
        insulin sensitivity, 122–123
        insulin uptake and action, 120
        lactate, 130–131
        temperature, 121
    severe hypoglycemia, prevention of
        intermittent high-intensity exercise,
            137–138
        record keeping, 137
        strategies, reducing risk, 134–136
        symptom identification improvement,
            134, 137
Hypoglycemia-associated autonomic failure
    (HAAF), 123–127

I

Impairment mechanism
    AMP-activated protein kinase, 129
    corticotrophin-releasing factor, 130
    gamma-aminobutyric acid, 129–130
    glucokinase, 128–129
    glucose-sensing neurons, 128
    lactate, 130–131
Insulin
    adverse effects, 188
    athletes abuse
        glucose metabolism, 187
        lipid metabolism, 187–188
        protein metabolism, 188
    and diabetes, 188
    prevalence of, 187
    synthesis, 186
Insulin-like growth factor-I
    adverse effects, 185
    athletes abuse
        carbohydrate metabolism, 184–185
        protein metabolism, 184
    and diabetes, 185–186
    prevalence of, 183–184
Intermittent exercise, 49–50
Interval sprint training, 39

K

Ketogenesis, 55

L

Late post-exercise hypoglycemia, 35–36
Leg glucose exchange, during exercise, 4, 5

M

MSNA. *See* Muscle sympathetic
            nerve activity (MSNA)
Muscle sympathetic nerve activity
        (MSNA), 116

N

Neurogenic symptoms,
        hypoglycemia, 116–117
Nocturnal hypoglycemia, 106–107

P

Phosphocreatine (PCr), 3
Physical activity. *See also* Exercise
    childhood diabetes
        assessment, 75–76

carbohydrate, 88–90
cardiovascular benefits, 79–80
competition and travel, 94–95
diabetes management, 82–83
endurance sports, 94
energy requirements, 86–88
fat, 91
fluid, hydration and thermoregulation,
    91–92
fluid management, 92
glucose and glycemic
    control, 80–82
management of, 84–86
nutrition and exercise, 83
patterns, 76–77
physical activity and developmental
    changes, 74–75
power/strength sports, 94
protein, 90–91
psychological well-being, 77–79
supplements and ergogenic aids, 93
team sports, 94
training/competitive sports, 86
unplanned and spontaneous, 83–84
vitamins and minerals, 93
    definition, 73
Post-exercise hypoglycemia
    carbohydrate intake and exercise, 57–60
    glycemic index, 60–61
    pre-exercise carbohydrate consumption and
            insulin administration, 61–63
    pre-exercise insulin dose efficacy
        basal insulins, 52
        rapid-acting insulins, 52–55
    preparatory insulin and carbohydrate
            strategies, 63–64
    rapid-acting insulin dose, safety
            strategies, 55–57
Power/strength sports, 94
Protein
    athletes
        insulin, 188
        insulin-like growth factor-I, 184
        with type 1 diabetes, 162–163
        without type 1 diabetes, 154
    in childhood diabetes, 90–91
Pyruvate dehydrogenase complex (PDC), 6–7

R

Rapid-acting insulins
    description, 52–55
    reduction of, 65
    safety strategies, 55–57
Resistance exercise, 50–51

S

Skeletal muscle
    acute exercise effect, on insulin
        action, 7–8
    exercise and hyperinsulinemia stimulate
        glucose uptake, 5–7
    fiber types, 3
Sodium/glucose co-transporter 1 (SGLT1), 57
Splanchnic glucose exchange,
        during exercise, 4, 5
Sprint exercise, 49

T

Therapeutic use exemption (TUE), 189–190
Total daily energy expenditure (TEE)
        estimation, 87
Type II fast-twitch fibers, 3
Type I slow-twitch fibers, 3

U

Unplanned and spontaneous physical activity,
        83–84

Printed by Printforce, the Netherlands